4/97

 St. Louis Community College

Forest Park
Florissant Valley
Meramec

Instructional Resources
St. Louis, Missouri

GAYLORD

ALCOHOL and AGING

ALCOHOL AND AGING

Edited by

THOMAS BERESFORD
EDITH GOMBERG

New York Oxford
OXFORD UNIVERSITY PRESS
1995

Oxford University Press

Oxford   New York
Athens   Auckland   Bangkok   Bombay
Calcutta   Cape Town   Dar es Salaam   Delhi
Florence   Hong Kong   Istanbul   Karachi
Kuala Lumpur   Madras   Madrid   Melbourne
Mexico City   Nairobi   Paris   Singapore
Taipei   Tokyo   Toronto

and associated companies in
Berlin   Ibadan

Library of Congress Cataloging-in-Publication Data
Alcohol and aging / edited by Thomas Beresford, Edith Gomberg.
p. cm.   Includes bibliographical references and index.
ISBN 0-19-508090-4
1. Aged—Alcohol use.   2. Middle aged persons—Alcohol use.
3. Alcohol—Physiological effect.   4. Alcoholism—Treatment.
I. Beresford, Thomas P. II. Gomberg, Edith Lisansky, 1920–
[DNLM: 1. Alcoholism—in old age.   2. Aging—drug effects.
3. Alcohol, Ethyl—metabolism.   WM 274 A34919 1995]
RC564.5.A34A43   1995
618.97′6861—dc20
DNLM/DLC
for Library of Congress   94-32853

1 3 5 7 9 8 6 4 2

Printed in the United States of America
on acid-free paper

Foreword

by MARC SCHUCKIT

This book combines information on two of the most important public health issues of our time—the growing population over age 65 and substance-use disorders, which are the most prevalent psychiatric diagnoses in most age groups. As a result, no health care provider in any service delivery system can confidently carry out a practice without a working knowledge of both areas—the elderly and problems associated with drugs and alcohol. At the same time, few clinicians who are not already schooled in these topics have the time to study the existing literature intensively. Most need some place to begin their readings.

Researchers, too, in the areas of substance-use disorders and geriatric psychiatry and psychology are becoming more aware of their need to keep up with the vast amount of research in both fields. Many drug actions change with increasing age, the usual clinical course or natural history of many substance-use disorders differs in various age groups, and it is difficult to conceive of appropriate diagnostic and treatment evaluations in any elderly individual without considering the possible ill effects of alcohol and drugs. While scientists are much more likely to feel comfortable in turning to the *Index Medicus*, few have the time to carefully review a multitude of articles.

For a long time I have searched for a single resource to which to refer the interested clinician and the researcher new to substance-use disorders and geriatrics. It is often too cumbersome to review my research files for overviews that meet their specific needs. It is, at the same time, inappropriate to try to introduce someone to a new field by focusing on methodologically correct but highly focused and complex individual research articles.

Finally, I have a way out. This text can meet some of the important needs of both researchers and clinicians, and is likely to help individuals who are expert in one but not in both fields. The book reviews a range of important issues: the problems associated with establishing proper diagnoses of substance-use disorders, the need to consider preexisting and comorbid psychiatric conditions, and data relating to the scope of substance-use problems among older men and women. For those asking questions about the specific vulnerabilities of older individuals to specific drugs, information is offered on neurochemical changes with aging as well as the predominant effects of specific substances, especially alcohol, on the brain. Of more direct clinical relevance are discussions of how physiological changes in older men and women increase their vulnerability to adverse reactions to alcohol, other drugs of abuse, and medications, as well as a presentation of the interaction between medical problems likely to be observed in older individuals and subsequent unique vulnerabilities to medical problems related to substance use. One special consideration is the need to understand more about how cognitive changes associated with aging might interact with vulnerabilities related to alcohol and other drugs. Those readers with a more immediate interest in rehabilitation options will also find important suggestions in several chapters. At the same time, there is a recognition that not all older men and women are identical in their treatment needs and required levels of support through the presentation of information related to special groups such as minorities and the homeless.

I believe most readers looking for a place to begin to enhance their understanding of substance-use problems in older men and women have come to the right place. Not only will the information offered in specific chapters be of direct relevance, but the reference sections in these thoughtful presentations can serve as guidelines for further reading.

Acknowledgments

With the greatest possible humility, the editors wish first to express their deepest thanks to each of the chapter authors. We view each of their contributions as original and of the highest quality. The breadth of perspective that each chapter adds to the volume has truly made this collaborative work much greater than the mere sum of its components. Credit for this is due to the efforts of the contributing authors.

Second, this work could not have been accomplished without research support from two primary sources: the National Institute on Alcohol Abuse and Alcoholism (NIAAA) and the Department of Veterans Affairs (DVA).

Both editors received funding through the NIAAA's center program during the planning phases of the volume with support continuing for Dr. Gomberg through the editing phase as well. Generous support was provided to Dr. Beresford by the Alcohol Research Center of the DVA, located at the Veterans Affairs Medical Center in Denver, during the editing phase. The editors wish to express special thanks to both these institutions.

Many of the chapter authors presenting their work in this volume have enjoyed individual funding from these institutional sources as well, reflecting the ongoing interests of both the NIAAA and the DVA in the growing health concerns raised by the convergence of alcoholism and an aging population. Those supported by the NIAAA include Drs. Beresford, Brennan and Moos, Bucholz and colleagues, Gomberg and Ms. Nelson, Lucey, Nair and colleagues, Schuckit, Tarter, S. Wilsnack and colleagues, and Wood. Those supported by the DVA include Drs. Atkinson, Beresford, Brennan and Moos, Korrapati and Vestal, Schuckit, Willenbring and colleagues, and Wood.

In addition, Drs. Bickford, McClearn, and Wood wish to acknowledge the support of the National Institute on Aging and Dr. McClearn that from the MacArthur Foundation and from the National Institute on Drug Abuse. Drs. Korrapati and Vestal thank the Merck Foundation which supported Dr. Korrapati as its fellow. Dr. Finlayson expresses his gratitude to the Mayo Clinic Foundation for its support. And Drs. Rubington and Glantz wish to thank their institutions, Northeastern University and the National Institute on Drug Abuse respectively, for their assistance in contributing to this work.

Third, the editors acknowledge a lasting debt to Joan Bossert of the Oxford University Press who believed in the usefulness of this project as a contribution to the scientific literature on alcoholism. Without her patience and steady encouragement through the months and the tribulations that threatened this project, it would simply not have been brought to a successful conclusion.

Finally, the editors wish to send special thanks to the Congress of the United States, particularly in memory of the late United States Representative, the Honorable Claude

Pepper of Florida. A long time advocate of the need for understanding and intervention in the problems of aging far before it became popular as an area of research, Congressman Pepper was instrumental in leading the research community into the more controversial area of alcoholism among the elderly. As we hope the information in this volume will demonstrate, Mr. Pepper's vision of this as a growing problem affecting our population's health was a more prescient one. *Alcohol and Aging* must be considered a part of his legacy to the nation. It is only fitting, therefore, that this volume be dedicated to his memory and to the continuing vision of the members of Congress who have succeeded him in their recognition of the growing magnitude of the health problems resulting from alcohol abuse and the aging process.

Contents

Contributors

Roland M. Atkinson, M.D.
Head, Division of Geriatric Psychiatry
School of Medicine, Oregon Health
Sciences University
Chief, Section on Geriatric and
Consultation Psychiatry
Veterans Affairs Medical Center
Portland, Oregon

Thomas P. Beresford, M.D.
Professor, Department of Psychiatry
University of Colorado School of
Medicine
University of Colorado Alcohol Research
Center
Department of Veterans Affairs Alcohol
Research Center
1055 Clermont Street
Denver, Colorado

Paula Bickford, Ph.D.
Assistant Professor, Department of
Pharmacology
University of Colorado School Of
Medicine and Research Service, Veterans
Affairs Medical Center
Denver, Colorado

John B. Bielinski, B.A.
Research Assistant
Addictive Disorders Section
Veterans Affairs Medical Center
Minneapolis, Minnesota

Penny Brennan, Ph.D
Research Health Scientist
Center for Health Care Evaluation
Department of Veterans Affairs and
Stanford University Medical Centers
Palo Alto, California

Kathleen Bucholz, Ph.D.
Research Assistant Professor of
Epidemiology in Psychiatry
Department of Psychiatry
Washington University School of
Medicine
St. Louis, Missouri

Kailash C. Chadha, Ph.D
Cancer Research Scientist
Associate Research Professor
SUNY at Buffalo
Roswell Park Memorial Institute
Buffalo, New York

Louise E. Diers, B.S.
Student Services Associate
Department of Neuroscience
University of North Dakota School of
Medicine
Grand Forks, North Dakota

Richard E. Finlayson, M.D.
Associate in Psychiatry
Mayo Medical School
Medical Director
Inpatient Addiction Program
Mayo Psychiatry and Psychology
Treatment Center
Rochester, Minnesota

Steven R. Gambert, M.D. FACP
Professor and Chairman (Acting)
Department of Medicine
Associate Dean for Academic Programs
New York Medical College
Valhalla, New York

Meyer D. Glantz, Ph.D
Director, Etiology Research Program
Associate Director, Division of
Epidemiology and Prevention Research
National Institute on Drug Abuse
Rockville, Maryland

Edith S. Lisansky Gomberg, Ph.D
Professor of Psychology, Alcohol
Research Center
Department of Psychiatry, University of
Michigan
400 E. Eisenhower Parkway, Suite A
Ann Arbor, Michigan

Debra Heller, Ph.D.
Research Associate
Center for Developmental and Health
Genetics
The Pennsylvania State University
University Park, Pennsylvania

John Helzer, M.D.
Professor and Chairman
Department of Psychiatry
University of Vermont College of
Medicine
Burlington, Vermont

Katherine Katsoyannis, M.D.
Faculty Attending
Division of Geriatrics and Gerontology
New Rochelle Hospital Medical Center
Assistant Professor of Clinical Medicine
New York Medical College
Valhalla, New York

Madhu R. Korrapati, M.D.
Merck International Fellow in Clinical
Pharmacology
Clinical Pharmacology and Gerontology
Research Unit
Department of Veterans Affairs Medical
Center
Boise, Idaho
Department of Medicine
University of Washington School of
Medicine
Seattle, Washington

Ziad A. Kronfol, M.D.
Associate Professor of Psychiatry
University of Michigan School of
Medicine
Ann Arbor, Michigan

Anya M.-Y. Lin, Ph.D
Institute of Biomedical Sciences
Academia Sinica, Nankang
Taipei, Taiwan

Michael R. Lucey, M.D.
Associate Professor of Medicine
Director of Hepatology
Medical Director of Liver
Transplantation
Associate Chief of the Division of
Gastroenterology
Deparment of Internal Medicine
University of Pennsylvania School of
Medicine
Philadelphia, Pennsylvania

John Lynch, M.S.W.
Social Work Service
Veterans Affairs Medial Center
Minneapolis, Minnesota

Gerald McClearn, Ph.D.
Evan Pugh Professor of Health and
Human Development
Director, Center for Developmental and
Health Genetics
The Pennsylvania State University
University Park, Pennsylvania

Rudolph Moos, Ph.D.
Director, Center for Health Care
Evaluation
Department of Veterans Affairs and
Stanford University Medical
Centers
Palo Alto, California

Madhavan P. Nair, Ph.D.
Research Professor of Medicine
SUNY at Buffalo
Buffalo General Hospital
Buffalo, New York

Belinda Nelson, M.S.W.
Research Assistant, Alcohol Research
Center
Department of Psychiatry, University of
Michigan
Ann Arbor, Michigan

Douglas H. Olson, Ph.D.
Coordinator, Alcohol Related Disorders
Clinic
Addictive Disorders Section
Veterans Affairs Medial Center
Assistant Professor
Department of Psychology
University of Minnesota
Minneapolis, Minnesota

Michael R. Palmer, Ph.D.
Associate Professor, Department of
Pharmacology
University of Colorado School of
Medicine
Denver, Colorado

Karen Parfitt, Ph.D
Assistant Professor, Department of
Biology
Pomona College
Claremont, California

Earl Rubington, Ph.D
Professor of Sociology
Northeastern University
Boston, Massachusetts

Marc A. Schuckit, M.D.
Professor of Psychiatry
University of California School of
Medicine and Veterans Affairs Medical
Center
San Diego, California

Stanley A. Schwartz, M.D., Ph.D.
Professor of Medicine
SUNY at Buffalo
Buffalo General Hospital
Buffalo, New York

Yvette Sheline, M.D.
Assistant Professor of Psychiatry

Department of Psychiatry
Washington University School of
Medicine
St. Louis, Missouri

Ralph Tarter, Ph.D.
Professor of Psychiatry and Neurology
Western Psychiatric Institute and Clinic
Pittsburgh, Pennsylvania

Robert E. Vestal, M.D.
Chief, Clinical Pharmacology and
Gerontology Research Unit
Department of Veterans Affairs Medical
Center
Director, Mountain States Medical
Research Institute
Boise, Idaho
Professor of Medicine and Adjunct
Professor of Pharmacology
University of Washington School of
Medicine
Seattle, Washington

Nancy D. Vogeltanz, Ph.D
Assistant Professor of Neuroscience
Department of Neuroscience
University of North Dakota School of
Medicine
Grand Forks, North Dakota

Mark L. Willenbring, M.D.
Chief, Addictive Disorders Section
Veterans Affairs Medial Center
Associate Professor
Department of Psychiatry
University of Minnesota School of
Medicine
Minneapolis, Minnesota

Richard W. Wilsnack, Ph.D
Professor of Neuroscience
Department of Neuroscience
University of North Dakota School of
Medicine
Grand Forks, North Dakota

Sharon C. Wilsnack, Ph.D.
Chester Fritz Distinguished Professor of
Psychology
Department of Neuroscience

University of North Dakota School of
Medicine
Grand Forks, North Dakota

W. Gibson Wood, Ph.D.
Associate Director for Education and
Evaluation
Geriatric Research, Education and

Clinical Center
Veterans Affairs Medial Center
Associate Professor
Department of Pharmacology
University of Minnesota School of
Medicine
Minneapolis, Minnesota

I

DIAGNOSIS AND EPIDEMIOLOGY

Alcoholic Elderly: Prevalence, Screening, Diagnosis, and Prognosis

THOMAS P. BERESFORD

Until recent times late life problem drinkers have suffered from the double stereotype of being both old and alcoholic. It has not been uncommon for health care professionals to think of elderly drinkers merely as survivors of a long, dissolute history of heavy alcohol use followed by predictably poor health and early demise (Clark, 1981; Geller et al., 1989). Persons living beyond age 65 with a history of heavy alcohol use have often been regarded merely as fortunate survivors. This stereotype, coupled with data from large survey studies (e.g., Cahalan, 1970), depicted alcohol problems in late life as rare and self-limited occurrences. This view was put in official terms as late as 1987 when the standard diagnostic manual for the American Psychiatric Association stated; "In males, symptoms of alcohol dependence or abuse rarely occur for the first time after age 45" (DSM-III-R, 1987). The few studies published on this topic over the past 20 years, however, suggest that late life problem drinkers are neither an infrequent phenomenon nor do they represent a homogeneous group. Rosin and Glatt's report (Rosin & Glatt, 1971) followed by Zimberg's (Zimberg, 1974), for example, gave evidence to suggest that up to one third of problem drinkers beyond age 65 may have begun their pathologic drinking in late middle age or after.

EPIDEMIOLOGICAL TRENDS

U.S. census figures forecast that the frequency of the population of this country older than 65 will double between the years 1980 and 2030 (Beresford et al., 1990). There is a wide range of estimates of late life problem drinking prevalence: from as little as 3 to 4% to as high as 10% in various studies looking at different elderly subject groups. If we hypothesize an estimated annual prevalence of alcoholism in the range of 5% for persons 60 years and older, Figure 1.1 (from Beresford et al., 1990) depicts a striking increase in the anticipated numbers of elderly alcoholic persons due to the sheer increase in the elderly population during the upcoming decades.

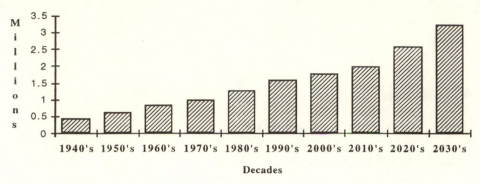

Figure 1.1. Estimated numbers of elderly alcoholics by decade (5% frequency; based on U.S. Census population projections).

In addition, however, there is evidence to suggest that the cohort effects operating among those who make up the elderly of today, those who were raised in the 1920s and 1930s when alcohol use carried a stigma of social opprobrium, have artificially lowered our current prevalence estimates. The large numbers of persons born after World War II, experiencing their formative years in times when the same social stigma was not present, will likely show a significantly higher prevalence of alcohol use disorders. This is already beginning to occur as documented in the Normative Aging Study (Glynn, Bouchard, LoCastro, & Laird, 1985).

SCOPE OF LATE LIFE ALCOHOL ABUSE

Rathbone-McCuan, in a community survey of 695 persons age 55 and older, first outlined the extent of elderly drinking (Rathbone-McCuan et al., 1976). In her sample, a total of 8% of subjects reported problem drinking defined as between one and six points scored on the Michigan Alcohol Screening Test (MAST), with another 4% reporting alcoholic drinking with a score greater than six. This contradicted earlier, less focused reports such as Cahalan's national telephone survey that noted only 6% of persons over 60 years as being heavy drinkers.

In a subsequent report, Barnes conducted a cross-sectional probability study of over 1,000 adults in western New York State (Barnes, 1979). Her findings were similar to Rathbone-McCuan's: 24% of males between 60 and 69 years of age could be classified as heavy drinkers. She characterized heavy drinkers as falling within a range of phenomena: from those who drank two or more drinks three or more times a day to those who drank two or more times a month but more than five standard beverages at a time. She also noted that males more than 60 years old who were heavy drinkers were nearly equally likely to be married (17%), widowed (14%), or never married (13%)—all of which differed from the non-heavy drinking sample, suggesting social isolation as a potential associated factor in late life alcohol abuse. Similarly, heavy drinking males over 60 years were slightly more likely to be employed (22%) than to be retired or unemployed (13%). This survey was one of the earliest studies to look into associated social phenomena as potentially causing or worsening heavy drinking in this age group.

No further large-scale community investigations were attempted for many years until the Environmental Catchment Area (ECA) study. Investigators from this project reported on the incidence of alcohol use disorders as defined by DSM-III (1980) by age (Eaton et al., 1989). While the group 65 and older witnessed an overall incidence that was about 20% of that among younger groups, the researchers nonetheless noted a steady frequency of new cases throughout the elderly cohort, with a gentle upswing in the incidence after age 75. Other researchers have noted that this upswing is based on data from very few cases and probably pertains generally to men (Atkinson, 1992a). The true importance of the ECA data lies in the continued incidence figures throughout late life, suggesting that the risk for alcohol dependence does not disappear after age 65.

A second community study, this time of prevalence of drinking problems among elderly persons, was recently conducted by Moos and colleagues, who reported on telephone interviews from over 1,800 persons between ages 55 and 65 (Moos et al., 1991). The investigators found one or more current alcohol problems in 37% of the respondents, and about one out of every three of the positive responders reported that they had not had alcohol problems 2 years before the survey. These data again point to the likelihood of an increase in drinking among some persons in late middle age and early old age, a phenomenon of some subtlety which may escape ordinary monitoring in health care centers.

CLINICAL SAMPLE PREVALENCE

Despite the fact that elderly persons visit general hospitals more frequently than younger people do and are prescribed more medicines than any other single age group, and despite the prior knowledge of the under-recognition of alcoholism among hospitalized patients of any age, we were surprised by our own findings of how infrequently elderly alcoholics were noticed in an early sample taken from the medical and surgical services of a university hospital. From a total of 5,962 discharges of patients 65 and above, only 87 (1,46%) merited a clinical diagnosis of alcoholism in the view of their physician (Beresford et al., 1988). Previous research, noted above, suggests that this figure should have been closer to 5%, the presumed rate in the general population.

Following this early study, we sought to establish the frequency of late life alcohol dependence likely to occur in inpatient health care settings. During a random sample study of screening measures for alcoholism among general hospital inpatients (Beresford et al., 1990), we provided a structured interview that elicited data on drinking style, alcohol problem symptomatology, and quantity and frequency of alcohol use, along with standard demographic descriptors. Table 1.1 lists our findings. Lifetime prevalence included those subjects who met alcohol dependence criteria (DSM-III-R, 1987) at any time in their lives, as judged by their history elicited by the study interview. Current prevalence required adherence to the DSM-3-R criteria for alcohol dependence as well as drinking three or more standard alcoholic beverages (12 oz. of beer, 4 oz. of table wine, or 1.5 oz. of spirits) on three or more occasions within the 30 days prior to the interview.

The figures demonstrate (1) a high lifetime prevalence of alcohol dependence after age 60, (2) a remarkably high prevalence of actively drinking elderly alcoholics, especially among those age 60 to 69, and (3) a sharp drop off after the eighth decade of

Table 1.1. Lifetime and Current Prevalence of DSM-III-R Alcohol Dependence for General Hospital Patients ($N = 1139$)

Age Group	n	Lifetime Prevalence (%)	Current Prevalence (%)
18–59	767	32.2	23.3
60–69	230	20.4	10.4
70–79	117	13.7	6.8
80+	25	0.0	0.0
60+ Overall	372	16.9	8.6

life. Recalling the earlier study on under-recognition, these data suggested that only one of every six active elderly alcoholic persons and only one of every 12 lifetime alcoholic persons were being recognized in acute medical settings when such knowledge could have materially affected the preservation of life and limb.

Because the total prevalence figures were in accord with previously published studies of alcoholism prevalence in this setting (Beresford, 1979), we believed the DSM-III-R criteria were adequate descriptors of alcohol dependence, although another analysis of these data demonstrated considerable theoretical variance in the application of the criteria to data upon which each of the nine DSM-III-R criteria are based (Beresford et al., 1991). While these criteria, and the later DSM-IV version, appear to be useful descriptors of alcohol dependence among aged persons, to our knowledge, no one has attempted a validity study of standard criteria in elderly subjects.

Stratification of this general hospital sample by age allowed comparison of standard alcohol screening examinations applied to elderly alcoholics as compared to the DSM-III-R (1987) frequency of alcohol dependence as a standard. Table 1.2 lists the data on screening as a function of the age of the study subjects. These data suggested (1) that all three of the brief screening interviews tested were sensitive to alcohol dependence in only 60% of elderly cases, (2) that the CAGE and the SAAST were highly specific, more so than the MAST, and (3) that the CAGE questions appeared to be the most sensitive for persons over 70. Nonetheless, these data suggested that there was room for a more sensitive age-specific screening instrument.

We proposed and developed an age-specific screening examination (Blow et al., 1992). This was derived from a 94-item inventory given to an initial sample of 840 older adults. Analysis of the sample data yielded a 32-item instrument that was tested on 305 elderly adults of varying alcohol histories from teetotalers to active dependent drinkers whose drinking histories and DSM-III-R diagnosis were ascertained through the Diagnostic Interview Schedule. The new screening interview yielded a sensitivity of 93.9%, specificity of 78.1%, positive predictive value of 87.2%, and negative pre-

Table 1.2. Validity Characteristics (%) of Alcohol Screening Interviews for Subjects Aged 60–69 Years ($N = 230$) versus 70+ Years ($N = 142$, values in parentheses)

Test	Sensitivity	Specificity	Positive Predictive Value
CAGE	59.3 (52.2)	94.7 (93.8)	79.6 (79.5)
MAST	59.3 (43.5)	86.5 (94.2)	60.3 (58.8)
SAAST	62.3 (28.6)	99.4 (99.7)	97.4 (99.4)

dictive value of 88.9% (Blow et al., 1992; see Appendix to this chapter). While these early data suggest a significantly more sensitive instrument for elderly drinking, further field testing will be required to verify these characteristics, especially in relation to setting.

For the present, the data mentioned above suggest (1) that large numbers of elderly drinkers exist in clinical settings, (2) that, as in younger age groups, elderly dependent drinkers are not recognized unless they are specifically looked for, (3) that the DSM-III-R and DSM-IV criteria appear to be adequate clinical descriptors of dependent alcohol use among the elderly, and (4) that methods are in hand that could allow for efficient recognition of elderly drinkers in efforts to refer for treatment.

RECENT VERSUS EARLY ONSET ALCOHOLISM AMONG ELDERLY IN CLINICAL SETTINGS

While screening methods can identify alcohol dependent persons, they do not tell of the onset or course of the dependence in any given case. As discussed above, recency of onset may be a significant, clinically useful distinction to make. In this context, we have compared two data sets in order to assess the early indications, discussed above, that socioeconomic characteristics are significantly associated with recency of use. We compared a state-supported, university general hospital sample and a sample from a private clinical facility.

General Hospital Sample

From the same study already mentioned, we analyzed the recency of onset character-istics presented in Table 1.3. We asked elderly dependent subjects to describe as spe-cifically as possible when their alcohol use accelerated to the point of tolerance acqui-sition and subsequent dependence symptomatology. Remarkably few in this sample reported beginning to drink within the five years previous to the survey. While the general hospital harbors many elderly dependent drinkers, it appears to be a reservoir of *early* onset elderly alcoholics who perhaps gain admission through the physical ravages of chronic alcoholism. This may also reflect the socioeconomic characteristics of the largely blue-collar population at this state-supported university hospital.

Table 1.3. Timing of Accelerated Alcohol Use among Elderly Drinkers (random general hospital admissions, > 60 years)

		Percent N	Percent n
Total N > 60 years	328	100.0	
Total n increase in use	64	19.5	100.0
Increased use within			
last 5 years	4	1.2	6.3
last 5–10 years	4	1.2	6.3
last 10–15 years	8	2.4	12.5
last 15+ years	48	14.7	75.0

Table 1.4. Characteristics of Elderly Private Rehabilitation Inpatients ($N = 47$)

	Males	Females
Total N	31	16
Onset in past 5 years	19 (61%)	10 (63%)
Average age (years)	68.7 ± 6.3	66.8 ± 3.9
Average length of stay (days)	20.5 ± 13.7	23.9 ± 12.5

Private Rehabilitation Unit Sample

In concert with the published reports on recent onset alcohol dependence in this age group, we retrospectively surveyed the experience of a privately supported community hospital. These data, representing three years in a newly established unit located in a city suburb, are listed in Table 1.4. Onset refers to the clinical history establishing the onset of pathological alcohol use. This sample includes all patients over 60 years of age. While the figures do not offer the confidence of systematically derived prospective data, they are consistent with survey reports (Moos et al., 1991) that suggest high frequencies of recent onset elderly alcoholics will be found among those who are economically more secure.

Comparison of the Two Settings

The comparison of the relative prevalence of alcohol dependent persons in these settings appears to give credence to the notion first articulated by Atkinson that recent onset elderly alcoholics are likely to have more social and economic resources and therefore are likely to be seen in private treatment facilities (Atkinson, 1990a). He reported, for example, that 24% of a sample of 54 patients seeking treatment in a VA alcohol clinic who were over 65 years of age had begun drinking within the previous 5 years. By contrast, Finlayson and colleagues (1988) reported that 41% of a sample of 211 elderly alcohol dependent patients seen at the Mayo Clinic had begun drinking after age 60. Reviewing this topic further, Atkinson (1990a) found an earlier study by Wiens and coworkers on a sample of 68 alcoholic persons over the age of 65 in a private alcohol rehabilitation facility (Wiens et al., 1982). Of these, fully 68% had begun drinking after the age of 60. Atkinson concluded that the increasing frequencies of late onset alcohol dependence in the three studies reflected a trend from lower to middle and upper middle class subjects in the respective studies. He observed that recent onset alcoholism may be more common among the relatively well off, while early onset alcohol dependence has more in common with the notion of a downhill, progressive course of alcoholism, outlined by Jellinek and others, that predicts a loss of personal resources because of uncontrolled alcohol use (Jellinek, 1960).

DIAGNOSTIC ACCURACY IN ELDERLY ALCOHOLISM

One fundamental question for any clinician is whether or not standard diagnostic schemes are adequate for elderly heavy drinkers in separating dependence from abusive or nonabusive alcohol use. Over the past 20 years, clinical researchers have become increasingly sophisticated in codifying pathologic drinking. In most diagnostic schema, two forms exist: abuse and dependence. The latter condition generally entails some evidence of physical dependence, usually either a tolerance to ethanol or withdrawal symptoms on cessation of use, along with some evidence of impaired control of drinking once begun or with evidence of social dysfunction attributable to drinking. Table 1.5 compares two standard schemes devised respectively in North America and in Europe. While many of the phenomena required by the DSM-IV (1994) on the one hand and the ICD-10 (WHO, 1992) on the other are held in common, several gaps occur, making it theoretically possible for a person to be declared an alcoholic in Europe but not in America, with the reverse case also possible. As a catalog of symptoms, both seem adequate for any age group.

When we consider the general symptom categories, however, such as tolerance, withdrawal symptoms, impaired control of drinking, and social decline, some clinical differences appear with respect to age. Considering tolerance as an example, a daily ethanol dose viewed, in some contexts, without alarm in a younger person may signal an ability to handle an increased ethanol load presented to the central nervous system in an older person. For instance, tolerating three rather than two standard drinks daily might not be considered a profound change to a 25-year-old but could represent a striking increase to a sexagenarian. No one knows whether tolerance to alcohol may be acquired more rapidly and with less total alcohol exposure among elderly persons than among younger persons. A related question is whether the same amounts of alcohol have measurably more debilitating effects in normal, nonalcoholic elderly persons than in younger persons. Precise knowledge of the levels at which this might occur, either by measurements of peak blood alcohol levels or areas under ethanol's metabolic curve, is lacking at the present time.

Similarly, very early studies noted below suggest that withdrawal symptoms are more severe and last for longer periods among elderly alcoholics than among their younger counterparts. Whether this is a function of the lifetime exposure to alcohol, exposure to repeated withdrawal episodes along the model of kindling, or merely the interaction of a toxin with an elderly nervous system is unknown. The only animal study of aging and withdrawal that exists, to the best of our knowledge, demonstrated that older rats trained to drink alcohol experienced more severe withdrawal symptoms than did younger animals given the same length of exposure to ethanol (Maler & Pohorecky, 1989). The fact that ethanol is more toxic to older animals was demonstrated when

Table 1.5. Comparison of Two Alcohol Dependence Criteria

DSM-IV Criteria	ICD-10 Criteria
1. Markedly increased tolerance	5. Evidence of tolerance
2a. Characteristic withdrawal symptoms	4. Physiological withdrawal state
2b. Alcohol use to treat withdrawal	3. Alcohol effective for withdrawal
3. Drinking more than intended	2. Awareness of impaired control
4. Unable to cut down/stop use	2. Awareness of impaired control
5. Much time used to get/use/recover	No counterpart
6. Activities given up due to drinking	7. Neglect of alternative pleasures
7. Continued use despite problems	8. Persistent use despite harm
No counterpart	1. Desire/compulsion to drink
No counterpart	6. Narrowing drinking pattern
No counterpart	9. Relapse leads to rapid return of symptoms

Source: Adapted from Atkinson (1990a).

researchers noted that the lethal dose (LD 50) for ethyl alcohol decreased as the animals aged (Wiberg et al., 1970).

But only brief, retrospective clinical reports discuss alcohol withdrawal phenomena and their severity in elderly persons. Liskow applied a withdrawal scale to young and old subjects and found that withdrawal symptoms were more severe and required more chlordiazepoxide for their control in the elderly subjects (Liskow et al., 1989). Brower and associates reviewed records of older and younger adults in a rehabilitation facility and found the same thing (Brower et al., 1994). Neither study controlled for the length or regularity of exposure to alcohol, the frequency of previous withdrawal episodes, or the recency of onset of alcohol addiction. No studies exist that compare withdrawal phenomena in samples of early onset versus recent onset alcoholic elderly patients. Severe withdrawal symptoms, especially delirium tremens, appear to worsen with age and often result in a remarkably prolonged period of cognitive impairment (Liskow et al., 1989). Instances of this may require extended treatment and hospitalization well beyond that normally required in middle-aged or younger persons similarly affected. For purposes of diagnosis, what little is known suggests that withdrawal symptoms may occur after less frequent or less heavy alcohol use among elderly persons, a possibility that must be accounted for in the clinical history.

In contrast to the symptomatology of tolerance to ethanol and withdrawal symptoms on ceasing its use, the symptoms of the impaired control phenomenon may appear very much the same in elderly dependent drinkers as in their younger counterparts. Impaired control is defined as an inability to predict the extent or amount of alcohol used in a consistent fashion from one drinking episode to the next. No present studies exist to suggest that alcoholic elderly are any less likely to experience characteristic symptoms. When control of alcohol use has been lost, dependent drinkers struggle to stop drinking after one or two standard drinks, report many attempts at cutting down or stopping alcohol use, and engage external means of trying to control this internally driven behavior. For example, a dependent drinker may attempt to limit pathologic drinking by using alcohol only at certain times of the day, in certain beverage forms, or within the constraints of a previously determined supply or amount of money to be spent on drink. While the nature of the loss of control phenomenon continues to elude those searching for the neural mechanisms that might account for it, its presence as a phenomenological entity remains at the center of our present conceptions of dependent drinking. By most definitions, dependent alcohol users are unable to control their drinking regardless of age (Schuckit, 1982).

As with the physiologic symptoms of addiction, however, social decline resulting from uncontrolled drinking does appear to be reflected, at least phenomenologically, in age-specific symptoms. For example, while frequent fist fights may commonly indicate uncontrolled alcohol use in a 25-year-old male, most male alcoholics at 65 do not report this as a frequent symptom. Conversely, present data suggest that threatened loss of a driver's license due to drinking carries with it a far greater impact at age 65, because of the loss of personal autonomy (Atkinson, 1990a), often already compromised by age, as compared to a similar threat at 25. It is important to assess age-specific phenomena when attempting to understand the social sequelae of drinking in an elderly person.

As the DSM-IV diagnostic scheme (APA, 1994) replaces its predecessors, no studies exits, to our knowledge, establishing the usefulness of the new diagnostic method in

Table 1.6. Comparison of Alcohol Dependence or Abuse Criteria by Prevalence among Hospitalized Patients ($N = 1,139$)

DSM-III (1980)	25%
DSM-III-R (1987)	34%
DSM-IV proposed (1994)	30%

the elderly. At present, we can offer only the following comparisons (Table 1.6) taken from our general hospital study, reflecting persons ranging from 21 to the late 80s in age. While differences exist in the prevalence rates of dependence and abuse in the three versions, we have no data to support any discrepancies associated with age. Further study of diagnostic criteria in the elderly age group is certainly warranted.

GENDER CONSIDERATIONS AMONG ELDERLY DRINKERS

The extent to which gender may affect the establishment and course of alcohol dependence among the elderly is unknown at the present time. The following, however, may offer clues for further inquiry and for clinical identification.

Treatment Center Samples of Elderly Drinkers

Alcoholism is generally regarded as a condition that affects four males for every female. But the data noted in the private rehabilitation unit sample above presents a 2:1 ratio. Similarly, the recent community telephone survey quoted above (Moos et al., 1991) noted a higher proportion of women in the recent onset alcohol problem group (39%) versus that seen in the early onset problem drinking group (22%). Very early data suggest that these observations may not be merely geographic or accidental.

In the only study of its kind, to the best of our knowledge, Dr. Gomberg (1992, 1993) surveyed elderly drinkers (> 60 years of age) from treatment units resembling the private unit noted above. Her sample included 83 males and 41 females and represented all of the elderly drinkers seen in those treatment centers during the study period. This represented a higher than expected number of females and is consistent with our findings noted above. The women reported the onset of alcohol problems at a much later age than did the men: 46.2 versus 27.0 years ($p < .015$). One quarter of the women (25%), but only 1% of the men reported that their first problem occurred after age 60. An additional 27% of the women, but only 1% of the men, reported their first alcohol problem between ages 50 and 59 years. Over one third (38%) of all the elderly women surveyed reported the onset of their dependence as having begun within the past ten years, as compared to only 4% of the men in the study. Dr. Gomberg noted several associated findings: Women were more likely to be widowed ($p < .003$), to have had a problem-drinking spouse ($p < 001$), to have experienced depression ($p < .05$), and to have been injured in falls ($p < .025$). This study suggests that alcohol dependence among the elderly may differ from that seen among younger subjects not only by age characteristics but by gender-specific phenomena as well.

Gender and Length of Stay of Elderly Alcoholics in Rehabilitation

One question about gender differences in this age group concerns whether or not severity of alcoholism or of its associated physical and social problems is related to age, to gender, or to recency of onset. If we view length of stay in a rehabilitation unit as a rough indication of severity, figures from the private rehabilitation unit noted above may provide a clue in beginning to answer this question. As depicted in Figure 1.2, there was no correlation between length of stay and either age or recency of onset among the male sample. In Figures 1.3 and 1.4, however, age was positively and significantly associated with length of stay both for early onset and recent onset alcohol dependent elderly females. The correlation appears stronger for the recent onset females, although the number of subjects is small and length of stay may be determined by many factors. Very preliminary data such as these, however, cause one to wonder whether the interaction of age with alcohol use differs, not only socially but perhaps biologically, between the genders.

COURSE AND PROGNOSIS

Any discussion of diagnosis and prevalence must be brought in relation to course since diagnosis is usually our first, and often our best, clue to prognosis. The now classic longitudinal study by Vaillant (Vaillant, 1983) of early onset, middle-aged (mean = 45 yrs, ± 10 years) alcoholics identified four prognostic factors that were associated with continued abstinence from alcohol beyond three years: (1) a substitute dependence or activity with which to structure the time previously spent drinking, (2) a significant

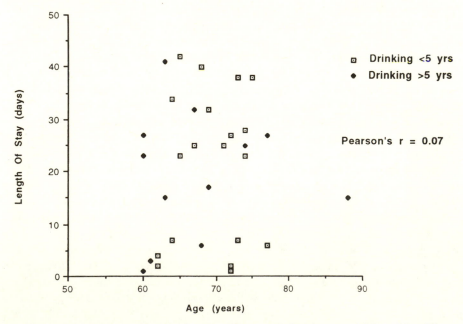

Figure 1.2. Age versus length of stay, male recent and early-onset drinkers ($N = 31$).

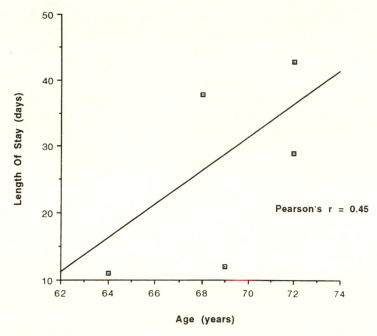

Figure 1.3. Age versus length of stay, female early-onset drinkers ($N = 6$).

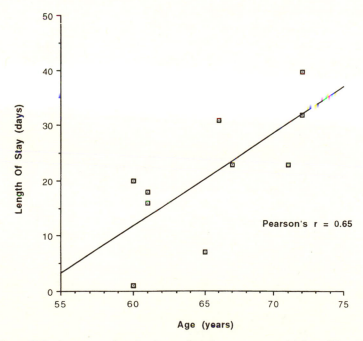

Figure 1.4. Age versus length of stay, female recent-onset drinkers ($N = 10$).

relationship with a caring person who was capable of drawing knowledgeable limits on drinking behavior, (3) a source of hope or improved self-esteem that served to counterbalance guilt due to drinking or related problems, and (4) a consequence of drinking that was both certain and noxious. Whether these factors apply, and to what extent they may apply to elderly alcoholic persons, remains an important question.

In a study of treatment of late life alcoholic persons, Atkinson demonstrated that the last of Vaillant's factors was useful when he showed that the revocation or impending revocation of a driver's license was one of the best predictors of treatment compliance in his sample of elderly VA outpatient alcoholics (Atkinson et al., 1993). Along similar lines, the short-term remission study noted above (Moos et al., 1991) reported that late life problem drinkers who remitted within one year of initial contact ''consumed less alcohol, reported fewer drinking problems, had friends who approved less of drinking, and were more likely to seek help from mental health practitioners.'' While Moos's first two factors may appear somewhat academic, the disapproval of friends and the seeking of help from another person both appear congruent with Vaillant's idea of a knowledgeable significant other whose concern is balanced by clear limits to tolerating drinking. In the Moos study as well, late onset problem drinkers were more likely to remit over the follow-up period than were early onset problem drinkers.

At first glance the remission Moos and coworkers observed might be ascribed to the brevity of problem drinking. It may also be the case, however, that if recent onset elderly drinkers remit more easily than do their younger recent onset counterparts, the intransigence of uncontrolled drinking characteristic of alcohol dependence at a young age may itself be altered in ways that could be traced to the alterations of an aging physiology. Moos and colleagues used very general language to conclude that late onset problem drinkers might be ''more reactive to physical health stressors and to social influences'' than are persons with long-standing alcoholism. While present data suggest that late life recent onset alcoholism may be less severe and more treatable than early onset alcoholism, they do not offer a view of a path to recovery so much as a list of the possible resources to be used in that cause. What course characterizes those who recover versus those who do not remains unknown at the present time. How best to approach recent versus early onset elderly alcoholism, if indeed a differential approach is required, has yet to be determined systematically.

SUMMARY

There can be little doubt that alcoholism among the elderly is a significant health problem that is likely to increase rather than decrease over the next three decades. While present screening and diagnostic methods appear adequate to the task of recognizing elderly alcoholics, it is important to know that neither has been tested rigorously in large samples of aged drinkers and nondrinkers. Similarly, little attention has been paid to the issues of (1) physiologic interaction with the aging metabolic and nervous systems as these apply to diagnosis and prognosis, (2) the characteristics of onset and course of alcoholism as they present uniquely among the elderly, and (3) specific problems related both to age and to gender among elderly alcoholics. While these are only a few of the issues needing attention, and while many more will become evident through the pages of this book, these seem to be some of the most salient clinically and most likely to yield immediate changes in both the prevention and the rehabilitation of alcohol use disorders among the elderly.

References

American Psychiatric Association. (1980). *Diagnostic and statistical manual of mental disorders* (3rd ed.). Washington, D.C.

American Psychiatric Association. (1987). *Diagnostic and statistical manual of mental disorders* (3rd ed. rev.). Washington, D.C.

American Psychiatric Association. (1994). *Diagnostic and Statistical Manual, Fourth Edition.* Washington, D.C.

Atkinson, R. M. (1990a). Aging and alcohol use disorders: Diagnostic issues in the elderly. *International Psychogeriatrics, 2*, 55–72.

Atkinson, R. M., Tolson, R. L., & Turner, J. A. (1990b). Late versus early onset problem drinking in older men. *Alcoholism: Clinical and Experimental Research, 14*, 574–579.

Atkinson, R. M. (1994). *Late onset problem drinking in older adults. International Journal of Geriatric Psychiatry*, in press.

Atkinson, R. M. & Tolson, R. L. (1992b). *Late onset alcoholism: Is it rare?* San Francisco: American Association For Geriatric Psychiatry.

Atkinson, R. M., Tolson, R. L., & Turner, J. A. (1993). Factors affecting outpatient treatment compliance of older male problem drinkers. *Journal of Studies on Alcohol, 54*, 102–106.

Barnes, G. M. (1979). Alcohol use among older persons: findings from a Western New York State general population survey. *Journal of the American Geriatric Society, 27*(6), 244–50.

Beresford, T. (1979). Alcoholism consultation and general hospital psychiatry. *General Hospital Psychiatry, 2*, 293–300.

Beresford, T. P., Blow, F. C., & Brower, K. J. (1988). Alcohol and aging in the general hospital. *Psychosomatics, 29*, 61–72.

Beresford, T. P., Blow, F. C., & Brower, K. J. (1990). Alcoholism in the elderly. *Comprehensive Therapeutics, 16*, 38–43.

Beresford, T. P., Blow, F. C., Hill, E. M., & Singer, K. (1991). When is an alcoholic an alcoholic? *Alcohol and Alcoholism, 26*(Suppl. 1), 487–488.

Beresford, T. P., Blow, F. C., Hill, E. Singer, K., & Lucey, M. R. (1990). Comparison of CAGE questionnaire and computer-assisted laboratory profiles in screening for covert alcoholism. *Lancet, 336*(8713), 482–85.

Blow, F. C., Brower, K. J., Schulenberg, J. E., Demo-Dananberg, L. M., Young, J. S., & Beresford, T. P. (1992). The Michigan Alcoholism Screening Test—Geriatric Version (MAST-G): A new elderly specific screening instrument. *Alcoholism: Clinical and Experimental Research, 16*, 372.

Brower, K. J., Mudd, S., Blow, F. C., Young, J. P., & Hill, E. M. (1994). Severity and treatment of alcohol withdrawal in elderly versus younger patients. *Alcoholism: Clinical and Experimental Research, 18*, 196–201.

Cahalan, D. (1970). *Problem drinkers: A national survey.* San Francisco: Jossey-Bass.

Clark, W. D. (1981). Alcoholism: blocks to diagnosis and treatment. *American Journal of Medicine, 71*, 275–86.

Eaton, W. W., Kramer, M., Anthony, J. C., et al. (1989). The incidence of specific DIS/DSM-III mental disorders: Data from the NIMH Epidemiological Catchment Area Program. *Acta Psychiatrica Scandinavia, 79*, 163–78.

Finney, J. & Moos, R. (1984). Life stressors and problem drinking among older adults. In M. Galanter (Ed.), *Recent Developments in Alcoholism, Vol 2*, (pp. 267–88). New York: Plenum.

Finlayson, R. E., Hurt, R. D., Davis, L. J., Morse, R. M. (1988). Alcoholism in elderly persons: A study of the psychiatric and psychosocial features of 216 inpatients. *Mayo Clinic Proceedings, 63*, 761–68.

Geller, G., Levine, D. M., Mammon, J. A., Moore, R. D., Bone, L. R., & Stokes, E. J. (1989). Knowledge, attitudes and reported practices of medical students and house staff regarding the diagnosis and treatment of alcoholism. *Journal of the American Medical Association, 261*, 3115–20.

Glynn, R. J., Bouchard, G. R., LoCastro, J. S., & Laird, N. M. (1985). Aging and generational effects on drinking behaviors in men: Results from the normative aging study. *American Journal of Public Health, 75*(12), 1413–9.

Gomberg, E. S. L. (1985). Gerontology and alcohol studies. In E. Gottheil Druley, K. A., Skoloda, T. E. (Ed.), *The combined problems of alcoholism, drug addiction and aging*. Springfield, IL: Charles C. Thomas.

Gomberg, E. S. L. (1992). Elderly alcoholic men and women in treatment. Research Society on Alcoholism. Annual Scientific Meeting, San Diego, CA.

Gomberg, E. S. (1993). Recent developments in alcoholism: Gender issues. *Recent Developments In Alcoholism, 11*, 95–107.

Jellinek, E. M. (1960). *The Disease Concept Of Alcoholism*. New Haven. Hillhouse Press.

Liskow, B. I., Rinck, C., Campbell, J., & DeSouza, C. (1989). Alcohol withdrawal in the elderly. *Journal of Studies on Alcohol, 50*(5), 414–21.

Maier, D. M., & Pohorecky, L. A. (1989). The effect of repeated withdrawal episodes on subsequent withdrawal severity in ethanol-treated rats. *Drug and Alcohol Dependence, 23*(2), 103–10.

Moos, R. H., Brennan, P. L., & Moos, B. S. (1991). Short-term process of remission and non-remission among late-life problem drinkers. *Alcoholism: Clinical and Experimental Research, 15*, 948–55.

Rathbone-McCuan, E., Lohn, H., Levenson, J., et al. (1976). *Community survey of aged alcoholics and problem drinkers, report to the NIAAA*. Baltimore: Levindale Geriatric Research Center.

Rosin, A. J. & Glatt, M. M. (1971). Alcohol excess in the elderly. *Quarterly Journal of Studies on Alcohol, 32*, 53–59.

Schonfeld, L. & Dupree, L. W. (1991). Antecedents of drinking for early- and late-onset elderly alcohol abusers. *Journal of Studies on Alcohol, 52*, 587–92.

Schuckit, M. A. (1982). A clinical review of alcohol, alcoholism, and the elderly patient. *Journal of Clinical Psychiatry, 43*, 396–99.

Spitzer, R., Williams, J. B. W., & Gibbon, M. (1987). *Structured clinical interview for DSM-3-R personality disorder (SCID-II)*. New York: New York State Psychiatric Institute, Biometrics Research.

Vaillant, G. E. (1983). *The natural history of alcoholism*. Cambridge, MA: Harvard University Press.

Wiberg, G. S., Trenholm, H. L., & Coldwell, B. B. (1970). Increases in ethanol toxicity in old rats: Changes in LD 50, *in vivo* and *in vitro* metabolism and liver alcohol dehydrogenase activity. *Toxicol Appl Pharmacol, 16*, 718–27.

Wiens, A. N., Miller, C. E., & Schmitz, R. E. (1982). Medical-behavioral treatment of the older alcoholic patient. *American Journal of Drug and Alcohol Abuse, 9*, 461–75.

Zimberg, S. (1974). Two types of problem drinkers: Both can be managed. *Geriatrics, 29*, 135–39.

APPENDIX

Michigan Alcoholism Screening Test—
Geriatric Version (MAST-G)

		Yes (1)	No (0)			Yes (1)	No (0)
1.	After drinking have you ever noticed an increase in your heart rate or beating in your chest?	—	—	10.	Does having a drink help you sleep?	—	—
2.	When talking with others, do you ever underestimate how much you actually drink?	—	—	11.	Do you hide your alcohol bottles from family members?	—	—
3.	Does alcohol make you sleepy so that you often fall asleep in your chair?	—	—	12.	After a social gathering, have you ever felt embarrassed because you drank too much?	—	—
4.	After a few drinks, have you sometimes not eaten or been able to skip a meal because you didn't feel hungry?	—	—	13.	Have you ever been concerned that drinking might be harmful to your health?	—	—
5.	Does having a few drinks help decrease your shakiness or tremors?	—	—	14.	Do you like to end an evening with a night cap?	—	—
6.	Does alcohol sometimes make it hard for you to remember parts of the day or night?	—	—	15.	Did you find your drinking increased after someone close to you died?	—	—
7.	Do you have rules for yourself that you won't drink before a certain time of the day?	—	—	16.	In general, would you prefer to have a few drinks at home rather than go out to social events?	—	—
8.	Have you lost interest in hobbies or activities you used to enjoy?	—	—	17.	Are you drinking more now than in the past?	—	—
9.	When you wake up in the morning, do you ever have trouble remembering part of the night before?	—	—	18.	Do you usually take a drink to relax or calm your nerves?	—	—
				19.	Do you drink to take your mind off your problems?	—	—
				20.	Have you ever increased your drinking after experiencing a loss in your life?	—	—

continued

APPENDIX (continued)

Yes No   *Yes No*
(1) (0)   (1) (0)

21. Do you sometimes drive when you have had too much to drink?   21. — —

24. When you feel lonely does having a drink help?   24. — —

22. Has a doctor or nurse ever said they were worried or concerned about your drinking?   22. — —

23. Have you ever made rules to manage your drinking?   23. — —

Scoring: 5 or more "yes" responses indicative of alcohol problem.

© The Regents of the University of Michigan, 1991

2

The Epidemiology of Alcohol Use, Problems, and Dependence in Elders: A Review

KATHLEEN K. BUCHOLZ, YVETTE I. SHELINE, AND JOHN E. HELZER

The study of elder alcohol practices, alcohol problems, and alcohol dependence is an idea whose time has come. Despite numerous calls in the literature for such studies (Gomberg, 1980; Atkinson, 1987), there has been relatively little alcohol research conducted on representative samples of elders. Rather than being sampled as a tenable and distinct study population, elders have been studied mainly as part of national or clinical populations or other types of samples in which they serendipitously appear. Those studies in which elders have been specifically targeted suffer from limited generalizability that results from the type of sample, which is often from a particular geographic region (for example, a single metropolitan area) or some other sample of convenience (e.g., clinic attenders or clients of social service agencies).

There are several compelling reasons for alcohol researchers to focus on the spectrum of alcohol use in a representative sample of elders. It is widely accepted that drinking in the elderly declines and therefore may merit less attention than drinking in a younger population. Results from some recent studies conducted both in clinical and community samples challenge this. A recent analysis of National Health Interview Survey data over an 11-year period showed an increase in average daily alcohol consumption among men 65 or older, and a slight increase in women between the ages of 65 and 74 (Malin et al., 1985). These data suggest the possibility of an increase in late-onset drinking problems in the 65 or older population.

Second, the increases both in drinking and in rates of alcohol consumption in the "pre-elder" groups (that is, those younger than 60) suggest that there will be an increase in alcohol dependent elders as these people age (Helzer et al., 1991; Reich et al., 1988). Studying elderly alcoholics today may help to anticipate the demands that these younger alcoholics will eventually place on our resources and society. Findings from a recent survey of the elderly in upstate New York underscore this point. The most important predictor of heavy drinking in late life was heavy drinking in early life (Welte & Mirand, 1992).

Finally, alcohol poses an important health risk to the elderly population through its direct toxic effects as well as in combination with other drugs that increase its toxic effects. With the rise in physical illness in the elderly population, the likelihood increases that alcohol will have an adverse impact on another medical condition. Moreover, undetected alcohol use in the elderly makes it particularly insidious.

This chapter will start by defining elders, categories of alcohol consumption, and alcohol dependence and then will review the epidemiology of alcohol consumption, alcohol problems, and alcohol dependence in elders. It will present some data on alcohol abuse and dependence disorder in a multi-site community survey conducted to estimate the prevalence of psychiatric disorder, including alcohol dependence (the NIMH Epidemiologic Catchment Area Program, Regier et al., 1985) in several age cohorts of elderly individuals. It will also suggest some areas for future research that would be particularly fruitful.

METHODOLOGICAL ISSUES

Who Are the Elderly and Why Should They Be Studied?

On an individual basis, the concept of "elderly" may be arbitrary, given the heterogeneity in rates of aging physically, psychologically, and socially. One of the most widely used definitions of elderly adults as "65 and older" is based on retirement or age of Social Security benefits. Some studies use 60 or even 50 as the entry point for studying the elderly, and distinctions have been made between the "young-old" (those younger than 80) and the "old-old" (80+) (Neugarten, 1976). Since there is no general agreement on specific age limits for "elderly," it is critical that research studies carefully define age groups.

Currently, Americans over the age of 65 represent 11% of the population, and they are expected to grow to 17% of the population by the year 2030. In 1984, they accounted for 31% of total health care expenditures, and as the number in the oldest age group grows, these expenditures will increase (USDHHS, 1986). In community samples, 80% of people over the age of 65 have at least one chronic illness and often more (Kovar, 1977).

Any factor such as alcohol use that adversely affects the health of the elderly will be important to understand, in terms of both its specific adverse effects and its interaction with other health factors. Illness per se can make the elderly more vulnerable to the toxic effects of alcohol. In addition, the elderly are often on a variety of medications, both prescription and over-the-counter, which can have dangerous or even lethal effects in combination with alcohol (Richelson, 1984). The elderly are prescribed a large number of drugs—four on average in one survey (Alexander et al., 1985). In addition, 69% of elders take over-the-counter drugs (Guttmann, 1978). Because chronic alcohol use may cause liver damage, there is morbidity not only from liver damage itself, but also from the diminished capacity to metabolize drugs. With the number of drugs that are prescribed for the elderly, a change in the physiology of the liver is an important risk. Potentially high or even fatal drug levels may result from inability to metabolize drugs, especially if there is liver damage that goes undetected. The normal aging process involves a 40% decrease in hepatic blood flow and liver size decreases in relation to body mass (Vestal, 1984).

Another physiological change occurring with aging that exacerbates the effect of alcohol is the change in body composition. The elderly have a decrease in body water content (Bruce et al., 1988), resulting in higher peak serum ethanol levels (Vestal et al., 1977) for a given intake of alcohol. This change in the effective alcohol content of a drink in combination with slowed reaction time (Salthouse, 1985) may account for some of the accidental injuries that are responsible for significant morbidity and mortality in the elderly (Ray, 1992). In addition, alcohol causes deranged bone mineral metabolism, which increases the already high risk of osteopenia and compression fractures in the elderly (Feitelberg et al., 1987).

The differential diagnosis in an elderly person who presents with confusion and depressive symptoms can be extremely complex and includes singly or in a combination physical illness, dementia, depression, drug and alcohol abuse, and prescription or non-prescription drug use. Alcohol is well known to have permanent adverse effects on cognitive functioning, especially memory (see Chapter 14). In addition, many of the elderly have primary dementing illnesses that can be further exacerbated by alcohol. It is estimated that 4 to 6% of the population over 65 have severe dementia (Weissman et al., 1985). In the age category ''80 and older,'' 20% of the population has dementia. The vulnerability of the brain to a wide array of insults increases with age. The concept of decreased cortical reserve with age helps to explain why nondemented elderly persons are more vulnerable to effects as different as intensive care unit psychosis and delirium secondary to infection or metabolic imbalance. Depression can present as pseudodementia, which may be indistinguishable from a progressive dementing illness other than by duration and course (Larson et al., 1985; Post, 1975). Physical illness can precipitate depression, and in the face of compromised health, depression is more common, more severe, more likely to result in suicide, and more refractory to treatment (Bulbena & Berrios, 1986; Himmelhoch et al., 1982; Snow & Wells, 1981; Meehan et al., 1991). Alcohol use is in itself a risk factor for depression and suicide (Blumenthal, 1988).

Understanding in more detail the specific health risks in elderly adults will become increasingly important in the future not only because of the sheer increase in numbers of the elderly, but also because of a longer life span. A larger number of people will live into their eighties and even nineties, resulting in their spending 20 to 30% of their lifespan in the ''over 65'' age category.

Who Is a Drinker?

A second methodological question concerns the definitions of *drinker, light drinker, moderate drinker*, and *heavy drinker*. In a comprehensive and thorough review (Room, 1991), the progression of measurement of types of alcohol consumption proceeded from the dichotomous separation of drinker and nondrinker (a distinction which itself was not necessarily simple) to assessment of actual amounts of drinking. In the latter, consumption of specific alcohol amounts would typically be calculated in a time frame that might vary from 1 week, 2 weeks, 4 weeks, 30 days, to the last year. Unfortunately, no single time frame has been used by alcohol researchers, which has complicated cross-study comparisons of drinking.

Furthermore, in some studies, heavy drinking has been assessed as well, often by the number (or proportion) of heavy drinking occasions, with *heavy* usually defined in terms of a threshold amount (for example, five or more drinks per occasion). Categories used in alcohol research have reflected researchers' objectives and interests, study hypotheses, and analytical strategies, which may explain the sometimes parochial nature of these categories. However, meaningful synthesis of the literature requires attention to these definitions.

Even the apparently straightforward term *abstainer* has differed from study to study (Hilton, 1986). In some, abstainers have been defined as current nondrinkers regardless of their prior drinking habits (see Malin et al., 1985), while in others, abstainers include only lifelong abstainers. Thus, the category of abstainers may reflect current nondrinkers and may include not only lifelong teetotalers but also recovering alcoholics who do not currently drink and infrequent drinkers. The issue of abstention is particularly germane to elders, of whom many are likely to be current nondrinkers, perhaps for health or economic reasons, but not necessarily lifelong abstainers. One illustration of the importance of precision in the term *abstainer* is the common finding that moderate drinking is beneficial, but abstention is deleterious, to cardiovascular health (Ellison, 1990). Imprecise classification of drinking status in some earlier studies left unresolved whether this finding pointed to a truly harmful effect of lifelong abstention from alcohol, or merely reflected the fact that some individuals were too sick to drink. Subsequent studies, with better definitions of abstention, suggest that the latter explanation does not hold (Boffetta & Garfinkel, 1990).

Definition of Alcohol Dependence and Its Application to Elders

From a psychiatric epidemiologic perspective where the focus is on alcohol diagnosis instead of alcohol use, the definition of alcohol dependence disorder is far less variable than that of alcohol consumption. In 1980, the American Psychiatric Association published the DSM-III classification system, which set forth diagnostic criteria for specific psychiatric disorders, including alcohol dependence and abuse. A major community survey of psychiatric disorder, the Epidemiologic Catchment Area Project, (Regier et al., 1985) was conducted, using the DSM-III criteria (1980) as operationalized in a structured psychiatric interview. Data from this study will be presented later in this chapter. The DSM-III criteria have since been revised twice, in 1987 with the DSM-III-R (1987), and most recently with the DSM-IV (1994). Each of these systems will be reviewed briefly.

Hallmark features of alcohol dependence disorder in the DSM-III diagnostic classification system include physiological dependence on alcohol as manifested by tolerance to alcohol or withdrawal symptoms when going without alcohol (e.g., shakes, anxiety, sweating, etc.), plus one of the following: evidence of impairment in social functioning (e.g., serious family problems, job or school problems, legal difficulties) or pathological use of alcohol (e.g., being unable to stop drinking, experiencing blackouts, or binge drinking where usual responsibilities were neglected).

It should be noted that alcohol researchers whose focus is on problem drinking rather than alcohol disorder have constructed measures to reflect dimensions of dependence on alcohol, including psychological dependence (e.g., escape drinking); symptomatic behaviors (e.g., morning drinking, shakes); loss of control (inability to abstain or to control the amount of drinking); and binge drinking (drinking steadily for 24 hours or longer). As can be seen, these overlap somewhat with the criteria for alcohol dependence disorder, but not entirely.

The DSM-III diagnostic system also allowed for a less severe form of alcohol disorder called *alcohol abuse*. To meet criteria for abuse, an individual must have evidence of both pathological use and social impairment, as described above for alcohol dependence disorder. Tolerance or withdrawal, necessary for the dependence diagnosis, is not required for abuse. Under the DSM-III criteria, an individual may meet criteria for alcohol abuse only, alcohol dependence only, or alcohol abuse and dependence. For the purposes of this paper, *alcohol disorder* will include individuals who meet criteria for either abuse or dependence. *Alcohol disorder* and *alcoholism* will also be used interchangeably.

In 1987, a revision of the DSM-III classification system was published (1987). Under the DSM-III-R system, criteria for substance dependence were changed to a count of symptom groups, with three out of nine symptom groups required, all of equal importance. New criterion items were added. Lastly, the concept of alcohol abuse was substantially reinterpreted, so that *abuse* and *dependence* were mutually exclusive diagnoses. Abuse was considered the residual diagnosis, available only for individuals who did not qualify for a diagnosis of dependence. This set of diagnostic criteria has been used in two national surveys (Grant, 1992), one of these an ongoing longitudinal study for which data are not yet available.

The DSM-III-R criteria have been replaced by DSM-IV. In the new criteria, the number of criterion symptoms for dependence has been reduced to seven (from nine) and clustering of three of these criterion groups within any 12-month period is required. The hierarchy of dependence and abuse will be maintained in the DSM-IV; only those who do not qualify for a diagnosis of alcohol dependence may be evaluated for a diagnosis of abuse. The number of criterion symptom groups for the abuse diagnosis will be increased from two to four, and clustering of symptom groups within any 12-month period will also be required. Data are not yet generally available that reflect the new DSM-IV criteria.

Although the appropriateness of these new criteria for the elderly has yet to be formally studied, the similarities to previous classification systems suggest that the objections to the old will apply to the new. These objections include the diminished occupational or familial responsibilities often experienced by elders that preclude the occurrence of many of the common social problems associated with alcohol dependence; increased memory problems that may confound recall of even recent alcohol consumption, as well as the more difficult task of long-term recall; the difficulty in differentiating the physical effects of alcohol consumption from those of the normal aging process; and the possibility that denial might be especially acute in an elderly population (Graham, 1986; Atkinson, 1990). Furthermore, thresholds of drinking set to define heavy or tolerant drinking (typically 5 to 7 drinks or more per drinking occasion) may not be appropriate for an older person in light of changing physiology and metabolism that diminish an older person's capacity to drink at this level. In the absence of empirical data, the existing diagnostic criteria should be applied to elders, but a study of the suitability of the criteria would make a welcome contribution to the field.

EPIDEMIOLOGIC STUDIES: OVERVIEW

Cross-Sectional Studies

Much of what is known about elderly drinking practices, drinking problems, and alcohol dependence is based on cross-sectional studies, also known as prevalence studies, that is, one-time surveys of samples of individuals. *Prevalence* is the proportion of individuals in a population with a particular disease, behavior, condition, or other characteristic of interest at a specific time. The time period defines the type of prevalence being estimated: Prevalence on a given day (like the day of the interview) is described as *point prevalence*; over a time interval, like one year, as *period prevalence*; over a lifetime as *lifetime prevalence*. Prevalence studies include only individuals who are available at the time of the study and so may be thought of as studies of survivors. Because information on the same individual is gathered only once in a prevalence study, these studies are primarily descriptive rather than analytic, meaning that etiologic hypotheses or causal relationships cannot be tested. This is so because in a prevalence study, it is not possible to distinguish precursors from consequences of the outcome of interest. For example, a common observation from cross-sectional studies is that alcoholics are less likely to complete their education (Helzer et al., 1991). At least two plausible interpretations may be posited, but not decided, by cross-sectional data: Alcoholism may have caused the failure to complete schooling; or the stress, disappointment, and possible humiliation of failure to complete an academic program may have provoked the alcoholism. Determining which is correct would require at least one other measurement, preferably before school failure had occurred, to determine whether alcoholism predated or postdated that event. Cross-sectional studies may lead to inferences that differ from those suggested by studies with multiple assessments of the same individuals over time, that is, longitudinal studies.

Longitudinal Studies on Drinking Behavior

Longitudinal, or incidence or cohort studies, include at least two data collection points (and often more), separated by a period of time (often least several years). The initial, or baseline, assessment (by personal interview, exam, or other method) at the start of the study permits identifying individuals who do not have a disease, or who have some behavior or characteristic of interest (like drinking behavior). Reassessments, then, permit analysis of changes in the behavior or in the disease status. Essential to longitudinal design is that the characteristic of interest be assessed at both points in time to detect the change from baseline.

There is a growing body of literature of longitudinal studies that provide information on the drinking practices and problems of the elderly. Some of these are offshoots of ongoing epidemiologic studies such as the Framingham study, a landmark study begun in 1948 to investigate the etiology of cardiovascular disease; its comprehensive baseline and subsequent multiple measurements have provided a wealth of information about other topics not part of the original proposal, such as the relationship between alcohol use, blood pressure, and uric acid (Gordon & Kannel, 1983). Because participants were 28 to 62 at entry, changes in drinking practices throughout the very long follow-up period can be observed among women and men of all ages. Another study providing information about drinking changes is the Albany Study (Gordon & Doyle, 1986), a longitudinal study to explore the predictors of cardiovascular disease began in 1953, with enrollment of male New York State civil service employees. Evidence is also accumulating from the Normative Aging Study (Glynn et al., 1986), a volunteer sample of healthy men from the Boston area of all ages who enrolled in the study in 1963 and have been followed by questionnaire (in 1973) and personal exam (in 1982).

Types of Populations Studied

In a 1982 monograph, Gomberg classified studies about drinking behavior and alcoholism in the elderly according to the type of population sampled. Her categorization included: national surveys, where individuals of all ages have been sampled and results reported by age groups (e.g., Clark & Midanik, 1982; Grant, 1992; Grant et al., 1991; Cahalan, Cisin, & Crossley, 1969; Smart & Adlaf, 1988); surveys conducted in a smaller geographic region, often restricted to a particular city or region (Barnes, 1979, 1982; Meyers et al., 1982); those directed specifically at elderly individuals, often in a particular region or city and rarely national (Saunders et al., 1991; Welte & Mirand, 1992; Douglas et al., 1988; Guttmann, 1978); elderly attenders at medical or specialty clinics or clients of elderly community outreach services (Iliffe et al., 1991; Jinks & Raschko, 1990; Bridgewater et al., 1987); participants in other elderly focused studies (Sulsky et al., 1990; Goodwin et al., 1987); elderly inpatients in medical or psychiatric wards (Schuckit & Miller, 1976; Rosin & Glatt, 1971).

Drinking Measure Used

Alcohol research may also be distinguished by the type of alcohol indicator analyzed: any alcohol use, heavy drinking, problem use, and alcohol dependence. Alcohol dependence has in the past been studied primarily in treated populations. Only recently, with the establishment of standard diagnostic criteria for alcohol dependence and instruments to operationalize that criteria, have researchers been able to study community samples using these criteria (Bucholz, in press). Some results about alcohol dependence in the elderly from the landmark ECA study of psychiatric disorder will be presented later in the chapter.

Although study of alcohol disorder is possible, a more common focus in alcohol research with the elderly has been on drinking practices. In many studies, the examination of drinking practices has centered on whether a subject has had something alcoholic to drink in a specified time period, usually a current measure, like the last week, the last 30 days, or the last 12 months. In addition, amount of alcohol consumed per drinking occasion and frequency of drinking occasions have also been queried. These assessments have been aggregated into an overall measure of drinking, usually with qualitative labels like light, moderate, and heavy. Even though it is part of the drinking spectrum, problem drinking has rarely been assessed in community surveys of elders; heavy drinking is more commonly examined.

Table 2.1. Sample of Cross-Sectional Findings Regarding Drinking, Heavy Drinking, Problem Drinking, and Alcohol Dependence in Elders

Study	Type of Sample	N	Age Range	Gender	Prevalence Estimate	Drinking Measures
Barnes (1979)	Community	237	60+	M 42% F 58%	69% 7% 9%	Any current drinking 3–5 drinks/day 1+ problem
Douglass et al. (1988)	2 samples: Community	207	60+	M 40% F 60%	58% 20% 31%	Drinking 2+ times/wk Drinking
	Low income	71	60+	M 15% F 85%	4%	2+ times/wk
Goodwin et al. (1987)	Community volunteer	270	65+	M 46% F 54%	66%	1 drink per month
Busby et al. (1988)	GP registry	774	70+	M 39% F 61%	71% 15%	Any drinking Daily drinking
Meyers et al. (1982)	Community	928	60+	M 36% F 64%	47% 6% 1%	Any drinking 2+ drinks/day Problem drinking
Welte & Mirand (1992)	Commuity	2,325	60+	M 34% F 66%	62% 6%	Any current drinking Current heavy (2+ drinks/day)
Iliffe et al. (1991)	Patients in GP registry	239	75+	M 35% F 65%	32% 3%	Any current drinking 4+ drinks/day
Smart & Adlaf (1988)	Comm—1976 National 1982	617 400	60+	M 49% F 51%	57% 10% 65% 14%	Any drinking—'76 Daily drinking—'76 Any drinking—'82 Daily drinking—'82

continued

EPIDEMIOLOGIC STUDIES: FINDINGS

Overall Estimates

Table 2.1 summarizes the overall findings of elderly alcohol use, problem use, and alcohol dependence. Time period is specified where known; other estimates should be considered a point prevalence. As can be seen, for community samples, the prevalence of current drinking in elders ranges from 31% (in a low-income sample in Detroit) to 71%. Drinking (*not* abstinence) is the predominant pattern among elders. The current prevalence of daily drinking ranges from 10 to 20%, and of heavy drinking (when it is assessed), defined variously, from 1% to about 6%. Problem use is rarely covered; the estimates provided in Table 2.1 are 9% (Barnes, 1979), 3% (men only in Hilton, 1987) and 1% (Meyers et al., 1982). Perhaps the best prevalence estimates of serious problem alcohol use are those for alcohol dependence or abuse. For those 65 or older, the one-year prevalence of alcohol dependence or alcohol abuse for males was 3.1%, for females

Table 2.1. (continued)

Study	Type of Sample	N	Age Range	Gender	Prevalence Estimate		Drinking Measures
Guttmann (1978)	Community	237	60+	M 40%		44%	Any drinking
				F 60%		20%	Daily use
Cahalan, Cisin, & Crossley	National all ages	624	60+	M 41%		51%	Current drinkers
				F 59%	M	13%	Heavy drinkers
					F	1%	Heavy drinkers
Sulsky et al. (1990)	Volunteer	586	60+	M 36%	M	53%	1 drinks/week
				F 64%	F	43%	1 drinks/week
					M	17%	7 drinks/week
					F	8%	7 drinks/week
Grant (1992)	National	43,809	18+	N/A	M	1.79%	DSM-IV, proposed
					F	0.21%	(1 yr)
							dependence & abuse
Grant et al. (1991)	National	43,809	18+	N/A	M	2.77%	DSM-III-R (1 year)
					F	0.37%	dependence & abuse
Helzer et al. (1991)	Community & institutional	19,182	18+	M 48%	M	3.10%	DSM-III
				F 52%	F	0.46%	Alc. abuse or
							dependence
Schuckit & Miller (1976)	Hospital inpatient	113	65+	Males only	M	18%	Current alcoholism
					M	10%	Past alcoholism
Hilton (1987)	National	5,221	18+	M 40%	M	58%	Percent drinkers
						4%	Freq. heavy
						3%	Problem drinkers
				F 60%	F	49%	Percent drinkers
						1%	Freq. heavy
						—	Problem drinking
Colsher & Wallace (1990)	Community	1,155	65+	M 100%		77%	Ever drinker
						10%	Ever heavy drinker

less than one-half percent (0.46%) (DSM-III criteria), 2.8% for males and 0.4% for females for DSM-III-R criteria (combined dependence and abuse); 1.8% for males and 0.2% for females for DSM-IV criteria (combining dependence and abuse).

Although the prevalence estimates may vary, what does not vary across numerous cross-sectional studies with different definitions is the fact that drinking declines with age. This generalization holds as well for recent cross-sectional studies measuring current alcohol abuse and/or dependence, and holds for both men and women (see Figures 2.1 and 2.2).

A different impression is formed from data from longitudinal studies (see Table 2.2). The inference from most of the follow-up studies is that drinking patterns have remained stable for the oldest groups. It is also true, as Table 2.2 indicates, that when change occurs in the older groups, it is overall a decrease rather than an increase. However, as some studies suggest, there are subgroups in the older population in which drinking has increased. Data from the Framingham study (Gordon & Kannel, 1983) suggested that over the approximately 20-year follow-up interval, the rate of increase was small in the oldest age groups in comparison to younger age groups but very large in elderly women compared to the small increase among elderly men. Because the Framingham study

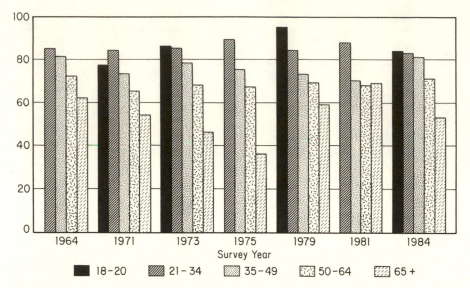

Figure 2.1. Proportion of drinkers, by age group, males only. Cross-sectional surveys from 1964 to 1984. (Adapted from Hilton, 1991.)

covered the years 1950 to 1982, its data are a microcosm of the changes in drinking in the United States as a whole, where marked increases were observed over that period, particularly for women (Helzer et al., 1992). In another study, although the percentage of the elderly who continued to drink decreased, alcohol consumption of those who continued to drink remained stable and, in fact, only decreased among heavy drinkers (Adams et al., 1990).

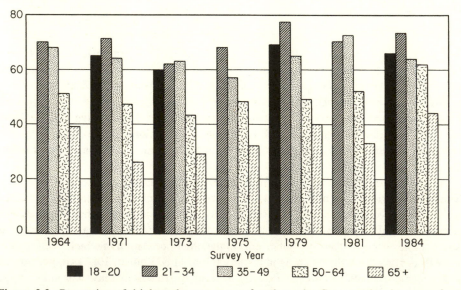

Figure 2.2. Proportion of drinkers, by age group, females only. Cross-sectional surveys from 1964 to 1984. (Adapted from Hilton, 1991.)

Table 2.2. Longitudinal Studies

Study	Type of Sample	N	Percent Followed	Duration	Entry Age	Gender	Outcome
Adams et al. (1990)	Volunteer	270	53%	7 years	60–86	M 46% F 54%	Stable consumption for all. Decline for heavy drinkers.
Glynn et al. (1986)	Volunteer	1,859	89% (to '73, '82 surveys)	9 years	21–81	Males only	Those 60+: Stable for 54%, for 46% decreased.
Ekerdt et al. (1989)	Volunteer	543	77%	2 years	55+	Males only	Some decrease in overall consumption. Increase in periodic heavy drinkers at time 2 among retired.
Gordon & Doyle (1986)	Civil Service Employees (Albany Study)	1,768	50%	18 years	38–55	Males only	12% increase in consumption for those 50+ at entry. Increase in proportion who drank heavily.
Gordon & Kannel (1983)	Community (Framingham)	5,209	59%	20 years	29–62	M 42% F 58%	Increase in average alcohol consumption in elders; for women (large) & men (small).

Gender

A consistent finding in alcohol research is that compared to women, more men drink, and drink heavily. This interpretation holds in both cross-sectional and longitudinal studies, and whether alcohol consumption or alcohol dependence is the variable of interest. One method of examining the relative excess of male over female drinking is to calculate a ratio of male to female rates. The larger the ratio, the greater the difference between men and women. Ratios close to 1 suggest equivalent rates, and ratios less than 1 indicate a higher rate among females. The male:female ratios among the elderly for current drinking calculated from studies examined in this chapter average about 1.2; male:female ratios for heavy drinking, on the other hand, are in the 4.5 to 6.5 range. These calculations support the interpretation that elderly women are as likely to drink alcohol as men, but are considerably less likely to drink heavily. One interesting finding from a telephone survey of elders in upstate New York found a steadily increasing ratio of male:female drinkers with age, suggesting that at least for that sample, even in the oldest age groups (80 or older), more men than women drink (Welte & Mirand, 1992). This observation merits further exploration in other data sets.

The male:female ratios for alcohol dependence are similar to those observed for heavy drinking, with a substantial excess in men over women: about 6.7:1 for the DSM-III definition from the ECA data, 7.5:1 for the DSM-III-R definition in the NHIS survey, and 8.5:1 for the then proposed DSM-IV definition (Grant, 1992). These male:female ratios in the older age groups are much larger than those observed for younger age groups, where several researchers (Helzer et al., 1991; Reich et al., 1988) have noted ratios that approach 1. Several explanations are possible. Rates of alcohol dependence may truly differ between older men and women. Women alcoholics may not survive as long as male alcoholics, which may account for lower alcohol dependence rates in older women. Older women may have been more influenced by cultural factors, which might tend to decrease drinking in this cohort. Resolution of this issue awaits further research.

Ethnicity

With the exception of data from national and multi-site samples from which little has been published directly on the elderly, nonwhite respondents have not been well represented in most studies of the elderly, thus limiting the applicability of findings. Data from one study found that compared to whites, blacks were less likely to be ever and current drinkers, but equally likely to be heavy drinkers (Welte & Mirand, 1992). This finding must be tempered by the fact that this survey occurred in a geographic area where nonwhites comprised a very small proportion of the overall population and therefore may not be generalizable to the nation as a whole. In the ECA study, where alcohol dependence, not drinking practices, was assessed, the lifetime prevalence of alcohol dependence among black males 65 or older was very high (21.6%), compared to their white (12.5%) counterparts, but current prevalence (2.9%) was comparable to that for whites (2.8%). The inference is that remission rates (that is, the proportion of lifetime cases that are currently active) are higher in older black, compared to older white, men. Whether this is a real finding or an artifact of the ECA data is another topic for future research.

Marital Status

The findings thus far have suggested that while there are more drinkers among the married, heavy drinking is not related to marital status. This is contrary to findings in younger age groups, where heavy drinking is disproportionately high among those who are separated or divorced. Smart and Adlaf (1988) reported that there were more daily drinkers among the married, but that there was no difference by marital status when drinking five or more drinks per occasion was the variable of interest. Barnes (1979) did not find a relationship between heavy drinking and marital status, although there was a suggestion that currently married individuals drank more heavily than those who were widowed or who were not currently married, but this difference did not reach statistical significance. In a telephone survey of residents of a geographic area similar to that studied by Barnes but about ten years later, Welte and Mirand (1992) again found that married individuals were more likely to be drinkers, but not heavy drinkers. There was a greater proportion of heavy drinkers among those ever separated or divorced, but this difference was not significant.

The relationship between marital status and alcohol consumption merits further examination. This may be a particularly important area of alcohol research for women, whose drinking might be greatly influenced by husbands' or partners' drinking (see Chapter 17 by Wilsnack in this volume).

Education, Income, and Socioeconomic Status

There is agreement in findings across studies of the elderly that education is positively associated with any drinking; that is, the proportion of drinkers increases with educational attainment. However, less well established is the relationship between education and amount of drinking. A report from one study indicated that those with a college education reported the highest mean alcohol consumption (Smart & Adlaf, 1988), but another study did not find this relationship (Goodwin et al., 1987).

As with education, most studies have found a positive relationship between any drinking and income (Goodwin et al., 1987; Douglass et al., 1988; Cahalan et al., 1969), but an inverse relationship with *heavy* drinking (that is, lower income individuals were more likely to be heavy drinkers). In a national survey of men (Cahalan et al., 1969), heavy drinking was inversely related to socioeconomic status (SES), with a lower proportion of high SES men who were classified as heavy drinkers compared to their lower SES counterparts. This finding held for men in two other studies (Goodwin et al., 1987; Welte & Mirand, 1992). Findings for women are less conclusive; there was only a slight tendency for women of lower SES to drink heavily (Welte & Mirand, 1992).

Regional Differences

Urban-rural contrasts in drinking practices among the elderly have rarely been available. Welte and Mirand (1992) reported, based on data from their telephone survey in upstate New York, that compared to urban residence, rural residence was positively associated with current drinking for both elderly men and women; however, elderly women who lived in rural areas were more likely than elderly men to be heavy drinkers. However, data from a national survey of Canadians did not find a relationship with rural dwelling status for either current drinking or current heavy drinking (Smart & Adlaf, 1988) among the elderly.

Multivariate Framework

Two studies have examined correlates of drinking behavior while simultaneously controlling for the effects of several variables (Welte & Mirand, 1992; Smart & Adlaf, 1988). For the most part, the bivariate findings have been borne out; correlates of current drinking included being male, Catholic, living in rural area, being currently employed, frequent attendance at church services, having an active lifestyle, being of higher socioeconomic status, not living alone, and smoking. These findings are consistent with the observation made by Gomberg (1990) that social drinking was related to good health, social contacts, and a sense of well-being. Current heavy drinking was correlated with similar variables, but there was evidence of an interaction between gender and rural or urban residence, with heavy drinkers more likely to be females in rural areas and males in urban area (Welte & Mirand, 1992).

Smart and Adlaf (1988), in their study of a national sample of Canadians, found that among males, being between 71 and 75, being Roman Catholic, and having some college education predicted daily drinking; while being male, younger, a native French speaker, and Roman Catholic predicted heavy drinking.

NEW ANALYSES OF DATA FROM THE EPIDEMIOLOGIC CATCHMENT AREA PROGRAM

Data from the ECA study have potential to shed light on the issue of alcohol dependence and drinking among the elderly. Previously published reports of these data had not provided more discrete stratifications of the elderly beyond 60 or older (Holzer et al., 1984), or 65 or older (Helzer et al., 1991). In this report, ECA data are presented for 10-year age categories up to 80+ and older. Data on DSM-III alcohol dependence disorder are presented, along with lifetime drinking patterns that are available from ECA data. Unfortunately, data on current alcohol consumption patterns are not available from the ECA study. All data are weighted, to take into account the sampling strategy employed in the survey (Leaf et al., 1991). Data from household samples from all five ECA sites are included.

Results

As shown in Table 2.3, there is a decrease in prevalence of DSM-III alcohol abuse/ dependence with age for all prevalence estimates: 2 week, 1 year, and lifetime. This is true for both males and females. The decrease in lifetime prevalence with age has been observed in the ECA study for psychiatric disorders other than alcohol abuse/dependence. While it may seem counterintuitive for lifetime prevalence to decrease among those who have been at risk for disorder the longest period of time, several explanations may account for this. One may be the effect of differential mortality: Alcoholics are more likely to die prematurely than their nonalcoholic peers. A second possibility is that older subjects may forget alcohol problems that occurred a long time ago. A third possibility allows that this is a true cohort effect: that there *is* less alcoholism in older age cohorts because of some unique exposure years ago (e.g., Prohibition, the Depres-

Table 2.3. Prevalence of DSM-III Alcohol Abuse/Dependence by Gender and Age (ECA Data)

Prevalence	18–29	30–39	40–49	50–59	60–69	70–79	80+
Male (N)[a]	1863	1419	729	749	1346	864	276
Two week	4.52	5.47	4.32	3.73	2.38	1.03	0.58
One year[b]	15.15	12.25	11.25	6.66	4.81	2.43	0.95
Lifetime[c]	23.57	23.33	24.38	19.40	14.44	11.22	5.72
Female (N)[a]	2407	1913	1058	1100	1844	1595	648
2 week	1.29	0.75	0.45	0.32	0.32	0.36	0
One year[b]	3.93	2.03	1.26	1.09	.63	.38	0
Lifetime[c]	6.49	4.80	4.45	2.71	1.91	1.10	0.29

[a]Prevalence estimates are weighted; N's are unweighted.

[b]Includes the last two weeks.

[c]Includes both two-week and one-year prevalence estimates.

Table 2.4. Male:Female Ratios of DSM-III Alcohol Abuse/Dependence by Age Group

Prevalence	18–29	30–39	40–49	50–59	60–69	70–79	80+
Two week	3.50	7.29	9.60	11.65	7.43	2.86	—[a]
One year	3.85	6.03	8.92	6.11	7.63	6.39	—[a]
Lifetime	3.63	4.86	5.48	7.16	7.56	10.18	19.72

[a]No alcoholics in this category

sion) that has protected them from alcoholism. However, as noted earlier, the decrease in lifetime prevalence with age is seen with other psychiatric disorders as well, so if this is a true cohort effect, it does not appear to be specific to alcohol abuse and/or dependence. The ECA data do not permit resolution of which explanation may be correct; for this, longitudinal data will be required.

From Table 2.4, the male:female ratios of alcohol abuse and dependence prevalence increase with age for lifetime prevalence, and they show a relatively steady increase up to the age of 60 to 69 for 1-year prevalence. The smallest ratios are seen in the youngest age group (18 to 29), an observation consistent with findings from other research that suggests rates of alcoholism in females are approaching those of males. However, one interesting observation in Table 2.4 is that the 2-week prevalence ratios appear to converge at both ends of the age spectrum, and in fact are smallest in the 70 to 79 age group. This is so because the 2-week prevalence for females remains constant from the age of 50 through old age, while the prevalence for men steadily decreases. This may reflect differential mortality among male alcoholics, with older alcoholic men dying off, or perhaps it indicates that older male alcoholics achieve remission more often than their female counterparts.

Table 2.5 summarizes lifetime prevalence data for various drinking patterns, problem drinking, and alcohol abuse/dependence. The categories are hierarchical. *Social drinker* (including abstainers, since in the ECA a separate question for "ever drinking" was not asked) consists of those who denied heavy or problem drinking. *Heavy drinker* includes those who reported ever having seven or more drinks per day for 2 weeks or ever drinking at least seven drinks one day a week for at least 3 months, but never having any problems. *Problem drinker* includes any one with any social, legal, or medical problems due to drinking, but not enough to qualify them for a diagnosis of

Table 2.5. Proportion of Lifetime Drinking Patterns among Men and Women by Age (ECA Data)

Alcohol level	18–29	30–39	40–49	50–59	60–69	70–79	80+
Males							
Social drinker	45.31	50.57	54.77	56.46	66.43	72.73	85.19
Heavy drinker	14.40	13.56	9.15	10.35	6.40	5.33	4.77
Problem drinker	16.71	12.54	11.70	13.80	12.74	10.71	4.33
Alcohol ab/dep	23.57	23.33	24.38	19.40	14.44	11.22	5.72
Females							
Social drinker	78.43	84.64	86.94	92.24	93.57	96.34	97.87
Heavy drinker	6.16	3.42	1.88	1.87	0.89	0.74	0.07
Problem drinker	8.92	7.14	6.74	3.18	3.62	1.82	1.77
Alcohol ab/dep	6.49	4.80	4.45	2.71	1.91	1.10	0.29

Table 2.6. Percentage of Lifetime Alcoholics Who Are Currently Active,[a] by Age and Gender

Gender	18–29	30–39	40–49	50–59	60–69	70–79	80+
Male	64%	53%	46%	34%	33%	22%	17%
Female	61%	42%	28%	40%	33%	34%	0

[a]Defined as one-year prevalence divided by lifetime prevalence.

alcohol abuse/dependence. Finally, *alcohol abuse and/or dependence* includes those individuals who met the criteria for a diagnosis of DSM-III alcohol abuse and/or dependence on a lifetime basis.

Some observations worthy of note are that non-problem, non-heavy drinking becomes more common with each 10-year increment in age. A sizeable percentage of older men who are not alcoholic have a history of heavy drinking. In contrast, women with histories of heavy drinking are rather rare in the 60 or older age groups. This suggests that it may be difficult for women to maintain heavy non-problem drinking, that almost all women who drink heavily eventually develop problems or outright alcohol abuse/dependence.

Table 2.6 displays the proportion of active alcoholics by gender and age group. Noteworthy is the steady decrease with age of the proportion of active male alcoholics compared to women, where the percentage is fairly stable from the age of 50. This may indicate a more intractable form of alcoholism among women compared to men.

Marital Status

Figure 2.3 displays data for the elderly ECA sample on the prevalence of alcohol abuse or dependence by marital status. There is a pronounced increase in prevalence for those

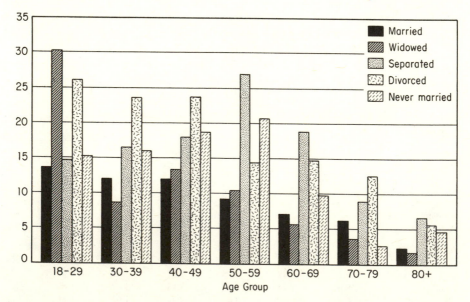

Figure 2.3. Lifetime prevalence of DSM-III alcohol abuse and/or dependence by marital status and age. ECA data from five sites, weighted.

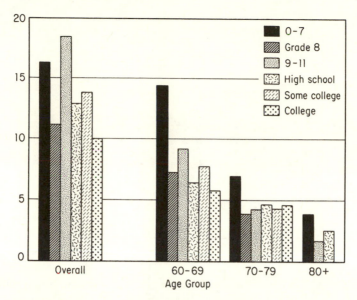

Figure 2.4. Lifetime prevalence of DSM-III alcohol abuse and/or dependence by age and completion of education. ECA data from five sites, weighted.

who are separated or divorced among the older age groups as well as the younger age groups, suggesting that disruption in marital status is associated with alcoholism regardless of age. However, rates of alcohol abuse/dependence are relatively low among those who are widowed, lower even than those who are currently married. While this may in part be gender-related (more women are widowed than men and women also have lower rates of alcoholism), it may be suggestive that being widowed may not be a risk factor for alcoholism as hypothesized in the literature.

Education

Previous data analyses from the ECA suggested a strong relationship between alcoholism and failure to complete education, regardless of the level left unfinished (Helzer et al., 1991). These earlier analyses did not examine data within age categories. We now present data for the elderly ECA sample in Figure 2.4. This finding appears to hold for those 60 to 69, but does not hold for those 70 or older. Moreover, there is a striking and consistent finding that those with very little education have high rates of alcoholism across all elderly categories. Further study will be required to determine whether this reflects a cohort effect, some form of selection bias, or simply small sample size in this very old cohort.

Late-Onset Alcoholics

A current and somewhat controversial research issue in the field of alcohol research on the elderly is the magnitude of late-onset alcoholism. *Late-onset* has been defined as after 40, after 45, after 50, and after 60 (Gomberg, 1985; Atkinson et al., 1990). Data from the ECA study provide some information about the occurrence of late-onset al-

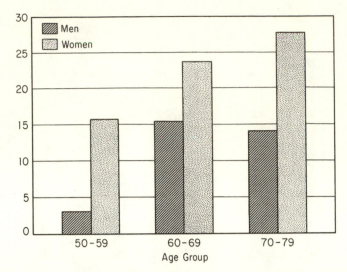

Figure 2.5. Proportion of late-onset (first criterion symptom after age 49) alcoholics of all alcoholics by age and gender. Data from five ECA sites.

cohol abuse and/or dependence. By late onset, here, we will adopt the age used by others (Schonfeld & Dupree, 1991) as the first criterion problem with alcohol occurring after age 49. Information on the age of occurrence of the first alcohol problem elicited in the ECA study was tabulated to produce Figure 2.5, the percentage of alcoholics in each age decade who reported that the first symptom of the disorder appeared after age 49. Three percent (6/177) of male alcoholics between 50 and 59 reported first having a symptom of alcoholism after 49, compared to 15% (33/215) of those between 60 and 69, and 14% (15/106) of those between 70 and 79. For women, 16% (7/45) between 50 and 59 report a first symptom of alcoholism after the age of 50, with 24% (9/38) of women between 60 and 69 and 28% (5/18) of women between 70 and 79 reporting first occurrence after 50. These percentages are not trivial and suggest that late-onset alcoholism is a problem meriting further investigation.

CONCLUSIONS

Data from literature surveys summarizing drinking patterns in the elderly have been presented. There are several findings about which there is good agreement across studies. These include the decline in drinking with age as measured by cross-sectional studies; consistent gender differences with a greater percentage of men drinking any alcohol and a greater percentage of men drinking heavily; a direct relationship between drinking and income, but an inverse relationship with heavy drinking. New analyses of data from the ECA have examined alcohol abuse/dependence in age deciles to the age of 80 or older. The major findings were that there is a decrease in prevalence of alcohol abuse/dependence for all prevalence measures, a steady increase in the male:female ratio of alcohol abuse/dependence with age for lifetime prevalence and a plateau at age 50 to 59 for 1-year prevalence, distinctive gender differences in remission rates and drinking patterns with age, and a pronounced increase in the prevalence of alcohol abuse/dependence among the elderly who have been separated or divorced, but no apparent increase in the widowed elderly.

FUTURE RESEARCH

Although this chapter has pointed out the considerable research that has been conducted on the elderly and alcohol use, it seems clear that there is still much that remains to be done. The issue is still debatable regarding how drinking changes with age. While cross-sectional research is consistent in its finding that alcohol consumption is lower among the elderly in comparison to their younger counterparts, whether this indicates that drinking declines with age seems to be an arguable point. The equivocal evidence from longitudinal studies would suggest that this is a topic meriting additional research. Future longitudinal studies may help to settle this issue. For the time being, it appears to be the case that drinking in late life is heavily influenced by drinking in early life, and that histories of heavy drinking appear to be important in maintaining heavy drinking in late life. Strategies for prevention of alcohol abuse ought to recognize the important influence of early-life drinking patterns.

Another underresearched topic is alcohol consumption patterns of representative samples of elderly nonwhites, primarily African Americans, Hispanic Americans, and Asian Americans. Very little representative work has been carried out on these groups.

As with ethnicity, drinking patterns of elderly women also deserve serious study. This seems particularly timely in light of the new initiative into women's health that has recently been launched by the NIH. There are several reasons that these patterns merit research. Alcohol consumption has been shown to have a beneficial effect on heart disease. Most of these studies have used predominantly male samples; it would be beneficial to know whether this finding would obtain in samples of women as well. A second reason for investigating alcohol consumption in elderly women is the fact that moderate drinking has been linked to breast cancer in postmenopausal women (Gapstur et al., 1992). Would the apparent increased risk of breast cancer be outweighed by the cardiovascular benefits of drinking? Finally, the interplay of alcohol and medication may be particularly important in women, who are perhaps more likely than males to be prescribed certain types of medication that may interact negatively with alcohol, and who may have different metabolic rates of drug metabolism as well.

Another productive research area would be intensive study of late-onset alcoholics to determine whether symptom patterns and course are similar to those whose alcoholism began much earlier, and to identify possible etiologic agents in producing alcoholism at such a late date. Such an investigation would inform prevention efforts.

Finally, the appropriateness of diagnostic criteria of alcohol abuse and dependence for an elderly population merits further investigation. Such an evaluation can be based on both physiological and sociological grounds, details of which may be found elsewhere in this volume. This evaluation may also take into account different measurement strategies that may have to be considered with an elderly population, where memory of past events may be poor. Attention to these suggestions will offer the possibility of improving the state of knowledge regarding epidemiology of alcohol use and abuse in the elderly.

Acknowledgments

The authors gratefully acknowledge the programming expertise of Joseph J. Shayka, expert manuscript preparation by Jan Konrad, and the support of the National Institute on Alcohol Abuse and Alcoholism by USPHS grants U10AA08401, U10AA08403, and R01 AA08752.

References

Adams, W. L., Garry, P. J., Rhyne, R., Hunt, W. C., & Goodwin, J. S. (1990). Alcohol intake in the healthy elderly: changes with age in a cross-sectional and longitudinal study. *Journal of the American Geriatrics Society, 38*, 211–216.

Alexander, N., Goodwin, J. S., & Currie, C. (1985). Comparison of admission and discharge medications in two geriatric populations. *Journal of the American Geriatrics Society, 33*, 827–832.

American Psychiatric Association. (1980). *Diagnostic and statistical manual of mental disorders (3rd ed.).* Washington, D.C.

American Psychiatric Association. (1987). *Diagnostic and statistical manual of mental disorders (3rd ed. rev.).* Washington, D.C.

American Psychiatric Association. (1994). *DSM-IV.* Washington, D.C.

Atkinson, R. M. (1990). Aging and alcohol use disorders: Diagnostic issues in the elderly. *International Psychogeriatrics, 2*, 55–72.

Atkinson, R. M. (1987). Alcohol problems of the elderly. (Editorial). *Alcohol and Alcoholism, 22*, 415–417.

Atkinson, R. M., Tolson, R. L., & Turner, J. A. Late versus early onset problem drinking in older men. *Alcoholism: Clinical and Experimental Research, 14*, 574–579.

Barnes, G. (1982). Patterns of alcohol use and abuse among older persons in a household population. In W. G. Wood & M. F. Elias (Ed.). *Alcoholism and aging: Advances in research*, (pp. 3–15). Boca Raton, FL: CRC Press.

Barnes, G. M. Alcohol use among older persons: Findings from a western New York State general population survey. *Journal of the American Geriatrics Society, 27*, 244–250.

Blumenthal, S. J. (1988). Suicide: A guide to risk factors, assessment and treatment of suicidal patients. *Medical Clinics of North America, 72*, 937–971.

Boffetta, P., Garfinkel, L. (1990). Alcohol drinking and mortality among men enrolled in an American Cancer Society prospective study. *Epidemiology, 1*, 342–348.

Bridgewater, R., Leigh, S., James, F., & Potter, J. (1987). Alcohol consumption and dependence in elderly patients in an urban community. *British Medical Journal, 295*, 884–885.

Bruce, A., Anderson, M., Arvidsson, B., et al. (1980). Body composition: Prediction of normal body potassium, body water and body fat in adults on the basis of body height, body weight and age. *Scandinavian Journal of Clinical Laboratory Investigation, 40*, 461–473.

Bucholz, K. K. (in press). Alcohol abuse and dependence from a psychiatric epidemiologic perspective. *Alcohol and Health Research World.*

Bulbena, H., & Berrios, G. E. (1986). Pseudodementia: Facts and figures. *British Journal of Psychiatry, 148*, 87–94.

Busby, W. J., Campbell, A. J., Borrie, M. J., & Spears, G. F. S. (1988). Alcohol use in a community-based sample of subjects aged 70 years and older. *Journal of the American Geriatrics Society, 36*, 301–305.

Cahalan, D., Cisin, I., & Crossley, H. (1969). *American drinking practices: A national study of drinking behavior and attitudes.* [Monograph 6]. New Brunswick, NJ: Rutgers University Press.

Clark, W. B., & Midanik, L. (1982). Alcohol use and alcohol problems among U.S. adults: Results of the 1979 survey. In *Alcohol consumption and related problems* (pp. 3–52). [Alcohol and Health Monograph 1]. DHHS Publication No. (ADM) 82-1190. Washington D.C.: USGPO.

Colsher, P. L., & Wallace, R. B. (1990). Elderly men with histories of heavy drinking: Correlates and consequences. *Journal of Studies on Alcohol, 51*, 528–535.

Douglass, R. L., Schuster, E. O., & McClelland, S. C. (1988). Drinking patterns and abstinence among the elderly. *International Journal of Addictions, 23*, 399–415.

Ekerdt, D. J., De Labry, L. O., & Glynn, R. J. (1989). Change in drinking behaviors with retirement: Findings from the Normative Aging Study. *Journal of Studies on Alcohol, 50*, 347–353.

Ellison, R. C. (1990). Cheers! (Editorial). *Epidemiology, 1*, 337–339.

Feitelberg, S., Epstein, S., Ismail, F., & D'Amanda, C. (1987). Deranged bone mineral metabolism in chronic alcoholism. *Metabolism, 36*, 322–326.

Gapstur, S. M., Potter, J. D., Sellers, T. A., & Folsom, A. R. (1992). Increased risk of breast cancer with alcohol consumption in postmenopausal women. *American Journal of Epidemiology, 136*, 1221–1231.

Glynn, R. J., Bouchard, G. R., LoCastro, J. S., & Hermos, J. A. (1986). Changes in alcohol consumption behaviors among men in the normative aging study. In G. Maddox, L. N. Robins, & N. Rosenberg (Ed.). *Nature and extent of alcohol problems in the elderly*, (pp. 101–116). New York: Springer.

Gomberg, E. L. (1980). Drinking and problem drinking among the elderly. Institute of Gerontology, University of Michigan.

Gomberg, E. S. L. (1990). Drugs, alcohol and aging. In L. T. Kozlowski (Ed.). *Research advances in alcohol and drug problems*, (pp. 171–213). New York: Plenum.

Gomberg, E. S. L. (1982). Alcohol use and alcohol problems among the elderly. In *Special Populations Issues*, (pp. 263–290). [NIAAA Research Monograph No. 4] DHHS Publ. No. (ADM) 82-1193. Washington DC: Gov. Printing Office.

Gomberg, E. S. L. (1985). Gerontology and alcohol studies. In E. Gottheil, K. A. Druley, T. E. Skoloda, & H. M. Waxman (Ed.). *The combined problems of alcoholism, drug addiction and aging*, (pp. 51–73). Springfield, IL: C. Thomas.

Goodwin, J. S., Sanchez, C. J., Thomas, P., Hunt, C., Garry, P. J., & Goodwin, J. M. (1987). Alcohol intake in a healthy elderly population, *American Journal of Public Health, 77*, 173–177.

Gordon, T., & Kannel, W. B. (1983). Drinking and its relation to smoking, blood pressure, blood lipids, and uric acid. *Archives of Internal Medicine, 143*, 1366–1374.

Gordon, T., & Doyle, J. T. Alcohol consumption and its relationship to smoking, weight, blood pressure and blood lipids. *Archives of Internal Medicine, 146*, 262–265.

Graham, K. (1986). Identifying and measuring alcohol abuse among the elderly: Serious problems with existing instrumentation. *Journal of Studies on Alcohol, 47*, 322–326.

Grant, B. F. (1992). Prevalence of the proposed DSM-IV alcohol use disorders: United States, 1988. *British Journal of Addiction, 87*, 309–316.

Grant, B. F., Harford, T. C., Chou, P., Pickering, R., Dawson, D. A., Stinson, F. S., & Noble, J. (1991). Prevalence of DSM-III-R alcohol abuse and dependence: United States, 1988. *Alcohol and Health Research World, 15*, 91–96.

Helzer, J. E., Burnam, M. A., & McEvoy, L. T. (1991). Alcohol abuse and alcoholism. In L. N. Robins & D. A. Regier (Ed.). *Psychiatric disorders in America*, (pp. 81–115). New York: The Free Press.

Helzer, J. E., Bucholz, K., & Robins, L. N. Five communities in the United States: Results of the Epidemiologic Catchment Area Survey. In J. E. Helzer & G. J. Canino (Ed.). *Alco-*

holism in North America, Europe and Asia, (pp. 71–95). New York: Oxford University Press.

Hilton, M. E. (1987). Drinking patterns and drinking problems in 1984; results from a general population survey. *Alcoholism: Clinical and Experimental Research, 11*, 167–175.

Hilton, M. E. (1986). Abstention in the general population of the USA. *British Journal of Addiction. 81*, 95–112.

Hilton, M. E. (1991). Trends in U.S. drinking patterns: Further evidence from the past twenty years. In W. B. Clark & M. E. Hilton (Ed.). *Alcohol in America: Drinking practices and problems,* (pp. 121–138). Albany, N.Y.: State University of New York Press.

Himmelhoch, J. M., Auchenback, R., & Fuchs, C. Z. (1982). The dilemma of depression in the elderly. *Journal of Clinical Psychiatry, 43*, 26–32.

Holzer, C. E., Robins, L. N., Myers, J. K., Weissman, M. M., Tischler, G. L., Leaf, P. J., Anthony, J., & Bednarski, P. B. (1984). Antecedents and correlates of alcohol abuse and dependence in the elderly. In G. Maddox, L. Robins, & N. Rosenberg (Ed.). *Nature and extent of alcohol problems among the elderly,* (pp. 217–244). [NIAAA Research Monograph No. 14]. USPHS, Washington D.C.

Iliffe, A., Haines, A., Boroff, A., Goldenberg, E., Morgan, P., & Gallivan, S. (1991). Alcohol consumption by elderly people: A general practice survey. *Age and Ageing, 20*, 120–123.

Jinks, M. J., & Raschko, R. R. (1990). A profile of alcohol and prescription drug abuse in a high-risk community-based elderly population. *DICP, 24*, 971–975.

Kovar, M. (1977). Health of the elderly and use of health services. *Public Health Report, 92*, 9–19.

Larson, E., Reifler, B., Sumi, S., et al. (1985). Diagnostic evaluation of 200 elderly outpatients with suspected dementia. *Gerontology, 40*, 536–543.

Leaf, P. J., Myers, J. K., & McEvoy, L. T. (1992). Procedures used in the Epidemiologic Catchment Area Study. In L. N. Robins & D. A. Regier (Ed.). *Psychiatric disorders in America,* (pp. 11–32). New York: The Free Press.

Malin, H., Wilson, R., Williams, G., & Aitken, S. (1985). 1983 Alcohol/health practices supplement. *Alcohol and Health Research World, 10*, 48–50.

Meehan, P., Saltzman, L., & Saltin, R. (1991). Suicides among older United States residents: Epidemiologic characteristics and trends. *American Journal of Public Health, 81*, 1198–1200.

Meyers, A. R., Hingson, R., Mucatel, M., & Goldman, E. (1982). Social and psychologic correlates of problem drinking in old age. *Journal of the American Geriatrics Society, 30*, 452–456.

Neugarten, B. L. (1976). The psychology of aging: An overview. *Journal Supplement Abstract Service of the American Psychological Association*, MS 1340.

Post, F. (1975). Dementia, depression and pseudo-dementia. In D. F. Benson & D. Rhiner (Ed.). *Psychiatric aspects of neurological disease,* (pp. 99–120). New York: Grune & Stratton.

Ray, W. A. (1992). Psychotropic drugs and injuries among the elderly: A review. *Journal of Clinical Psychopharmacology, 12*, 386–396.

Regier, D. A., Myers, J. K., Kramer, M., Robins, L. N., Blazer, D. G., Hough, R. L., Eaton, W. W., & Locke, B. Z. (1985) Historical context, major objectives and study design. In W. W. Eaton & L. G. Kessler (Ed.). *Epidemiologic field methods in psychiatry: The NIMH Epidemiologic Catchment Area Program,* (pp. 3–19). New York: Academic Press.

Reich, T., Cloninger, C. R., Van Eerdewegh, P., Rice, J. P., & Mullaney, J. (1988). Secular trends in the familial transmission of alcoholism. *Alcoholism: Clinical and Experimental Research, 12*, 458–464.

Richelson, E. (1984). Psychotropics and the elderly: Interactions to watch for. *Geriatrics, 39*, 30–42.

Room, R. (1991). Measuring alcohol consumption. In W. B. Clark & M. E. Hilton (Ed.). *Alcohol* in America: Drinking practices and problems, (pp. 26–50). Albany: State University of New York Press.

Rosin, A. J., & Glatt, M. M. (1971). Alcohol excess in the elderly. Quarterly Journal of Studies on Alcohol, 32, 53–59.

Salthouse, T. A. (1985). Speed of behavior and its implications for cognition. In J. E. Birren & K. W. Schaie (Ed.). Handbook of the psychology of aging, (pp. 400–426). New York: Van Nostrand and Reinhold.

Saunders, P. A., Copeland, J. R. M., Dewey, M. E., Davidson, I. A., McWilliam, C., Charma, V., & Sullivan, C. (1991). Heavy drinking as a risk factor for depression and dementia in elderly men. British Journal of Psychiatry, 159, 213–216.

Schonfeld, L., & Dupree, L. W. (1991). Antecedents of drinking for early and late onset elderly alcohol abusers. Journal of Studies on Alcohol, 52, 587–592.

Schuckit, M. A., & Miller, P. L. (1976). Alcoholism in elderly men: A survey of a general medical ward. Annals of the New York Academy of Science, 273, 559–571.

Smart, R. G., & Adlaf, E. M. (1988). Alcohol and drug use among the elderly: Trends in use and characteristics of users. Canadian Journal of Public Health, 79, 236–242.

Snow, S. S., & Wells, C. E. (1981). Case studies in neuropsychiatry: Diagnosis and treatment of coexistent dementia and depression. Journal of Clinical Psychiatry, 42, 439–441.

Sulsky, S. I., Jacques, P. F., Otradovec, C. L., Hartz, S. C., & Russell, R. M. (1990). Descriptors of alcohol consumption among nonalcoholic elderly. Journal of the American College of Nutrition, 9, 326–331.

U.S. Department of Health and Human Services, American Association of Retired Persons and the Administration on Aging. (1986). A profile of older Americans. Program Resources Department. PF3049 (1086) D996.

Vestal, R. E. Geriatric clinical pharmacology: An overview. In R. E. Vestal (Ed.). Drug treatment in the elderly, (pp. 12–28). Boston: ADIS Health Science Press.

Vestal, R. E., McGuire, E. A., Tobin, J. D., et al. (1977). Aging and ethanol metabolism. Clinical Pharmacology and Therapeutics, 21, 343–354.

Weissman, M. M., Myers, J. K., & Harding, P. S. (1980). Prevalence and psychiatric heterogeneity of alcoholism in a United States urban community. Journal of Studies on Alcohol, 41, 672–681.

Weissman, M. M., Myers, J. K., Tischler, G. L., et al. (1985). Psychiatric disorders (DSM-III) and cognitive impairment among the elderly in the U.S. urban community. Acta Psychiatrica Scandinavica, 71, 366–379.

Welte, J. W., & Mirand, A. L. (1992). Alcohol use by the elderly: Patterns and correlates. A Report on the Erie County elder drinking survey. Research Institute on Addictions, Buffalo, New York, October.

3

Alcohol and Medications in the Elderly: Complex Interactions

MADHU R. KORRAPATI AND ROBERT E. VESTAL

The shift in the age distribution around the world has been persistent and dramatic since the turn of the century. By 1992 there were 342 million people age 65 or older, constituting about 6.2% of the population. By 2050 the number of people 65 years or older will expand to at least 2.5 billion people, or about 20% of the world's projected population (Olshansky et al., 1993). This fastest growing segment of the population uses drugs and other health services to a greater extent and more often than any other segment of the population (Brock et al., 1990). Elderly people are more susceptible to multiple chronic diseases. These include diseases of the cardiovascular system such as coronary artery disease, hypertension, and stroke; diseases of endocrine function such as diabetes; bone and joint diseases such as arthritis and osteoporosis; chronic obstructive pulmonary diseases; and psychiatric diseases. Multiple pathologic states most likely will lead to considerable disturbances in physiologic function, which further cause modifications in both organ function and handling of the drugs by the body. Because of these multiple pathologies, physicians often prescribe multiple drugs to treat them. Although they comprise only 12% of the U.S. population in 1988, the elderly accounted for 35% of prescription drug expenditures (Health Care Financing Administration, 1988). This, together with the effects of aging per se, could account for at least part of the heterogeneity of drug response in elderly patients.

COMMONLY USED MEDICATIONS IN THE ELDERLY

With increasing age, there is increasing use of prescription drugs, both for the treatment of chronic age-related disease, and also for the treatment of acute intercurrent disease. The elderly are also more likely to take over-the-counter drugs in order to obtain relief, both from disease-related symptoms and from other health problems. Hale et al. (1987)

Table 3.1. Commonly Used Prescription and Nonprescription Drugs in the Elderly

Commonly prescribed drugs	Commonly used nonprescription drugs
Diuretics	Analgesics
hydrochlorothiazide	aspirin
triamterene	acetaminophen
furosemide	ibuprofen
Cardiovascular drugs	Multiple vitamins with
digoxin	minerals
nitroglycerin	iron
propranolol	vitamin E
dipyridamole	vitamin C
isosorbide dinitrate	zinc
methyldopa	Vitamin E
nifedipine	Vitamin C
quinidine	
	Laxatives
Sedative-hypnotics	psyllium
diazepam	
flurazepam	Others
	antacids containing magnesium
Others	hydroxide, aluminum hydroxide
H$_2$ blockers	and simethicone
theophylline	
chlorpropamide	cold medications containing
	anti-histamines

Source: Adapted from Hale, W. E., May, F. E., Marks, R. G. & Stewart, R. B. (1987).

studied the pattern of drug usage in an ambulatory elderly population in Dunedin, Florida, and found that among prescription drugs, cardiovascular drugs, diuretics, and sedative-hypnotic drugs accounted for 75% of the total prescriptions (Table 3.1). The most commonly used nonprescription drugs were analgesics, nutritional supplements, and laxatives (Hale et al., 1987).

ALTERED DRUG RESPONSE IN THE ELDERLY

One of the goals of gerontology is not necessarily to increase the life span, but rather to increase the health span, that is, the number of years that an individual will enjoy the function of all body parts and processes. Aging results from multiple ongoing processes, and understanding of aging is further complicated by disease and disability. Several age-related changes once thought to be manifestations of normal human aging have now been shown to be due to disease. Some drugs act differently in older people than they do in young or middle-aged people (Table 3.2) (Cusack & Vestal, 1986). The pharmacokinetics of many drugs in the elderly are characterized by prolonged half-life and delayed clearance. Pharmacodynamic changes are more ambiguous, with an increased sensitivity to some drugs and decreased sensitivity to others (Cusack & Vestal, 1986). Also, errors in compliance, from whatever cause, can lead to unpredictable intake of drugs. Psychological and socioeconomic factors contribute to compliance errors and no doubt also lead to increased intake of combinations of drugs.

Table 3.2. Effect of Aging on Response to Drug Effect

Drug	Action	Effect of Aging
Analgesics		
Aspirin	Acute gastroduodenal mucosal damage	No change
Morphine	Acute analgesic effect	Increased
Pentazocine	Analgesic effect	Increased
Anticoagulants		
Heparin	Activated partial thromboplastin time	No change
Warfarin	Prothrombin time	Increased
Bronchodilators		
Albuterol	Bronchodilation	No change
Ipratropium	Bronchodilation	No change
Cardiovascular drugs		
Adenosine	Minute ventilation and heart rate	No change
Diltiazem	Acute antihypertensive effect	Increased
Enalepril	Acute antihypertensive effect	Increased
Isoproterenol	Chronotropic effect	Decreased
Phenylephrine	Acute vasoconstriction	No change
	Acute antihypertensive effect	No change
Prazocin	Chronotropic effect	Decreased
Timolol	Chronotropic effect	No change
Verapamil	Acute antihypertensive effect	Increased
Diuretics		
Furosemide	Latency & size of peak diuretic response	Decreased
Psychotropics		
Diazepam	Acute sedation	Increased
Diphenhydramine	Psychomotor function	No change
Haloperidol	Acute sedation	Decreased
Midazolam	EEG activity	Increased
Temazepam	Postural sway, psychomotor effect, and sedation	Increased
Triazolam	Psychomotor activity	Increased
Others		
Levodopa	Dose elimination due to side effects	Increased
Tolbutamide	Acute hypoglycemic effect	Decreased

Source: Adapted from Cusack, B. J., & Vestal, R. E. (1986).

ALTERED PHARMACOKINETICS

Drug Absorption

Drug absorption has not been a clinical problem in the elderly despite some evidence for a decrease in gastric acid secretion, reduced splanchnic blood flow, reduced gastrointestinal motility, and a decline in the absorptive capacity with aging. This is because absorption is dependent on passive diffusion. In general, data do not show that there is an age-related change in the intestinal absorption of drugs, especially those that exhibit high lipid solubility and are absorbed via passive diffusion (Schmucker, 1985).

Drug Distribution

Changes in body composition with age may influence drug distribution. Generally, with aging, the percentage of water and lean tissue (mainly muscle) in the body decreases, while the percentage of fat tissue increases. These changes can affect the distribution and the length of time that a drug stays in the body, as well as the amount that is absorbed by body tissues (Vestal et al., 1977). In this situation, drugs that are more lipid soluble such as diazepam, alprazolam, propranolol, and lidocaine are extensively distributed in the elderly, and drugs such as acetaminophen, antipyrine, lithium, and ethanol that are more water soluble tend to have a smaller volume of distribution, which results in higher plasma concentrations (Greenblatt et al., 1982).

Changes in binding of drugs to plasma proteins, red blood cells, and other body tissues may cause an altered distribution and clearance of drugs in the elderly. Several studies have shown an age-related decrease (10 to 20%) in serum albumin and probably an increase in α_1 acid glycoprotein. Acidic drugs such as salicylic acid, phenytoin, and tolbutamide bind to plasma albumin. The principal binding protein for several basic drugs including propranolol, lidocaine, verapamil, meperidine, and tricyclic antidepressants is α_1 acid glycoprotein (Loi & Vestal, 1988). These findings have important clinical implications for highly protein-bound drugs, particularly if additional drugs or diseases alter binding and change the free fraction. Increases in free drug will increase transiently the pharmacological response and could result in drug toxicity. Changes in binding also affect the interpretation of serum drug concentrations if only the total drug concentration is measured.

Drug Elimination

Most drugs are eliminated from the body by metabolism in the liver and excretion by the kidney. Metabolism occurs to a limited extent in other organs as well, including the gastrointestinal tract, kidneys, and lungs. Although the intrinsic activity of drug-metabolizing enzymes in general does not decline with age, liver mass as a percentage of body weight and liver blood flow both decrease with aging (Montamat et al., 1989). As a result, the overall capacity of the liver to convert some drugs to their inactive metabolites declines with age. For example, some studies show that drugs such as diazepam, alprazolam, chlordiazepoxide, propranolol, lidocaine, and theophylline are metabolized at a slower rate in older people than in younger people (Lamy, 1982). This is highly variable, however, and not all drugs metabolized by the liver show an age-related decline in the rate of metabolism. In fact, the metabolism of alcohol by the liver does not decline with age (Vestal et al., 1977).

The most consistent physiologic change with aging is a decline in renal function. Both glomerular filtration rate (GFR) and the renal blood flow decline with age. GFR can fall as much as 50% from the third to the eighth decade. The fall in GFR may not be accompanied by a rise in serum creatinine because muscle mass also declines with age (Schmucker, 1985). As a result, drugs that are substantially excreted by the kidney regularly exhibit decreased plasma clearance in the elderly. This is particularly important for drugs with narrow therapeutic indices (a ration of effective to toxic drug levels) such as digoxin, aminoglycoside antibiotics, lithium, and chlorpropamide (Greenblatt et al., 1982).

ALTERED PHARMACODYNAMICS

Pharmacodynamic properties of a drug refer to the type, intensity, and duration of the effect of a given concentration of a drug at its site of action. In essence, this depends on the processes involved in the interaction between a drug and the effector organ, resulting in a change in the functional state of that organ. This change constitutes the response. Alterations in physiologic and homeostatic systems, including the autonomic system, baroreceptors, thermoregulation, and balance may explain the propensity of the elderly to postural hypotension, falls, hypothermia, and confusion, particularly following drug-induced decrements in these systems (Vestal et al., 1992). An increased sensitivity that increases the susceptibility to adverse drug reactions is observed particularly with drugs acting on the central nervous system. Any drug that affects alertness, coordination, and balance will likely cause more falls and accidents in elderly people than in younger people. Hangover effects of sedative-hypnotic drugs and other psychotropics (e.g., antipsychotics, antidepressants, anxiolytics, metoclopramide, and narcotic analgesics) are common and often more prominent in the elderly (Lamy, 1991). This can lead to serious consequences, such as falls and hip fractures. Cook et al. (1984) found that the dose of diazepam or nitrazepam required to produce sedation in the elderly is twofold less than that of young individuals. This suggests in part that neurotransmitter receptors are more sensitive in the elderly. This increase in sensitivity may account for the observation that adverse reactions to benzodiazepines occur more frequently in the elderly patients. When compared to young persons, narcotic analgesics cause more sedation, respiratory depression, and confusion in the elderly. While most medications rarely lead to severe central nervous system toxicity in younger patients, problems such as confusion, depression, anxiety, insomnia, and sedation are common in the elderly.

Catecholamines have an important endocrine and neuroendocrine role in mediating a variety of autonomic functions. One consequence of normal aging, in particular in the cardiovascular system, is a decline in beta-adrenergic function associated with an alteration in responsiveness to beta-adrenergic therapy. Plasma norepinephrine concentration increases with age. The reduced high-affinity receptors and the reduced hormone-stimulated adenylyl cyclase activity with age may be explained by receptor desensitization due to increased plasma norepinephrine concentration (Scarpace et al., 1991). The elderly are less sensitive to some drugs. For example, sensitivity of the beta-adrenoreceptor for both agonist and antagonist molecules diminishes with aging. Thus, heart rate slows less with propranolol and accelerates less with epinephrine and there may be less bronchodilatation with isoproterenol, suggesting that the elderly may experience side effects before achieving the therapeutic concentrations in the plasma (Vestal et al., 1979). Not only is there reduced beta-adrenergic receptor responsiveness, but reduced baroreflex function also occurs with age. These changes lead to increased sensitivity to the therapeutic and postural hypotensive effects of diuretics and vasodilators (Phillips et al., 1991).

ADVERSE DRUG REACTIONS IN THE ELDERLY

In general, the elderly have more health problems than their younger counterparts. Because of multiple and chronic diseases, geriatric patients often take multiple prescription and OTC drugs. Persons over the age of 65 years may take as many as seven or more prescription drugs in addition to OTC drugs. Multiple drug therapy predisposes the elderly to an increased risk of adverse drug reactions (ADR). Previous studies used the method of intensive inpatient monitoring and identified digoxin, diuretics, aspirin, psychotropics, and cytotoxins as drugs of concern (Lindley et al., 1992). Nonsteroidal anti-inflammatory drugs (NSAIDs) have been added to the list that cause hospital admissions related to adverse drug reactions. ADRs in the elderly may result from drug overuse or misuse, slowed drug metabolism or elimination secondary to aging or to age-related chronic diseases, intake of alcohol, and food-drug incompatibilities. Furthermore, ADRs are more severe. The overall incidence of ADRs is two to three times that of young adults. Although the results of studies vary, about 20% of all adverse drug reactions occur in the elderly (Korrapati et al., 1992). Risk factors include female gender, living alone, multiple diseases, multiple drugs, poor nutritional status, and impaired sensorium. Some of the age-related physiologic causes for increased plasma levels and examples of altered receptor sensitivity to drugs have already been discussed. Elderly persons who drink alcohol regularly, even if they are not alcoholic, place themselves at risk for drug-alcohol interactions. Since the elimination capacity of both the kidneys and the liver can be reduced in old age, in general, drugs should be prescribed at lower initial doses to geriatric patients.

ALCOHOL USE AND THE ELDERLY

Prevalence of Alcohol Use in the Elderly

Alcohol abuse remains a public health problem in the elderly. It is estimated that among those 65 to 74 years of age, 42% are users of alcohol. This figure falls to 30% after age 75 years. About 6% of the elderly are considered heavy drinkers (more than two drinks per day) and about 5% to 12% of men and 1% to 2% women in their sixties are problem drinkers (Atkinson, 1984). Alcohol is a drug that has addictive properties in susceptible individuals, and alcoholism is a disease with diverse and highly destructive pathological effects. Although its victims often do not recognize that alcoholism is a disease, it does meet the criteria for a disease. It has definite symptoms, and it is chronic, progressive, fatal, and treatable. It destroys the person not only physically, but mentally, emotionally, and spiritually. Many people with this disease die from accidents, suicide, or physical complications. In Western society, excessive consumption of alcohol and of tobacco are two of the most insidious forms of drug abuse. Yet, they are often considered socially acceptable. In the United States, two-thirds of all adults use alcohol occasionally. If cigarette smoking is excluded, alcoholism is by far the most serious drug problem in the United States and most other countries in the world.

Effects of Alcohol Use in the Elderly

A number of studies have shown that alcohol in moderate amounts is a useful therapeutic agent for the elderly and improves social interaction, alertness, and a variety of physical indices. Alcohol is primarily a depressant drug in the central nervous system

(CNS), although in small to moderate doses it has mood elevating effects that account for its popularity. The CNS depression and disinhibition it causes contribute to feelings of relaxation, confidence, and euphoria.

In general, the medical complications of alcohol abuse observed in older individuals are the same as in younger alcoholics. These include alcoholic liver disease, acute and chronic pancreatitis, gastrointestinal bleeding and other gastrointestinal tract diseases, and susceptibility to infections and other metabolic disturbances. The elderly tolerate gastrointestinal bleeding and infection less well than do younger individuals. In a recent study, Beresford et al. (1993) observed age differences in reaction time and cognition at baseline, upon which the intoxication effect of alcohol was superimposed. They concluded, therefore, that physical changes related to age, rather than a direct effect of alcohol, make the elderly appear to be more sensitive. At low doses (the equivalent of one to two drinks) relative to baseline, older social drinkers probably are at no greater risk of performance impairment than are younger social drinkers. However, the effect at higher doses may not reflect this equivalency. One reason that alcohol might be expected to have a greater dose-related effect in the elderly is because of a smaller volume of distribution (total body water), resulting in higher blood alcohol levels than in the young at an equivalent dose (Vestal et al., 1977). Finally, alcohol-induced peripheral neuropathy and cerebral degeneration (brain atrophy with dementia, cerebellar ataxia) are more common in the elderly because they are superimposed on the normal loss of neurons that occurs with age.

Problems of Alcohol and Drug Interactions in the Elderly

Alcohol use can impair the effectiveness of routine drug therapy, or can create new medical problems requiring additional therapy. Excessive alcohol use in association with medications in the elderly can severely compromise and complicate a well-planned therapeutic program. Even casual use of alcohol may be a problem for the elderly, particularly if they are taking medications that interact with ethanol. Difficulties can also arise from the interaction of alcohol and OTC medications. It is very difficult to determine the actual incidence of combined drug and alcohol use by the elderly, but it is likely to be reasonably high for the following reasons:

1. The average adult over 65 takes two to seven prescription medicines daily in addition to OTC medications.
2. Most elderly persons do not view alcohol as a drug and assume that modest amounts of alcoholic beverages can do little harm to an already aged body.
3. Few elderly persons hold to the traditional notion that mixing alcohol and medications will have deleterious consequences.

Acutely ingested, alcohol impairs the clearance of some drugs by the liver. In contrast, chronically ingested alcohol induces the synthesis of enzymes, leading to enhanced metabolism and increased clearance of some drugs including anticonvulsants, anticoagulants, and oral hypoglycemic agents. These drugs can become less effective, which increases the need for monitoring.

Alcohol-drug interactions do not generally result in death. However, there is evidence for a contributory role of alcohol in drug-related fatalities. Kurfees and Dotson in a study on drug interactions in the elderly attributed one-third (316 of 1052) of the drug interactions to an interaction with alcohol (Kurfees & Dotson, 1987). Anyone who drinks even moderately should inquire with a physician or pharmacist about possible alcohol-drug interactions.

Certainly not every medication interacts with alcohol; however, a variety of drugs interact consistently. Psychotropic drugs (antipsychotics, antidepressants, anxiolytics, and sedative-hypnotics) commonly are prescribed for the elderly, and studies suggest that the benzodiazepines or other sedative-hypnotics are the most commonly prescribed classes of these drugs. Alcohol impairs judgment and reduces alertness when taken with drugs such as antipsychotics, sedative-hypnotics, anxiolytics, opioid analgesics, antihistamines, and certain antihypertensive drugs (Table 3.3) (Rizack & Hillman, 1987). Frequent presentations include confusion, falls, emotional instability, and adverse drug interactions. The effects of these drugs are additive to those of alcohol. These factors together (alcohol, old age, multiple diseases, and medications) can lead to complications including toxic alcohol-drug interactions. The most dangerous of these reactions occurs when alcohol is combined with another central nervous system (CNS) depressant. In one study, diazepam, codeine, meprobamate, and flurazepam were the top four agents responsible for alcohol-drug interactions (Jinks & Raschko, 1990). Antihistamines including diphenhydramine, dimenhydrinate, and most cold medications, and anticholinergics such as scopolamine, which are found in OTC medications, can also cause confusion in the elderly. An important consideration in the elderly is the confused and altered behavior that so often follows excessive consumption of alcohol. Many times elderly alcoholics present with symptoms of falls, confusion, and self-neglect. Such changes may impair the elderly patient's ability to adhere to a prescribed treatment regimen, and the risks of mistakes or mishaps in dosage are far increased (Gerbino, 1982). Some of the well-described specific interactions are discussed below.

Psychotropic Drugs

When alcohol is combined with psychotropic drugs such as antipsychotics and antidepressants, the effects are less predictable than with other drugs. Antipsychotic drugs inhibit the metabolism of alcohol and may markedly enhance its effects on the CNS in the elderly. Antidepressants exaggerate the response to alcohol and impair motor skills. This could be a significant hazard in the elderly. Depression of the CNS may range from drowsiness to coma, because acute alcohol consumption may increase the CNS effects of antidepressants. Alcohol may also increase the risk of hypothermic reactions in the elderly taking tricyclic antidepressants. The avoidance of alcohol in elderly patients taking any of these drugs is a prudent recommendation (Scott & Mitchell, 1988).

Much controversy exists as to whether the observed enhancement of CNS depression from combined use of alcohol and psychotropics is simply additive or synergistic. When combined with members of this class of drugs, alcohol even in small quantities produces undesirable and sometimes dangerous additive effects. The interaction of alcohol with benzodiazepine drugs, however, may be much greater in the elderly than in the other age groups. This is especially true for diazepam and chlordiazepoxide. Commonly observed side effects include hypotension, sedation, confusion, and CNS depression that may progress to respiratory depression. Alcohol increases the clinical effects of these drugs, which already are especially hazardous in a segment of the population with decreased agility and greater danger of serious complications from falls and accidents. Two or more drinks can be enough to induce a drug-alcohol interaction with a CNS depressant medication (Hartford & Samorajski, 1982). As a general rule, elderly patients

Table 3.3. Drug-Alcohol Interactions and Adverse Effects

Drug	Adverse effect with alcohol
Acetaminophen	Severe hepatotoxicity with therapeutic doses of acetaminophen in chronic alcoholics
Anticoagulants, oral	Decreased anticoagulant effect with chronic alcohol abuse
Antidepressants, tricyclic	Combined CNS depression decreases psychomotor performance, especially in the first week of treatment
Aspirin and other nonsteroidal anti-inflammatory drugs	Increased the possibility of gastritis and gastrointestinal hemorrhage
Barbiturates	Increased CNS depression (additive effects)
Benzodiazepines	Increased CNS depression (additive effects)
Beta-adrenergic blockers	Masked signs of delirium tremens
Bromocriptine	Combined use increases gastrointestinal side effects
Caffeine	Possible further decreased reaction time
Cephalosporins and Chloramphenicol	Antabuse-like reaction with some cephalosporins and chloramphenicol
Chloral hydrate	Prolonged hypnotic effect and adverse cardiovascular effects
Cimetidine	Increased CNS depressant effect of alcohol
Cycloserine	Increased alcohol effect or convulsions
Digoxin	Decreased digitalis effect
Disulfiram (Antabuse)	Abdominal cramps, flushing, vomiting, hypotension, confusion, blurred vision, and psychosis
Guanadrel	Increased sedative effect and orthostatic hypotension
Glutethimide	Additive CNS depressant effect
Heparin	Increased bleeding
Hypoglycemics, sulfonylurea	Acute ingestion-increased hypoglycemic effect of sulfonylurea drugs
	Chronic ingestion-decreased hypoglycemic effect of these drugs
(Tolbutamide, chlorpropamide)	Antabuse-like reaction
Isoniazid	Increased liver toxicity
Ketoconazole, griseofulvin	Antabuse-like reaction
Lithium	Increased lithium toxicity
Meprobamate	Synergistic CNS depression
Methotrexate	Increased hepatic damage in chronic alcoholics
Metronidazole	Antabuse-like reaction
Nitroglycerin	Possible hypotension
Phenformin	Lactic acidosis (synergism)
Phenothiazines	Additive CNS depressant activity
Phenytoin	Acutely ingested, alcohol can increase the toxicity of phenytoin and Chronically ingested, alcohol can decrease the anticonvulsant effect of phenytoin
Quinacrine	Antabuse-like reaction
Tetracyclines	Decreased effect of doxycycline

Source: Adapted from Rizack, M. A., and Hillman, C. D. M. (1987).

should be instructed to refrain from alcohol while taking CNS depressant medications, including benzodiazepines, barbiturates, muscle relaxants, and antihistamines (both by prescription and in the form of OTC cold remedies or sleeping aids).

Cardiovascular Drugs

Alcohol is a vasodilator that enhances the absorption of nitroglycerin. Use of alcohol when there is a need for vasodilation with nitrates may cause severe hypotension. As stated earlier, alcohol use in the elderly can cause gastrointestinal bleeding, red blood cell and platelet abnormalities, anemia, and hepatic enzyme induction. When taken in combination with warfarin, alcohol can contribute to the risk of severe bleeding or facilitate alterations in the patient's anticoagulant stability. Extra care should be taken before prescribing drugs like digitalis, diuretics, antihypertensives, and antiarrhythmic agents (Gerbino, 1982).

Analgesics

The increase in morbidity associated with aging may result in consumption of a wide range of drugs including the nonsteroidal anti-inflammatory drugs (NSAIDs), which are most commonly prescribed worldwide when grouped by generic categories and account for 3 to 9% of total prescription numbers in various countries (Johnson & Day, 1991). Aspirin is the active ingredient in many OTC arthritis pain formulas and in numerous nonprescription combination headache and minor pain products. The ability of aspirin to cause gastric inflammation, gastrointestinal erosion, and frank gastrointestinal bleeding is well recognized. Alcohol not only produces gastritis, but also increases the risk of gastrointestinal bleeding caused by aspirin and other NSAIDs (Bush et al., 1991). The use of NSAIDs is accompanied by a two- to fivefold risk of serious complications of peptic ulcer disease, particularly hemorrhage or perforation, which increase in the elderly, particularly women. Elderly people at high risk for bleeding are best advised to avoid regular use of either alcohol or aspirin.

Chronic alcohol abuse can cause hepatotoxicity in a patient taking acetaminophen, probably due to enzyme induction leading to formation of toxic intermediary metabolites of acetaminophen. Age-related alterations in pharmacokinetics may influence the handling of NSAIDs in the elderly. In particular, dosage reduction is appropriate for azapropazone, naproxen, ketoprofen, and salicylates administered to healthy aged patients, whereas the presence of renal disease may also necessitate dosage reduction of diflunisal, indomethacin, sulindac, and mefenamic acid. Changes in NSAID pharmacodynamics with aging, such as increased CNS sensitivity to NSAIDs and impaired homeostasis, also predispose the elderly to NSAID-related adverse effects.

Other Therapeutic Agents

Many elderly patients with adult onset diabetes take sulfonylureas, which are orally effective antidiabetic agents. When alcohol is taken concomitantly with sulfonylureas, it may cause additive hypoglycemia, especially in patients with restricted carbohydrate intake. Another problem associated with this combination is the infrequent potential for an antabuse-like reaction, which is usually mild and characterized by nausea, vomiting, headache, blurred vision, and flushing. Symptoms of severe antabuse-like reactions include tachycardia, abdominal distress, sweating, hypotensive episodes, myocardial infarction, and laceration of the esophagus induced by vomiting. Psychosis may occur as well, and fatal reactions have been reported. Concomitant use of a variety of other drugs (Table 3.4) can also lead to an antabuse-like reaction.

Cough medicines may contain a narcotic analgesic such as codeine in combination with antihistamines. When taken together with alcohol, these drugs are hazardous and can cause altered sensorium and respiratory depression.

Despite the fact that cardiac disorders are very common in older individuals, few of

Table 3.4. Drugs Producing Antabuse-Like Reactions with Alcohol

Disulfiram (Antabuse)
Hypoglycemic agents
   chlorpropamide (Diabinese)
   tolbutamide (Orinase)
Other drugs
   chloramphenicol (Chloromycetin)
   griseofulvin (Fulvicin)
   ketoconazole (Nizoral)
   furazolidone (Furoxone)
   metronidazole (Flagyl)
   cefoperazone (Cefobid)
   cefamandole (Mandole)
   moxalactam (Moxam)
   cefotetan (Cefotan)
   cefmetazole (Zefazone)
   procarbazine (Matulane)
   monoamine oxidase inhibitors
   (eg. phenelzine and tranylcypromine)
   quinacrine (Atabrine)
Alcohol sensitizing mushrooms
   coprinus atrmentarius (inky-cap mushroom)
   clitocybe clavipes

those who suffer from these problems modify their drinking patterns. This may be dangerous, since as little as one cocktail can adversely affect cardiac efficiency in the presence of heart disease. For example, alcohol consumption in a person suffering from angina (cardiac pain on exertion) can mask the pain that might otherwise serve as a warning signal (Horowitz, 1975).

Illicit Drugs

Abuse of hallucinogens, illicit psychomotor stimulants and sedatives, and cannabis is very uncommon in old age. The low incidence of this type of substance abuse in old age may be because of early mortality and under-reporting. However, problem drinkers may abuse drugs such as sedatives, opioids, marihuana, and amphetamines. Sometimes these drugs are used in combination with alcohol. At other times, such drugs are taken in preference to alcohol, and alcohol is used only when the drug of choice is not available.

PRINCIPLES FOR PRESCRIBING MEDICATIONS AND USE OF ALCOHOL IN THE ELDERLY

1. Insist that the patient bring in whatever drugs he is taking at each visit. Evaluate the need for each drug and discontinue those that are unnecessary.
2. Patients with hepatic disease, peptic ulcer disease, and alcoholic skeletal or cardiac

Table 3.5. Guidelines for Use of Alcohol by the Elderly

1. Alcohol when taken in moderation may be useful.
2. Elderly patients are advised to avoid alcohol consumption immediately prior to going to bed in order to avoid sleep disturbances.
3. Alcohol ingestion must be avoided prior to driving.
4. Abstinence from alcohol by elderly patients receiving CNS depressants, analgesics, anticoagulants, antidiabetic drugs, and some cardiovascular drugs is recommended.
5. Older individuals who want to drink an alcoholic beverage, have no medical contraindications, and take no medications that interact with alcohol may consider one drink a day to be a prudent level of alcohol consumption.
6. A doctor or pharmacist should be consulted about alcohol-drug interactions.
7. Any side effect or loss of energy should be immediately reported to the physician.

Source: Adapted from Dufour, M. C., Archer, L., & Gordis, E. (1992).

myopathy should be advised to avoid alcohol. Clearly, it should be taken only in strict moderation or not at all.

3. As a general rule, a benzodiazepine should not be used on a long-term basis (not more than few months) without attempting to discontinue the drug. This rule does not apply when these drugs are used as anticonvulsants. The probability and intensity of the withdrawal effects are greatest with short-acting benzodiazepines. Intermediate-acting drugs may be tapered at a rate of 5 to 10% every 5 days, and long-acting preparations can be tapered more quickly. When a benzodiazepine is to be discontinued, taper the dose slowly. For example, an appropriate schedule would be to decrease the dose by one-half, wait 5 half-lives, and then discontinue the drug completely or reduce the dose by half again before discontinuing it.
4. Administration of drugs with anticholinergic effects (antipsychotics, antidepressants, and atropine derivatives) should be titrated carefully in elderly patients, because they cause urinary retention, constipation, blurred vision, and dry mouth.
5. In many cases, very low doses of medication may be effective. For example, 12.5 to 25 mg hydrochlorothiazide daily has been shown to be effective in treating hypertension. Initial doses of 0.25 mg of haloperidol or 10 mg of imipramine per day are appropriate in the elderly. Unless the clinical situation requires otherwise, drugs should be started at low doses in the elderly and titrated carefully upward during frequent early follow-up visits.
6. Every elderly patient should be encouraged to be aware of the guidelines for the appropriate use of alcohol (Table 3.5) (Dufour et al., 1992).

SUMMARY

Elderly people are the fastest growing segment of the population and consume more than one-fourth of all the drugs prescribed. The capacity to handle some drugs in the old differs from the young due to age-related physiologic and pathologic changes in various systems of the body. Such alterations in pharmacokinetics may result in a reduction in the dose required to achieve the optimum pharmacodynamic effect. Although alcohol metabolism is unchanged in healthy elderly people, the volume of distribution is smaller, which means that at equivalent doses peak concentrations will be higher in this age group. Alcohol abuse among the older individuals can lead to falls, fractures, and other similar medical complications. The combined use of medications (both prescribed and OTC) and alcohol can lead to serious complications. However, in the absence of any contraindications or concomitant medications, a small quantity of alcohol consumption may be beneficial in some elderly persons. In general, the use of multiple drugs creates a situation favorable to drug interactions and adverse reactions. Also, since old people are more sensitive to the effects of psychotropics, it is wise to reduce the dosage of drugs such as the benzodiazepines, analgesics, and sedative-hypnotics in the elderly, and concomitant use with alcohol should be discouraged.

References

Atkinson, R. M. (1984). Substance use and abuse in late life. In *Alcohol and drug abuse in old age.* (pp. 2–21.). Washington, DC: American Psychiatric Press, Inc.

Beresford, T. P., Demo-Dananberg, L., Schwartz, J., Young, J., Hill, E., & Lucey, M. R. (1993). Age, gastric function and ethanol metabolism. *Alcoholism: Clinical and Experimental Research, 17,* 446.

Brock, D. B., Guralnik, J. M., & Brody, J. A. (1990). Demography and epidemiology of aging in the United States. In E. L. Schneider & J. W. Rowe (Eds.). *Handbook of the Biology of Aging* (3rd ed.) (pp. 3–23). San Deigo: Academic Press, Inc.

Bush, T. M., Shlotzhauer, T. L., & Imai, K. (1991). Nonsteroidal anti-inflammatory drugs. Proposed guidelines for monitoring toxicity. *Western Journal of Medicine, 155,* 39–42.

Cook, P. J., Flanagam, R., & James, I. M. (1984). Diazepam tolerance: Effect of age, regular sedation and alcohol. *British Medical Journal, 289,* 351–353.

Cusack, B. J., & Vestal, R. E. (1986). Clinical pharmacology: Special consideration in the elderly. In E. Calkins, P. J. Dovin, & A. B. Ford (Eds.). *Practice of Geriatric Medicine.* (pp. 115–136). Philadelphia: W. B. Saunders Co.

Dufour, M. C., Archer, L., & Gordis, E. (1992). Alcohol and the elderly. *Clinical Geriatric Medicine, 8,* 127–141.

Gerbino, P. P. (1982). Complications of alcohol use combined with drug therapy in the Elderly. *Journal of the American Geriatrics Society, 30,* S88–S93.

Greenblatt, D. J., Sellars, E. M., & Shader, R. I. (1982). Drug disposition in old age. *New England Journal of Medicine, 306,* 1081–1088.

Hale, W. E., May, F. E., Marks, R. G., & Stewart, R. B. (1987). Drug use in an ambulatory elderly population: A five year update. *Drug Intelligence and Clinical Pharmacy, 21,* 530–535.

Hartford, J. T., & Samorajski, T. (1982). Alcoholism in the geriatric population. *Journal of the American Geriatrics Society, 30,* 18–24.

Health Care Financing Administration, Office of National Cost Estimates. (1990). National health expenditures, 1988. *Health Care Financing Review, 11,* 1–41.

Horowitz, L. D. (1975). Alcohol and heart disease. *Journal of the American Medical Association, 232,* 959–960.

Jinks, M. J., & Raschko, R. R. (1990). A profile of alcohol and prescription drug abuse in a high-risk community-based elderly population. *Drug Intelligence and Clinical Pharmacy, 24,* 971–975.

Johnson, A. G., & Day, R. O. (1991). The problems and pitfalls of NSAID therapy in the elderly (Part I). *Drugs and Aging, 1,* 130–143.

Korrapati, M. R., Loi, C. M., & Vestal, R. E. (1992). Adverse drug reactions in the elderly. *Drug Therapy, 22,* 21–30.

Kurfees, J. F., & Dotson, R. L. (1987). Drug interactions in the elderly. *Journal of Family Practice, 25*, 477–488.

Lamy, P. P. (1982). Comparative pharmacokinetic changes and drug therapy in an older population. *Journal of the American Geriatrics Society, 30*, S11–S19.

Lamy, P. P. (1991). Physiological changes due to age. Pharmacodynamic changes of drug action and implications for therapy. *Drugs and Aging, 1*, 385–404.

Lindley, C. M., Tully, M. P., Paramsothy, V., & Tallis, R. C. (1992). Inappropriate medication is a major cause of adverse reactions in elderly patients. *Age and Ageing, 21*, 294–300.

Loi, C. M., & Vestal, R. E. (1988). Drug metabolism in the elderly. *Pharmacology & Therapeutics, 36*, 131–149.

Montamat, S. C., Cusack, B. J., & Vestal, R. E. (1989). Management of drug therapy in the elderly. *New England Journal of Medicine, 321*, 303–309.

Olshansky, S. J., Carnes, B. A., & Cassel, C. K. (1993). The aging of the human species. *Scientific American, 268(4)*, 46–52.

Phillips, P. A., Hodsman, G. P., & Johnston, C. I. (1991). Neuroendocrine mechanisms and cardiovascular homeostasis in the elderly. *Cardiovascular Drugs and Therapy, 4(Suppl 6)*, 1209–1213.

Rizack, M. A., & Hillman, C. D. M. (1987). Adverse interactions of drugs. In *The Medical Letter Handbook of Adverse Drug Interactions*, (pp. 7–10). New York: The Medical Letter.

Scarpace, P. J., Tumer, N., & Mader, S. L. (1991). Beta-adrenergic function in aging. Basic mechanisms and clinical implications. *Drugs and Aging, 1*, 116–129.

Schmucker, D. L. (1985). Aging and drug disposition: An update. *Pharmacological Reviews, 37*, 133–148.

Scott, R. B., & Mitchell, M. C. (1988). Aging, alcohol, and the liver. *Journal of the American Geriatrics Society, 36*, 255–265.

Vestal, R. E., McGuire, E. A., Tobin, J. D., et al. (1977). Aging and ethanol metabolism. *Clinical Pharmacology and Therapeutics, 21*, 343–354.

Vestal, R. E., Montamat, S. C., & Nielson, C. P. (1992). Drugs in special patient groups. In K. L. Melmon, H. F. Morrelli, B. B. Hoffman, & D. W. Nierenberg (Eds.). *Clinical Pharmacology* (3rd ed.) (pp. 851–874). New York; McGraw Hill

Vestal, R. E., Wood, A. J. J., & Shand, D. J. (1979). Reduced β-adrenoceptor sensitivity in the elderly. *Clinical Pharmacology and Therapeutics, 26*, 181–186.

4

Comorbidity in Elderly Alcoholics

RICHARD E. FINLAYSON

In the substance use disorders field, the term *comorbidity* usually refers to psychiatric comorbidity. The term *dual diagnosis* has been adopted to describe the coexistence of a disorder and alcoholism. There are limitations to this term, however, especially for the elderly in whom it often fails to describe adequately the extent of clinical heterogeneity. Overall, the trend toward recognizing comorbidity in alcoholics has been useful. It raises interesting questions about etiology, pathogenesis, and natural history. Shaffer and Burglass (1981) expressed the opinion that the addictions field is struggling to develop paradigms. The interest in and emphasis on comorbidity have raised healthy doubts about the nature of alcoholism, thereby challenging monolithic dogmas and opening new paths of inquiry.

We should be interested in comorbidity in our patients for practical clinical reasons. Data from the Medical Outcomes Study (Stewart et al., 1989) revealed that patients with multiple conditions showed greater decrements in functioning and well-being than those with only one condition. There is evidence that the phenomenon of psychiatric disorders complicating the course of alcoholism is common (Regier et al., 1990). Relatively little research on this topic has been focused on older persons. This chapter reviews some of the literature pertaining to psychiatric comorbidity in elderly alcoholics, with a focus on epidemiology, diagnosis, and treatment. Although alcoholism may coexist with any other psychiatric disorder, the discussion will be limited to the most common, broad categories of mental illness.

MULTIPLE SUBSTANCE ABUSE

Several factors contribute to the phenomenon of combined drug and alcohol use and abuse in older persons. Although illicit drug use is unusual in the elderly (Cisin et al., 1977; Norton and Colliver, 1988; Bailey, 1990), the elderly use prescription drugs at two to three times the rate of the general population (Report to the Chairman, Special Committee on Aging, U.S. Senate, 1987). Additionally, the use of alcohol by the ''young old'' remains fairly high in the sixth and seventh decades of life (Atkinson,

1990). This increases the potential for combined drug and alcohol use in many elderly persons. Alcohol abusers (recognized or hidden) who present to physicians with various somatic, mood, and sleep complaints may receive psychoactive drugs as treatment for these symptoms. Community-based studies suggest that many older persons consume drugs in combination with alcohol (Butler et al., 1990; Jinks & Raschko, 1990).

Women are more likely to visit physicians and to receive prescriptions for psychoactive drugs than are men and are more likely than men to take these drugs on a chronic basis (Cafferata et al., 1983; Baum et al., 1985; Mossey & Shapiro, 1985). There is evidence that this may translate into drug-alcohol comorbidity. Schuckit and Morrissey (1979) reported that, among women in alcoholism treatment, two-thirds had received drugs of potential abuse and one-third of these admitted to abuse of the drugs. In a study comparing drug use in alcoholic and nonalcoholic women (Gomberg, 1990), the data revealed that when matched for age and social class, alcoholic women used significantly more psychoactive drugs both over their lifetimes and during the previous year. Women alcoholics have been reported (Ross, 1989) to be more frequent users of prescription drugs than male alcoholics.

The elderly are heavy consumers of over-the-counter medications (Kofoed, 1984; Dufour et al., 1992). Some of these medications are former prescription drugs such as antihistamines, which may interact with alcohol in harmful ways. Many antihistamines are sedating and, when used in combination with alcohol, can produce excessive sleepiness and even confusional states. Prescription medications such as tricyclic antidepressants, antipsychotics, and antiparkinsonian drugs also have anticholinergic properties, and, when used by the elderly person, add to the anticholinergic medication ''load'' and the danger of serious side effects, such as excessive water consumption, dry mouth, visual disturbance, cardiac arrhythmias, constipation, urinary retention, and confusion. It is important that the clinician include the over-the-counter-drug group when taking a history from the elderly alcoholic, especially when a cause for impaired cognitive symptoms is being sought.

Nicotine dependence, widely recognized as a persistent addiction, is apparently common in alcoholics of all ages. The literature relating to nicotine dependence in elderly alcoholics, however, is sparse. Nakamura et al. (1990), in a study of 1034 older persons, found that alcohol consumption before age 40 years, smoking, male sex, and marital status were predictors of severe drinking. Jensen and Bellecci (1987) reported nonagenarian men to have a higher prevalence of alcohol abuse, higher current alcohol intake, and greater smoking of cigarettes compared with men age 65 to 75 years. A study of elderly alcoholics (70% males) hospitalized for treatment of their alcoholism reported a prevalence rate of active tobacco dependence of 52% (Finlayson et al., 1988). The prevalence of smoking in alcoholics overall is more than 80% (Battjes, 1988; Istvan & Mararazzo, 1984). The prevalence of smoking addiction may decline in later years, perhaps due to health consequences and demographic factors.

The diagnosis of this addictive disorder is not difficult. Few people, including the elderly, deny their use of tobacco. Some, however, may identify themselves as nonsmokers but not mention that a lengthy smoking history was recently interrupted for health reasons. There is a new trend in substance abuse treatment for smoke-free treatment settings (for example, smoke-free Alcoholics Anonymous groups). In some programs, smoking cessation is offered to patients undergoing treatment for other addictions. We await data concerning the responsiveness of the elderly to this approach.

ORGANIC MENTAL DISORDERS

The literature describing the neuropsychiatric complications of alcoholism is extensive and will be discussed here only as it relates to aging and the elderly. Cognitive impairment is the most prevalent neuropsychiatric disorder of old age. It increases in prevalence with advancing age, whereas most other psychiatric disorders decrease (Kramer et al., 1985; Weissman et al., 1985; Bland et al., 1988).

One idea advanced in this area was the premature-aging theory of alcoholic dementia. Goldstein (1985) noted that clinical observations led to this theory. The decrements in problem solving, abstraction, judgment, and learning ability frequently seen in chronic alcoholics appeared analogous to the characteristics of the normal aged population. But the premature-aging theory has not been sustained, in part because of the growing evidence that aging per se does not typically lead to serious cognitive impairment.

The most commonly recognized cognitive disturbance is that of *age-associated memory impairment* (Crook et al., 1986). This term was proposed by a National Institute of Mental Health workgroup and is applied to people older than age 50 years who have complaints of memory impairment in tasks of daily life. It is not used to describe cognitive deterioration that goes beyond this point. Studies comparing alcoholism and aging have tended to suggest that both factors are relatively independent variables in their effects on cognitive impairment (Oscar-Berman & Bonner, 1985; Burger et al., 1987; Kramer et al., 1989; Oscar-Berman et al., 1990).

Although alcoholism does not seem to cause premature aging of the brain, there is ample evidence that both alcoholism and aging contribute to the risk of cognitive impairment. The heavy drinking, according to Saunders et al. (1991), need not occur in late life to increase the risk of dementia. In a random community sample of subjects age 65 years and older in Liverpool, England, men with a history of heavy drinking for 5 years or more at some time in their lives had a greater than fivefold risk of suffering from a psychiatric disorder, including dementia.

In a review, Dufour et al. (1992) cited evidence that alcohol is associated with impairment that increases with age in certain types of task performance and can also exacerbate cognitive impairment in dementias from other causes. In a Japanese study (Ikeda, 1991), age and chronicity of drinking correlated positively with a diagnosis of alcoholic dementia. Evidence for age as a factor in brain alteration in drinkers was provided by Pfefferbaum et al. (1988) from a controlled study of brain changes seen on computed tomograms in male alcoholics. Sulcal enlargement in alcoholics was found across all ages. In contrast, ventricular enlargement was apparent only in older alcoholics and became increasingly exaggerated with age.

Dementia associated with alcoholism (American Psychiatric Association, 1987) is recognized as a disorder of multifactorial origin involving alcohol neurotoxicity, head trauma, cardiovascular disease, hepatic dysfunction, and malnutrition (Goldstein, 1985). Aging may enhance these factors, thereby placing the elderly alcoholic at increased risk for dementia.

The diagnosis of dementia is typically made in older persons, although the introduction of acquired immunodeficiency syndrome into our culture has made us more aware of dementia as a problem in younger persons as well (Oechsner et al., 1993). The clinical history, including substance use history, physical examination, mental status examination, and appropriate laboratory tests (Table 4.1), constitutes the initial work-up for the elderly alcoholic. Screening for cognitive impairment should be done early in this process with an instrument such as the Folstein Mini-Mental State Examination (Folstein et al., 1975). This screening process is not, in itself, adequate for making the diagnosis of dementia.

The problems encountered in diagnosing this disorder in elderly alcoholics include denial by the patient and others, distortions caused by the memory loss itself, assessing the nature of emotional and behavioral symptoms, and uncertainty as to the reversibility of the condition. Intoxication and delirium may be confused with dementia, but a careful clinical evaluation usually makes the distinction possible. The patient's symptoms may be due not only to alcohol use but also to other drugs and various medical disorders such as congestive heart failure and renal insufficiency. Although cognitive impairment is the hallmark of dementia, some cases are initially manifested by changes in emotions or personality (Albert et al., 1974; Cummings & Benson, 1984). A firm diagnosis of dementia is usually not made until the patient has been abstinent for a few weeks. Even then the degree of reversibility is difficult to assess.

In this age group, other types of dementia may coexist with dementia associated with alcoholism. Multi-infarct dementia, occurring in about 15% of cases, is diagnosed by evidence of cerebrovascular disease and a stepwise clinical course, although some cases follow a progressive course similar to Alzheimer's disease, which is responsible for about two-thirds of the cases of dementia in old age. Even after the elderly alcoholic has achieved abstinence, the persistence of cognitive problems may remain a mystery. Although alcoholic dementia does not progress when alcohol use stops, the presence of a language disorder may suggest Alzheimer's disease. One Australian study did not implicate alcoholism as a risk factor for Alzheimer's disease, however (Broe et al., 1990).

Treatment of dementia associated with alcoholism is based on maintaining abstinence from alcohol and related drugs while taking measures to minimize the other factors that contribute to the cognitive, affective, and behavior disturbances. Management strategies do not differ greatly from those for nonalcoholic types of dementia. Early administration of thiamine may be particularly important for prevention of Wernicke-Korsakoff syndrome in chronic alcoholics and the demented elderly (Jeyasingham et al., 1987). The combination of aging and hepatic insufficiency may lead to a protracted recovery of

Table 4.1. Standard Diagnostic Studies for New-Onset Dementia

Complete blood cell count
Electrolyte panel
Screening metabolic panel
Thyroid function tests
Vitamin B_{12} and folate levels
Tests for syphilis and, depending on history, for human immunodeficiency virus
Urine screen for substances of abuse
Urinalysis
Electrocardiogram
Chest radiograph

Source: Modified from Office of Medical Applications of Research, National Institutes of Health (1987). Differential diagnosis of dementing disease. *JAMA*, 258, 3411-6.

cognitive functioning in those cases in which the liver disease itself or associated drug abuse (for example, benzodiazepines) has contributed to the problem. Close medical follow-up and social support are required.

In the long-term management of elderly patients with dementia associated with alcoholism, agitation may often become a problem as it does with other demented persons. The use of benzodiazepines for control of agitation should be avoided when possible because of their potential for impairing cognition and interacting unfavorably with the person's alcohol addiction. Low doses of neuroleptic agents may be the best choice in this circumstance.

DEPRESSIVE DISORDERS

Alcoholism and depression are common in the elderly. In a study by Schuckit et al. (1975), 24% of elderly medical-surgical patients had unrecognized mental illness, primarily depression and alcoholism. Kukull et al. (1986) found an association between alcoholism and depression in elderly general medical clinic patients. Although alcoholism and depressive states commonly coexist, the rates for both disorders probably decrease with age (Reifler et al., 1982). There is a gender differential, however, in that elderly women appear more likely to be depressed and elderly men more likely to suffer from alcoholism (Liptzin, 1987).

There may be some association between alcoholism and depression with respect to onset. In a report from Schonfeld and Dupree (1991), depression, loneliness, and lack of social support were frequently reported antecedents to alcohol abuse in elderly groups, but early-onset cases of alcoholism had more severe levels of depression and anxiety. Heavy drinking at some time in life seems to be a risk factor for depression in older men (Saunders et al., 1991), and according to a report from Cook et al. (1991), a past history of alcoholism is a risk factor for chronicity of depression in elderly men.

The difficulty in diagnosing affective illness in drinking alcoholics is well known. Consider the following case history of an older person whose long-standing dual disorder was not successfully treated until relatively late in life.

First contact with this now 75-year-old woman occurred after she had attempted suicide by ingesting cleaning fluid. A diagnosis of alcoholism had been made 3 years earlier. She had received the diagnosis of depression ten years before, which was variously modified as being situational depression, psychoneurotic depression, cyclothymia, and major depression. Her course was unstable and was marked by recurrent episodes of relapsing alcoholism and suicide attempts. Although she had been admitted many times to psychiatric units, inpatient addiction treatments, and for a 1-year stay at a psychiatric institute, her course remained unstable.

Six years after first contact, she was readmitted to an alcohol and drug dependence unit where several observations were made. Over the years, her treatments had, at any one time, tended to focus on either the depressive disorder or the alcoholism. Many physicians had been involved, and opinions differed as to the nature of the problem. Did she drink because she was depressed, or did she become depressed because she drank? Her own lack of understanding of the alcoholism was striking, as was her physician's, who continued well-meaning treatment of her anxiety with benzodiazepines—a recognized risk factor for relapse of alcoholism. This admission focused on improving her understanding of her alcoholism, and for the first time, she participated in a recovery program that acknowledged both disorders.

Some months later, while abstinent from alcohol and tranquilizers, she experienced a typical major depressive episode, after which she began to drink. After a brief psychiatric hospitalization she was stabilized with psychotherapy and treatment with an antidepressant.

Seventeen years after initial contact, she has continued to cooperate with a two-track program: participation in Alcoholics Anonymous and outpatient psychiatric treatment. The operating principle of her treatment can be stated simply. Both of her disorders must be treated fully and successfully; to fail in one is to increase the risk of a relapse of the other.

The potential for alcohol to mimic, precipitate, or set the stage for major depression is of great current interest and clinical importance. Alcohol is a central nervous system depressant that has potent effects not only on mood but also on sleep, appetite, and other basic "vegetative" functions. In the treatment of alcoholism it is common practice to withhold antidepressant therapy for newly abstinent, depressed alcoholics in order to allow the chemical depression to be reversed. In most cases, the patient improves, but affective disorders have been reported as being common intercurrent or persistent problems in alcoholics during recovery (Pottenger et al., 1978; Behar et al., 1984). Long-term follow-up may be necessary to clarify this issue. In elderly patients with complex medical conditions, clarification can be particularly difficult. Various disorders can contribute to depressive states (for example, endocrinopathies, cancer, or dementia), as can medications, in addition to alcoholism and primary affective illness.

Much has been written about the atypical nature of depression in elderly persons, but stereotypes that can be misleading have been created in the process. Musetti et al. (1989) failed to confirm stereotypes of elderly depressives as having somatization, hypochondriasis, agitation, psychotic tendencies, and chronicity. Caine et al. (1993), in a review of the literature pertaining to depression in the elderly, observed that "current sample selection procedures minimize the variability of the very phenomenon under study" and argued for study of a wider range of comorbid conditions. Depression in the elderly, with or without alcoholism, may occur in a wide variety of patterns.

A thorough general medical evaluation is particularly important for the depressed elderly alcoholic. One frequently uncovers multiple factors that could be contributing to the patient's state of poor health, and each should be addressed by the physician in the manner and sequence indicated by the examination. Detoxification, restoration of fluid and electrolyte balance, treatment of ketoacidosis in diabetics, nutritional therapy, and treatment of infections are examples of this strategy and are usually first-priority items. Severely depressed, psychotic, or suicidal elderly alcoholics should be admitted into a primary psychiatric setting.

Whether an antidepressant should be used depends on the past history (for example, prior depression or mania), family history of mental illness, and the nature of the patient's persistent symptoms. Psychotherapy is the bedrock of treatment for virtually all depressions and should not be withheld because the patient is elderly.

ANXIETY DISORDERS

Abrams (1991), in a review and discussion of anxiety in the elderly, noted that anxiety syndromes have their onset in early life and have lower reported prevalence in old age. Older women are more likely to receive an anxiety disorder diagnosis than are older men. Phobias remain quite common in later life, whereas the rate for panic disorder decreases considerably. Table 4.2 is a summary of conditions associated with anxiety in the elderly.

Alcoholism has the potential for increasing anxiety throughout the life span. Biologic factors such as an abstinence syndrome, organic mental disorders, and other organ damage syndromes may directly threaten homeostasis and survival. Elderly alcoholics in treatment have been reported to be more physically ill than their nonalcoholic counterparts in the community (Hurt et al., 1988). Bruce and McNamara (1992), in their study of noninstitutionalized elderly in the greater New Haven, Connecticut, area, noted that physical health status in elderly persons is related to the rate of anxiety disorders: Among homebound and nonhomebound elderly people the rates of anxiety disorders were 2.2% and 0.4%, respectively.

In addition to the direct physical effects of alcoholism, reactive psychologic factors play a powerful role in producing anxiety. The alcoholic is prone to self-medicate for anxiety; for example, the alcoholic may drink to relieve guilt and anxiety only to experience more guilt and anxiety as a result of the drinking (Davis, 1971). Thus, the elderly alcoholic's drinking may damage the body and disrupt interpersonal relationships, work performance, social standing, and economic survival.

The literature dealing with anxiety and anxiety disorders in elderly alcoholics is sparse. In the sample from the Mayo Clinic (Finlayson et al., 1988), fewer than 1% of elderly alcoholics in treatment were reported to have an anxiety disorder. Jinks and Raschko (1990), in their study of a high-risk community-based elderly population in Spokane, Washington, noted that 0.2% were diagnosed as having a primary anxiety disorder with secondary alcohol abuse.

The diagnosis of a primary anxiety disorder may be particularly difficult to make in the elderly alcoholic. Such disorders usually start early in life and the historical details are often not easily recalled. If the elderly person has been drinking from an early age, the primacy of the anxiety and the alcoholism are not readily determined. The history

Table 4.2. Summary of Conditions Associated with Anxiety in the Elderly

---

DSM-IV anxiety disorders (e.g., panic disorders, agoraphobia, social phobias, simple phobia, obsessive-compulsive disorder, post-traumatic stress disorder, generalized anxiety disorder)

Other Axis I syndromes: major depression, dementia

Personality disorders

Alcoholism; benzodiazepine abuse and dependence

Chronic pain syndromes

Chronic insomnia

Transient anxiety associated with negative life events

Medical conditions (e.g., cardiovascular disease, chronic respiratory disease, Parkinson's disease, movement disorders, thyroid dysfunction)

Pharmacologic treatments (e.g., corticosteroids, theophylline, thyroid replacement therapies, antipsychotic and antidepressant medications)

Source: Adapted from R. Abrams (1991).

taker should seek out symptoms not only of generalized anxiety but also of phobic anxiety, panic attacks, obsessive thinking, and rituals as indicators of an anxiety disorder. The spouse and other family members can be helpful in this process. The information is important in making the decision to supplement the recovering alcoholic's treatment program with therapy aimed specifically at an anxiety disorder.

Abstinence from alcohol and related drugs and sobriety are essential to the long-term management of an anxiety disorder. Specific strategies and techniques used to treat anxiety include biofeedback and relaxation training, systematic desensitization, group therapy for anxiety disorders, and pharmacotherapy. The use of benzodiazepines in the treatment of anxiety disorders in alcoholics (e.g., generalized anxiety disorder) is generally not advised because of the risk of dependence on the drug and reactivation of alcoholism. Allgulander et al. (1984), in a 4- to 6-year follow-up of 50 patients treated at the Karolinska Institute in Stockholm, Sweden, reported that most abusers of sedative-hypnotic drugs had high rates of primary alcoholism, and in many patients secondary alcoholism developed. This close association of addictive potential between alcoholism and sedative drug abuse is a cause for great caution in the use of benzodiazepines in the recovering alcoholic. However, a recent study by Adinoff (1992) demonstrated continued abstinence from alcohol in seven male alcoholic patients treated with benzodiazepines for an anxiety disorder or sleep disturbance.

The use of sedative drugs remains relatively contraindicated in recovering alcoholics. Other drug treatments are available for the treatment of anxiety. Buspirone is a relatively safe and efficacious treatment for generalized anxiety in elderly persons. In patients with phobic anxiety and obsessive-compulsive disorder, the tricyclic antidepressants, serotonin reuptake inhibitors, and monoamine oxidase inhibitors are generally used. In each case, agents that are well tolerated by the particular elderly person should be selected.

SCHIZOPHRENIC DISORDERS AND OTHER PSYCHOSES

The topic of schizophrenia in later life is probably a more compelling topic than alcoholism in elderly schizophrenics because it has only recently begun to gain acceptance as a diagnostic entity of much importance. The prevalence of schizophrenia in the general population is about 1%. The lifetime prevalence data from the Epidemiologic Catchment Area Study (Robins et al., 1984) recorded a prevalence rate for schizophrenia for those age 65 years and older in three communities as ranging from 0.0% to 0.7%. Two groups of schizophrenics are recognized in late life: early onset and late onset (≥ age 45 years for late onset). Medical comorbidity, accidents, suicide, and homicide are factors contributing to the deaths of early-onset schizophrenics who do not survive to old age (Waxman et al., 1982; Cavanaugh, 1986; McGlashan, 1986; Allgulander et al., 1992). The DSM IV defines late-onset schizophrenia as schizophrenia that begins after age 45 years. High female:male ratio, intense affective features, bizarre delusions (often persecutory), auditory hallucinations, favorable response to antipsychotic medication, and prevalence of schizophrenia in probands higher than in the general population have been described as characteristic of late-onset schizophrenia (Harris & Jeste, 1988; Flor-Henry, 1990). The report based on chart review of psychiatric inpatients by Craig and Bregman (1988) revealed that only 25% of the patients diagnosed as having late-onset schizophrenia followed a clinical course and responded to treatment unequivocally schizophrenic in pattern. This seems consistent with the general pattern of diversity and clinical heterogeneity observed in the elderly.

The literature comparing schizophrenia in different age groups of alcoholics is sparse. In a Canadian study of schizophrenic patients referred to a dual diagnosis clinic for substance abuse, the schizophrenia group was younger on average and had the highest proportion of males. There were fewer regular and former drinkers among the schizophrenics compared with a population of a similar age (el-Guebaly & Hodgins, 1992). Blow et al. (1992) reported data from the Veterans Affairs mental health care system indicating that rates for post-traumatic stress disorder, schizophrenia, and personality disorder peaked in younger alcoholics and declined in older alcoholics. Although the prevalence of schizophrenia declines in old age, it is important for the clinician to be aware of this disorder as one cause of psychotic states seen in association with alcoholism in elderly persons. In addition to schizophrenia, one may encounter late-life delusional disorder, psychoses associated with affective disorders, psychosis associated with dementia, and several other categories of DSM-IV defined psychotic disorders.

Alcoholic hallucinosis, which is characterized by either auditory or visual hallucinations and an absence of delirium, usually develops soon after the cessation of drinking (within 48 hours). In its more chronic form in which hallucinosis persists and other psychotic features develop, it may be clinically indistinguishable from schizophrenia.

Alcohol withdrawal delirium (also known as Delirium Tremens) is to be differentiated from other psychoses on the basis of the alteration in level of consciousness, autonomic signs, and a confusional state. The onset is usually on the second or third day after cessation of drinking or a reduction in alcohol intake.

Treatment of the various psychoses occurring in elderly alcoholics does not differ greatly from those encountered in younger persons. The schizophrenic person with alcoholism may have great difficulty handling the intense feelings and other relationship issues encountered in a group setting. A study by Panepinto et al. (1970) revealed that schizophrenics with alcoholism maintained longer treatment relationships with individual therapists than did other alcoholics. Although information concerning this combined disorder in elderly persons is extremely limited, one could infer that it would be even more difficult to manage in group settings in old age. Individual therapy is probably indicated as the primary strategy in most cases.

Antipsychotic drugs play a role in the treatment of elderly schizophrenics, particularly those with late-onset schizophrenia, in whom surprisingly small doses often produce a good result. These drugs have also been effective for treatment of the psychotic symptoms in persons with alcoholic hallucinosis. Selection of drugs and dosages should follow the general guidelines for antipsychotics in the elderly; small doses are often effective even when the psychotic symptoms are bizarre and intense.

PERSONALITY DISORDERS

Abrams (1991) observed that there is little cross-sectional information on personality disorders in the older age groups Information concerning the frequency and types of personality disorders in elderly alcoholics is equally sparse and not in agreement. Lamy (1984), in a review, concluded that the typical alcoholic male has had a reasonably stable life with little evidence of personality disorder. Speer and Bates (1992), in a study of psychiatric patients age 55 years and older, reported the triple occurrence of alcoholism, personality disorder, and depression along with finding personality disorders in 60% of patients with a diagnosis of both alcohol dependence and depression.

Until we know more about the longitudinal course of personality disorders in general, it will be difficult to understand the meaning of disordered personality in elderly alcoholics. As with other comorbid conditions, accurate assessment is not usually possible until the individual has been abstinent for weeks or months. In making this assessment, the clinician must consider the other factors that may modify personality and behavior in the elderly, such as bereavement, depressive disorders, dementia, and other physical disorders.

The literature in recent years has been encouraging with respect to the efficacy of psychotherapy in the elderly. Sadavoy (1987) discussed the use of psychotherapy for personality disorders in the elderly. The psychologic treatment of personality disorders is difficult at any age and, by inference, most difficult in late life. For most elderly alcoholics, the recovering community (Alcoholics Anonymous with its 12-step program and currently available elderly Alcoholics Anonymous groups) may provide many of the necessary tools for the management of alcoholism and its associated personality problems. Focused individual or group therapy is often indicated for such issues as bereavement and coping with physical illness.

References

Abrams, R. (1991). Anxiety and personality disorders. In J. Sadavoy, L. W. Lazarus, & L. F. Jarvik (Eds.), *Comprehensive review of geriatric psychiatry*, (pp. 369–386). Washington, DC, American Psychiatric Press.

Adinoff, B. (1992). Long-term therapy with benzodiazepines despite alcohol dependence disorder: Seven case reports. *American Journal on Addictions, 1*, 288–293.

Albert, M. L., Feldman, R. G., & Willis, A. L. (1974). The "subcortical dementia" of progressive supranuclear palsy. *Journal of Neurology, Neurosurgery and Psychiatry, 37*, 121–130.

Allgulander, C., Borg, S., & Vikander, B. (1984). A 4- to 6-year follow-up of 50 patients with primary dependence on sedative and hypnotic drugs. *American Journal of Psychiatry, 141*, 1580–1582.

Allgulander, C., Allebeck, P., Przybeck, T. R., & Rice, J. P. (1992). Risk of suicide by psychiatric diagnosis in Stockholm County: A longitudinal study of 80,970 psychiatric inpatients. *European Archives of Psychiatry and Clinical Neuroscience, 241*, 323–326.

American Psychiatric Association. (1987). *Diagnostic and statistical manual of mental disorders*, (3rd ed.). p. 107. Washington, DC: Author.

Atkinson, R. M. (1990). Aging and alcohol use disorders: Diagnostic issues in the elderly. *International Psychogeriatrics, 2*, 55–72.

Bailey, D. N. (1990). Drug use in patients admitted to a university trauma center: Results of limited (rather than comprehensive) toxicology screening. *Journal of Analytical Toxicology, 14*, 22–24.

Battjes, R. J. (1988). Smoking as an issue in alcohol and drug abuse treatment. *Addictive Behaviors, 13*, 225–230.

Baum, C., Kennedy, D., Knapp, D., & Faich, G. (1985). *Drug utilization in the U.S.—1985. Seventh annual review*. Rockville, Maryland: Food and Drug Administration.

Behar, D., Winokur, G., & Berg, C. J. (1984). Depression in the abstinent alcoholic. *American Journal of Psychiatry, 141*, 1105–1107.

Bland, R. C., Newman, S. C., & Orn, H. (1988). Prevalence of psychiatric disorders in the elderly in Edmonton. *Acta Psychiatrica Scandinavica, 77 Suppl. 338*, 57–63.

Blow, F. C., Cook, C. A., Booth, B. M., Falcon, S. P., & Friedman, M. J. (1992). Age-related psychiatric comorbidities and level of functioning in alcoholic veterans seeking outpatient treatment. *Hospital and Community Psychiatry, 43*, 990–995.

Broe, G. A., Henderson, A. S., Creasey, H., McCusker, E., Korten, A. E., Jorm, A. F., et al. (1990). A case-control study of Alzheimer's disease in Australia. *Neurology, 40*, 1698–1707.

Bruce, M. L., & McNamara, R. (1992). Psychiatric status among the homebound elderly: An epidemiologic perspective. *Journal of the American Geriatrics Society, 40*, 561–566.

Burger, M. C., Botwinick, J., & Storandt, M. (1987). Aging, alcoholism and performance on the Luria-Nebraska Neuropsychological Battery. *Journal of Gerontology, 42*, 69–72.

Butler, E. W., Schuller-Friedman, S., & Shichor, D. (1990). Alcohol and drug use among impaired and non-impaired elderly persons. In B. Forster & J. C. Salloway (Eds.), *The sociocultural matrix of alcohol and drug use: a source of patterns and factors*, (pp. 163–190). Lewiston, New York: Edwin Mellen Press.

Cafferata, G. L., Kasper, J., & Bernstein, A. (1983). Family roles, structure, and stressors in relation to sex differences in obtaining psychotropic drugs. *Journal of Health and Social Behavior, 24*, 132–143.

Caine, E. D., Lyness, J. M., & King, D. A. (1993). Reconsidering depression in the elderly. *American Journal of Geriatric Psychiatry, 1*, 4–20.

Cavanaugh, S. V. (1986). Psychiatric emergencies. *Medical Clinics of North America, 70*, 1185–1202.

Cisin, I., Miller, J. D., & Harrell, A. V. (1977). *Highlights from the National Survey on Drug Abuse: 1977*. Rockville, Maryland: National Institute on Drug Abuse, U.S. Department of Health, Education, and Welfare, Public Health Service.

Consensus conference (1987). Differential diagnosis of dementing diseases. *Journal of the American Medical Association* (Dec 18), *258(23)*, 3411–3416.

Cook, B. L., Winokur, G., Garvey, M. J., & Beach, V. (1991). Depression and previous alcoholism in the elderly. *British Journal of Psychiatry, 158*, 72–75.

Craig, T. J., & Bregman, Z. (1988). Late onset schizophrenia-like illness. *Journal of the American Geriatrics Society, 36*, 104–107.

Crook, T., Bartus, R. T., Ferris, S. H., et al. (1986). Age-associated memory impairment: Proposed diagnostic criteria and measures of clinical change—report of a National Institute of Mental Health work group. *Developments in Neuropsychology, 2*: 261–276.

Cummings, J. L., & Benson, D. F. (1984). Subcortical dementia: Review of an emerging concept. *Archives of Neurology, 41*, 874–879.

Davis, D. (1971). Mood changes in alcoholic subjects with programmed and free-choice experimental drinking. In *Recent advances in studies of alcoholism*. Washington, DC: Government Printing Office.

Dufour, M. C., Archer, L., & Gordis, E. (1992). Alcohol and the elderly. *Clinics in Geriatric Medicine, 8*, 127–141.

el-Guebaly, N, & Hodgins, D. C. (1992). Schizophrenia and substance abuse: Prevalence issues. *Canadian Journal of Psychiatry, 37*, 704–710.

Finlayson, R. E., Hurt, R. D., Davis, L. R., Jr., & Morse, R. M. (1988). Alcoholism in elderly persons: A study of the psychiatric and psychosocial features of 216 inpatients. *Mayo Clinic Proceedings, 63*, 761–768.

Flor-Henry, P. (1990). Influence of gender in schizophrenia as related to other psychopathological syndromes. *Schizophrenia Bulletin, 16*, 211–227.

Folstein, M. F., Folstein, S. E., & McHugh, P. R. (1975). "Mini-mental state": A practical method for grading the cognitive state of patients for the clinician. *Journal of Psychiatric Research, 12*, 189–198.

Goldstein, G. (1985). Dementia associated with alcoholism. In R. E. Tarter and D. H. Van Thiel (Eds.), *Alcohol and the brain: Chronic effects*, (1st ed.), (pp. 283–294). New York: Plenum Medical.

Gomberg, E. S. L. (1990). Drugs, alcohol, and aging. *Research Advances in Alcohol and Drug Problems, 10*, 171–213.

Harris, M. J., & Jeste, D. V. (1988). Late-onset schizophrenia: An overview. *Schizophrenia Bulletin, 14*, 39–55.

Hurt, R. D., Finlayson, R. E., Morse, R. M., & Davis, L. J., Jr. (1988). Alcoholism in elderly persons: Medical aspects and prognosis of 216 inpatients. *Mayo Clinic Proceedings, 63*, 753–760.

Ikeda, H. (1991). [Clinical and epidemiological studies of alcoholic dementia.] *Arukoru Kenkyuto Yakubutsu Ison, 26*, 341–348.

Istvan, J., & Matarazzo, J. D. (1984). Tobacco, alcohol and caffeine use: A review of their interrelationships. *Psychological Bulletin, 95*, 301–326.

Jensen, G. D., & Bellecci, P. (1987). Alcohol and the elderly: Relationships to illness and smoking. *Alcohol and Alcoholism, 22*, 193–198.

Jeyasingham, M. D., Pratt, O. E., Burns, A., Shaw, G. K., Thomson, A. D., & Marsh, A. (1987). The activation of red blood cell transketolase in groups of patients especially at risk from thiamin deficiency. *Psychological Medicine, 17*, 311–318.

Jinks, M. J., & Raschko, R. R. (1990). A profile of alcohol and prescription drug abuse in a high-risk community-based elderly population. *Annals of Pharmacotherapy, 24*, 971–975.

Kofoed, L. L. (1984). Abuse and misuse of over-the-counter drugs by the elderly. In R. M. Atkinson (Ed.), *Alcohol and drug abuse in old age*, (pp. 50–59). Washington, DC: American Psychiatric Press.

Kramer, J. H., Blusewicz, M. J., & Preston, K. A. (1989). The premature aging hypothesis: Old before its time? *Journal of Consulting and Clinical Psychology, 57*, 257–262.

Kramer, M., German, P. S., Anthony, J. C., Von Korff, M., & Skinner, E. A. (1985). Patterns of mental disorders among the elderly residents of eastern Baltimore. *Journal of the American Geriatrics Society, 33*, 236–245.

Kukull, W. A., Koepsell, T. D., Inui, T. S., Borson, S., Okimoto, J., Raskind, M. A., et al. (1986). Depression and physical illness among elderly general medical clinic patients. *Journal of Affective Disorders, 10*, 153–162.

Lamy, P. P. (1984). Alcohol misuse and abuse among the elderly. *Drug Intelligence and Clinical Pharmacy, 18*, 649–651.

Liptzin, B. (1987). Mental health and older women. *Public Health Reports, 102 Suppl.*, 34–38.

McGlashan, T. H. (1986). Predictors of shorter-, medium-, and longer-term outcome in schizophrenia. *American Journal of Psychiatry, 143*, 50–55.

Mossey, J. M., & Shapiro, E. (1985). Physician use by the elderly over an eight-year period. *American Journal of Public Health, 75*, 1333–1334.

Musetti, L., Perugi, G., Soriani, A., Rossi, V. M., Cassano, G. B., & Akiskal, H. S. (1989). Depression before and after age 65: A re-examination. *British Journal of Psychiatry, 155*, 330–336.

Nakamura, C. M., Molgaard, C. A., Stanford, E. P., Peddecord, K. M., Morton, D. J., Lockery, S. A., et al. (1990). A discriminant analysis of severe alcohol consumption among older persons. *Alcohol and Alcoholism, 25*, 75–80.

Norton, R., & Colliver, J. (1988). Prevalence and patterns of combined alcohol and marijuana use. *Journal of Studies on Alcohol, 49*, 378–380.

Oechsner, M., Möller, A. A., & Zaudig, M. (1993). Cognitive impairment, dementia and psychosocial functioning in human immunodeficiency virus infection: A prospective study based on DSM-III-R and ICD-10. *Acta Psychiatrica Scandinavica, 87*, 13–17.

Oscar-Berman, M., & Bonner, R. T. (1985). Matching- and delayed matching-to-sample performance as measures of visual processing, selective attention, and memory in aging and alcoholic individuals. *Neuropsychologia, 23*, 639–651.

Oscar-Berman, M., Pulaski, J. L., Hutner, N., Weber, D. A., & Freedman, M. (1990). Cross-modal functions in alcoholism and aging. *Neuropsychologia, 28*, 851–869.

Panepinto, W. C., Higgins, M. J., Keane-Dawes, W. Y., & Smith, D. (1970). Underlying psychiatric diagnosis as an indicator of participation in alcoholism therapy. *Quarterly Journal of Studies on Alcohol, 31*, 950–956.

Pfefferbaum, A., Rosenbloom, M., Crusan, K., & Jernigan, T. L. (1988). Brain CT changes in alcoholics: Effects of age and alcohol consumption. *Alcoholism: Clinical and Experimental Research, 12*, 81–87.

Pottenger, M., McKernon, J., Patrie, L. E., Weissman, M. M., Ruben, H. L., & Newberry, P. (1978). The frequency and persistence of depressive symptoms in the alcohol abuser. *Journal of Nervous and Mental Disease, 166*, 562–570.

Regier, D. A., Farmer, M. E., Rae, D. S., Locke, B. Z., Keith, S. J., Judd, L. L., et al. (1990). Comorbidity of mental disorders with alcohol and other drug abuse: Results from the Epidemiologic Catchment Area (ECA) study. *Journal of the American Medical Association, 264*, 2511–2518.

Reifler, B., Raskind, M., & Kethley, A. (1982). Psychiatric diagnoses among geriatric patients seen in an outreach program. *Journal of the American Geriatrics Society, 30*, 530–533.

Report to the Chairman, Special Committee on Aging, U.S. Senate. (July 1987). Medicare: Prescription drug issues. Washington, DC: United States General Accounting Office.

Robins, L. N., Helzer, J. E., Weissman, M. M., Orvaschel, H., Gruenberg, E., Burke, J. D., Jr., et al. (1984). Lifetime prevalence of specific psychiatric disorders in three sites. *Archives of General Psychiatry, 41*, 949–958.

Ross, H. E. (1989). Alcohol and drug abuse in treated alcoholics: A comparison of men and women. *Alcoholism: Clinical and Experimental Research, 13*, 810–816.

Sadavoy, J. (1987). Character disorders in the elderly: An overview. In J. Sadavoy & M. Leszcz (Eds.), *Treating the elderly with psychotherapy: The scope for change in later life*, (pp. 175–229). Madison, Connecticut: International Universities Press.

Saunders, P. A., Copeland, J. R. M., Dewey, M. E., Davidson, I. A., McWilliam, C., Sharma, V., et al. (1991). Heavy drinking as a risk factor for depression and dementia in elderly men: Findings from the Liverpool Longitudinal Community Study. *British Journal of Psychiatry, 159*, 213–216.

Schonfeld, L., & Dupree, L. W. (1991). Antecedents of drinking for early- and late-onset elderly alcohol abusers. *Journal of Studies on Alcohol, 52*, 587–592.

Schuckit, M. A., & Morrissey, E. R. (1979). Drug abuse among alcoholic women. *American Journal of Psychiatry, 136*, 607–611.

Schuckit, M. A., Miller, P. L., & Hahlbohm, D. (1975). Unrecognized psychiatric illness in elderly medical-surgical patients. *Journal of Gerontology, 30*, 655–660.

Shaffer, H., & Burglass, M. E. (Eds.). (1981). *Classic contributions in the addictions.* New York: Brunner/Mazel Publishers.

Speer, D. C., & Bates, K. (1992). Comorbid mental and substance disorders among older psychiatric patients. *Journal of the American Geriatrics Society, 40*, 886–890.

Stewart, A. L., Greenfield, S., Hays, R. D., Wells, K., Rogers, W. H., Berry, S. D., et al. (1989). Functional status and well-being of patients with chronic conditions: Results from the Medical Outcomes Study. *Journal of the American Medical Association, 262*, 907–913.

Waxman, H. M., Carner, E. A., Dubin, W., & Klein, M. (1982). Geriatric psychiatry in the emergency department: Characteristics of geriatric and non-geriatric admissions. *Journal of the American Geriatrics Society, 30*, 427–432.

Weissman, M. M., Myers, J. K., Tischler, G. L., Holzer, C. E., III, Leaf, P. J., Orvaschel, H., et al. (1985). Psychiatric disorders (DSM-III) and cognitive impairment among the elderly in a U.S. urban community. *Acta Psychiatrica Scandinavica, 71*, 366–379.

5

Alcohol-Related Medical Disorders of Older Heavy Drinkers

STEVEN R. GAMBERT
AND KATHERINE K. KATSOYANNIS

Although alcoholism and the effects of chronic alcohol consumption are not generally thought of as common problems affecting the elderly, "problem drinking" is present in 5 to 12% of men and 1 to 2% of women in their sixties (Atkinson, 1984). Overall, the lifetime prevalence of alcoholism for all persons age 65 or older ranges from 4.1 to 8.3% (Robins et al., 1984). The elderly are possibly more susceptible to substance abuse because of numerous social, physical, and emotional changes that occur during later life. These changes may impact negatively on well-being and include deaths of loved ones, loss of independence, reduced income, change in job status, and poor health.

Interestingly, such changes may explain an observation in the study of elderly alcoholics. That is, it appears that this population may be made up of two groups, early-onset alcoholics who continue to drink to excess and late-onset alcoholics. Most studies use a broad range of ages, 40 to 60 years, to delineate these groups. If late-onset alcoholism results at least in part from reaction to life changes, it is clear that major life stresses occur with increasing frequency by age 60. Although these studies have consistently reported that the majority of elderly alcoholics are early-onset drinkers, between 35 to 40% of this group began drinking in their later years (Hartford & Thien-haus, 1984; Hurt et al., 1988; Zimberg, 1978). The former group would be considered "survivors" in that they have achieved old-age status despite chronic alcohol ingestion and its subsequent sequelae. This group of patients will undoubtedly grow in number as health care professionals and technology continue to make advances in the care of ill patients.

Seventy percent of all elderly alcoholics are men and 30% are women. The early-onset alcoholic more commonly has a family history of alcoholism and suffers from disturbed psychosocial functioning, including a greater prevalence of psychiatric illness and lower socioeconomic status and a poor work history. The early-onset alcoholic is also more likely to live alone, suffer from malnutrition, and have a history of multiple physical injuries (Gambert, 1992).

Whichever group the elderly alcoholic belongs to, they all share some unfortunate characteristics. Both groups have an increased morbidity and mortality in relation to control groups of elderly persons. In one study of 216 patients over the age of 65 seeking inpatient treatment for alcohol abuse, serious medical conditions were significantly more common than is generally noted in the elderly population (Hurt et al., 1988). This study also found a larger percentage of these patients had died at the time of follow-up (32%); 47% of these deaths were attributed to the patient's alcoholism. Although this investigation did have a longer follow-up period than most studies, and the subjects studied may have been selectively more ''ill,'' it does emphasize the scope and serious nature of alcoholism in the elderly.

Both acute and chronic alcohol consumption have significant effects on physiologic function, leading to diverse medical disabilities. In addition to causing disease, chronic alcoholism may accelerate the otherwise normal age-related decline in physiologic functioning. In this chapter, the medical complications associated with chronic alcohol consumption will be discussed.

EFFECT OF CHRONIC ALCOHOL ABUSE
ON THE CENTRAL NERVOUS SYSTEM

Ethanol is a very potent neurotoxin. Acutely, alcohol exerts an immediate depressant effect on the central nervous system, primarily acting at subcortical areas. This effect may alter behavioral, psychomotor, and cognitive function. Alcohol consumption can lessen inhibition and in some individuals may allow decreased feelings of self-consciousness (Dufour et al., 1992). While one individual may become more boisterous and talkative, another may become verbally and physically abusive. Psychomotor function evidenced by cognition, peripheral organization, and visual motor skills all decline with alcohol consumption. Evidence suggests that age and even low-dose ethanol use may have a synergistic negative effect on subject performance on continuous tracking tasks (Linnoila et al., 1986). Alcohol can also alter sleep. Acutely, sleep latency is affected, making it difficult for people to fall asleep; REM sleep is depressed. With continued use, a phenomenon known as *REM rebound* may be observed, causing abnormal sleep cycles and deficiency in deep sleep (Roth et al., 1985).

Excessive alcohol intoxication and/or withdrawal can cause a delirium that can be a medical emergency. The Wernicke-Korsakoff syndrome is a severe neurologic disorder caused by a nutritional deficiency, specifically thiamine. Wernicke's encephalopathy presents acutely in chronic alcoholics as a triad of mental confusion, cerebellar ataxia, and occulomotor dysfunction. The patient's sensorium may become so clouded as to lead to stupor and even coma, which may be an undiagnosed presentation of Wernicke's encephalopathy. This condition is a medical emergency and carries an estimated mortality rate of 17% (Victor, 1976), although this rate may be declining as awareness has increased. It is especially important to recognize this entity in the elderly, as it is a potentially reversible cause of mental changes and delirium. Treatment consists of parenteral administration of thiamine. Particular attention should be given to replacing thiamine *prior* to glucose administration in any patient suspected of having this form of encephalopathy to avoid a worsening of the delirium state. Additional attention should be directed toward magnesium replacement, as hypomagnesemia may result in a resistance to thiamine replacement therapy.

Chronic alcoholics may go on to develop Korsakoff's psychosis. This is characterized by preservation of intellectual function with the exception of periodic severe retrograde and anterograde amnesia. While the most obvious symptom exhibited by these patients is confabulation, this may only be apparent in the late stages of the disease. This syndrome is also potentially reversible by early intervention with thiamine. The exact relationship between thiamine deficiency and Korsakoff's psychosis has not yet been established, over 50% of patients treated with thiamine achieve only a partial recovery, and 25% show no improvement at all.

The above neurologic complications in which intellectual functioning is maintained contrasts sharply with the syndrome of alcoholic dementia. Although there remains controversy regarding the exact etiology of this syndrome, it is an important consideration in the context of the elderly alcoholic. Computed tomography (Cala et al., 1980) and brain weight comparison studies (Torvik et al., 1982) have shown a higher incidence of cerebral cortical atrophy in alcoholic patients as compared to nondemented age-matched controls. It is currently thought that this syndrome is caused by a combination of progressive Wernicke's encephalopathy, other nutritional deficiencies, and direct toxic effects of alcohol on brain neurons. This syndrome is characterized by diffuse cognitive dysfunction. New studies have also implicated underlying liver disease (Arria et al., 1991) and associated abnormalities of regional cerebral blood flow (O'Caroll et al., 1991) as possible contributing factors.

Pathologically, one portion of the brain may be more sensitive to the effect of nutritional deficiencies and the toxicity of ethanol. Chronic alcoholics, especially men, are at significant risk for developing alcoholic cerebellar degeneration (Torvik & Torp, 1986), though those men over age 70 have a less clear causal relationship. Clinically, these patients exhibit gait and truncal ataxia; there is a relative sparing of upper extremity coordination. Once the Purkinje cells have been completely destroyed, the symptoms will remain unchanged. Fortunately, this syndrome may improve with abstinence from alcohol use and correction of any nutritional deficiency.

Another very common neurologic complication of chronic alcoholism is symmetric polyneuropathy. This usually affects the lower extremities first and may remain exclusive to them. This is again felt to be a result of a nutritional deficiency, specifically vitamin B complex. Unfortunately, recovery with supplementation is often incomplete. Usual symptoms include paresthesias, weakness, and pain. The pain may sometimes be excruciating, and in severe cases motor deficits and muscle atrophy may be noted. This axonal degeneration may also be noted in autonomic nerves, leading to bladder and bowel dysfunction, orthostatic hypotension, and impotence (Victor, 1975). Treatment, consisting of abstinence, vitamin supplementation, and general nutritional support, is often unsuccessful in improving the symptoms.

Although most of the neurologic complications of chronic alcoholism are directly related to poor nutritional status, one traumatic etiology must also be considered. Alcoholics suffer from falls, whether in the acutely intoxicated state or as a result of poor coordination and ataxia. These patients are at risk for developing subdural hematomas, both acute and chronic. It must be emphasized that detection is the key step to treatment; surgical intervention may be required.

ALCOHOL USE AND NUTRITION

In general, the elderly person experiences a decline in caloric expenditures; no significant change occurs, however, in nutritional requirements (Food and Nutrition Board, 1980). There are changes in body composition that may reflect a decline in physical activity. Overall, there is a reduction in lean body mass expressed as muscle and bone. Total body water, both extracellular and intracellular volume, lessens. These changes result in a reduction in the reserves of protein, water, sodium, potassium, calcium, phosphate, and magnesium in the older person's body stores. An older person is therefore much more sensitive to possible nutritional deficiencies associated with chronic alcohol consumption.

As a rule, complications resulting from malnutrition would depend on the direct toxic effect of alcohol on organ function and the extent to which alcohol replaces other nutrients in the diet. Chronic alcohol ingestion is a major cause of malnutrition because calories derived from ethanol have little to no nutritional value. At high levels of consumption, alcohol inhibits the absorption of thiamine, riboflavin, niacin, and folic acid from the intestine. Fat absorption is also impaired, and alcohol promotes loss of magnesium, calcium, and zinc (Lieber, 1982). With age, there is also an increase in body fat. This change, resulting in more fat and less body water, reduces the volume of distribution for alcohol and thus increases the potential for toxicity.

Fortunately, severe malnutrition is not common and is only reported to affect a minority of alcohol abusers in the United States. Because of body composition changes mentioned above, the elderly alcoholic may be more at risk. Marasmus malnutrition, manifested as a result of severe inadequacy of all forms of energy, is relatively rare in the alcoholic. Kwashiorkor malnutrition, or primarily protein energy deficiency, is the most common form of malnutrition seen in this group. Protein malnutrition is evidenced by muscle wasting, hypoproteinemia, and edema. Lack of protein intake coupled with impaired hepatic albumin synthesis may worsen malabsorptive syndromes by decreasing oncotic pressure and disrupting passive intestinal water and solute transport (Gambert et al., 1984). These changes can cause an abnormal distribution of fluids and electrolytes. The elderly are particularly sensitive because of their inability to adapt quickly and because of their reduced reserve capacity.

As noted, the vitamin and mineral deficiencies resulting from poor dietary intake and malabsorption can have debilitating effects on most of the body's organ systems. The central nervous system is particularly vulnerable to vitamin B complex deficiencies. Thiamine deficiency may result from poor intake, as well as malabsorption, chronic diarrhea, and folate deficiency. Hypomagnesemia and hypocalcemia are sometimes seen in chronic alcohol abusers and can precipitate neurologic dysfunction and cardiac arrhythmias. Hypophosphatemia may present with proximal myopathy, acute respiratory failure, congestive cardiomyopathy, hemolysis, and rhabdomyolysis.

Acutely, the elderly alcoholic may be extremely vulnerable to the debilitating effect of electrolyte disturbances. Alcoholic ketoacidosis may cause a range of neurologic complications including frank coma. Severe hypoglycemia must also be considered as an end result of both decreased dietary intake and the effect of prolonged alcohol consumption on hepatic function. Clearly, correction of nutritional deficiencies by supplementation becomes very important in this group of patients.

EFFECT OF ALCOHOL ON THE SKIN

Although frequently not noted, an alcoholic patient may be recognized by changes in the skin. These largely result from liver dysfunction and hyperestrogenism, in addition to nutritional deficiency. The patient may exhibit the abnormally dilated capillaries of palmar erythema. Cutaneous arterial ''spider'' angiomas can also be found on the face and trunk. These are the result of fragile blood vessel walls and are a marker for alcoholic liver disease.

EFFECT OF CHRONIC ALCOHOL USE
ON CARDIOVASCULAR FUNCTION

Over the past two decades, there have been a number of studies that have shown reduced coronary artery disease and occlusion in subjects who consume moderate quantities of alcohol (Anderson et al., 1978; Yano et al., 1977). This seemingly ''protective'' effect may be mediated by an increase in high density lipoprotein (HDL) cholesterol and apolipoprotein-a-1. Changes in clotting mechanisms have also been implicated.

The chronic alcohol abuser subjects the cardiovascular system to significant physiologic damage through a variety of mechanisms, resulting in serious complications. More recent epidemiologic studies have found a loss of any protective effect at higher levels of consumption (Crigui, 1987). It now appears that alcohol itself has a direct toxic effect on the myocardium. Pathologically, the heart develops areas of fibrosis and hypertrophy, and microvascular infarctions have been seen (Factor, 1976). The cells exhibit varying degrees of mitochondrial damage and lipid accumulation in addition to interstitial fibrosis and loss of myofibrils (Urbano-Marquez, 1989). These changes lead to congestive cardiomyopathy. The alcoholic may also develop beri-beri disease. This is a high-output cardiomyopathy that is easily distinguished. The electrical system of the heart is also sensitive to the effects of alcohol. Cardiac arrhythmias are not infrequent in alcoholics and include atrial and ventricular conduction defects (Ettinger et al., 1976). Potassium or magnesium imbalance may also create or facilitate arrhythmias.

Treatment of cardiovascular complications may include digitalis, diuretics, and antiarrhythmic agents. Unfortunately, as the cardiomyopathy progresses, the accompanying cardiomegaly and conduction disturbances become more refractory to therapy. One very important distinction is cardiac beri-beri disease, which is thiamine responsive and must be considered early.

Alcohol also has been reported to have an effect on blood pressure. Ethanol in low doses can cause a mild acute drop in blood pressure. More significant intake, three or more drinks a day, reportedly results in a dose-dependent increase leading to frank hypertension. Chronic alcohol consumption is therefore an important factor in the development of mild to moderate hypertension. This phenomenon is reversible with abstinence (Criqui, 1986).

EFFECT OF CHRONIC ALCOHOL USE ON THE
GASTROINTESTINAL SYSTEM

It is not surprising that alcohol exerts both direct and indirect effects on the gastrointestinal tract. This organ system comes into direct contact with ethanol and is responsible for transporting it into the bloodstream. The oropharynx is the first portion of the body to come into contact with alcohol, and chronic alcoholics have a higher incidence of glossitis and stomatitis. This may be due to poor nutrition and/or vitamin deficiency. The most significant risk, however, is for the development of squamous cell carcinoma. The increased risk of head and neck cancer has been extensively studied in alcoholics. Although alcohol is considered a cocarcinogen with tobacco, there is enough evidence to link alcohol use alone as a significant risk factor for the development of this form of cancer (Rothman & Keller, 1972).

The esophagus is also greatly affected by alcohol use. Here again alcoholics have an increased risk of developing cancer separate from the risk associated with tobacco use (Tuyms, 1979). Acute ingestion of alcohol reduces peristalsis and also impairs upper and lower esophageal sphincter function (Hogan et al., 1972). This may explain the high incidence of reflux esophagitis following alcohol ingestion. While chronic alcoholics with polyneuropathy appear to have intact upper esophageal sphincter functioning, there is a decrease in peristalsis in the distal esophagus (Winship et al., 1968). This motor dysfunction places the patient at increased risk for developing gastroesophageal reflux, which may then lead to esophagitis and even pulmonary aspiration. Treatment consists of abstinence and antireflux medications.

The alcoholic, both acutely and chronically, is at an increased risk for bleeding from the esophagus. Prolonged and violent retching may induce tears in the lower esophageal mucosa, known as the *Mallory-Weiss syndrome*. Chronic alcoholism may result in the development of gastroesophageal varices secondary to increased portal circulation pressures. Both of these conditions can lead to massive and ultimately fatal gastrointestinal hemorrhage. This type of hemorrhage is usually managed conservatively with supportive treatment including intensive care monitoring and fluid and blood replacement. Unfortunately, about 50% of variceal bleeds require aggressive therapy, including selective administration of vasopressin to stimulate vasoconstriction, balloon tamponade, and finally emergent endoscopy. Endoscopy allows localization of the area of hemorrhage and treatment by injection of a sclerosing agent or by laser coagulation. Sclerosing therapy has a reported success rate as high as 90% and may be employed repeatedly to prevent recurrent bleeds (Cello et al., 1984). One of the newest methods of treating emergent gastrointestinal bleeding involves transjugular intrahepatic porto-caval shunt (TIPS) placement. In one recent study, this modality reduced portal vein pressure and reduced or eliminated endoscopically viewed gastrovarices (Bilodeau et al., 1992).

It has long been known that alcohol exerts a direct toxic effect on gastric mucosa. While the exact mechanism remains unclear, there appears to be an acute effect in increased gastric acid production and disruption of the gastric mucosal barrier (Fromm & Robertson, 1976). Chronic alcohol abuse may in turn lead to lower basal acid output and an increase in the likelihood of developing chronic atrophic gastritis. Erosive gastritis, with the potential for inducing upper gastrointestinal hemorrhage, is also common in chronic alcohol abuse. This may be aggravated by use of aspirin or other nonsteroidal anti-inflammatory medications.

Although there is much evidence supporting the link between alcohol use and gastritis, a causal relationship to peptic ulcer disease remains controversial. In fact, a large epidemiologic study found no direct correlation between the prevalence of peptic ulcer disease and alcohol consumption (Friedman et al., 1979). In the alcoholic population, tobacco use and hepatic cirrhosis are much more common and are clearly associated with peptic ulcer disease.

Acute ingestion of alcohol directly affects the duodenum and jejunum through intraluminal transport and back diffusion from the blood. Chronic alcoholism also affects the intestinal mucosa by associated nutritional deficiencies of vitamins, particularly folate and thiamine. A common complaint is diarrhea; the etiology of this symptom is multifactorial, including decreased peristalsis and increased permeability to water and solutes. Pancreatic exocrine dysfunction may also contribute to the development of diarrhea and malabsorption. This further compromises the nutritional status of the patient.

There is a well-established link between alcohol abuse and pancreatitis. In fact, alcohol is capable of causing a variety of pancreatic disorders including acute necrotizing pancreatitis and subclinical chronic calcific pancreatitis on which acute recurrent attacks are superimposed. Chronic alcohol ingestion causes an already malfunctioning pancreas to produce a pancreatic juice that is high in protein and low in bicarbonate. The protein may then precipitate in the pancreatic ducts and subsequently calcify. An alcoholic patient may then go on to develop acute pancreatitis, but even in this population it appears that this is a randomly occurring event and other factors may influence the development of acute and fulminant disease. These factors include the general constitution of the patients and their nutritional status. Complications of acute pancreatitis include fluid and electrolyte imbalances, hypocalcemia, hypomagnesemia, hypoxemia, cardiovascular abnormalities, and blood coagulation disturbances. Finally, the patient may develop sepsis and shock. Increasing age is a significant risk factor for mortality. It is clear that in the elderly patient who may already be compromised in organ system function, early recognition of alcoholic pancreatitis is imperative. Therapy remains mainly supportive with close monitoring and correction of fluid and electrolyte disturbances. In the past, nasogastric suction and hormonal manipulation using glucagon, calcitonin, and somatostatin have been employed, but these measures are not currently recommended.

The exact pathogenesis of ethanol-induced pancreatitis remains unclear, but inappropriate activation of zymogens appears to be the most likely factor, acting through a variety of biochemical pathways. The patient with chronic pancreatitis may experience a wide spectrum of illness. With advanced destruction of the pancreas, islet-cell function may be compromised and diabetes mellitus may result. Treatment is much the same for the superimposed acute events, including pain control and fluid and electrolyte management. Pancreatic insufficiency, both exocrine and endocrine, requires lifelong therapy. Fortunately, most studies have not found any significant association between alcohol use and the development of pancreatic cancer (Monson & Lyon, 1975).

Unlike pancreatic disease, hepatic damage and dysfunction is directly related to the duration and dose of ethanol consumption. Although there is a large range of pathologic findings from fatty metamorphosis to cirrhosis (Sherlock, 1981), there is, as yet, no proof of progression from one problem to the other. It is also apparent from a number of studies that the clinical presentation, or lack thereof, is not always indicative of the extent of the liver damage that has occurred. It is known that the earliest pathologic changes, the so-called fatty liver evidenced by lipid laden hepatocytes, can be reversed by cessation of drinking. This condition is usually benign and does not predispose to cirrhosis; alcoholics with fatty livers nevertheless have a significant risk of developing alcoholic hepatitis if they continue to drink to excess.

Acute alcoholic hepatitis can be life threatening, particularly in the elderly population.

Although the presentation may be quite variable, the illness usually presents with an insidious onset of abdominal discomfort, nausea, vomiting, anorexia, weight loss, fever, and jaundice. The diagnosis of alcoholic liver disease may be difficult to make because of difficulty in obtaining a history of alcohol use or abuse. The extra-hepatic manifestations of alcohol abuse, such as the associated neurologic syndromes, gastrointestinal complications, and skin changes mentioned above, can all point to alcohol as the etiologic factor. As noted, the illness may range from a mild episode of abdominal discomfort to fulminant hepatic failure. It may be complicated by the development of portal hypertension and hepato-renal failure. Infections, including spontaneous bacterial peritonitis and aspiration pneumonia, can, and frequently do, occur. Supportive therapy is aimed at correction of fluid and electrolyte imbalances, maintaining hepatic function, and antibiotic use as necessary.

Cirrhosis is an irreversible stage in alcoholic liver disease and fortunately occurs in only a minority of alcoholic patients. Once again, the spectrum of illness is broad, ranging from asymptomatic disease discovered fortuitously to complete hepatic failure and its complications. The patient may present with nonspecific complaints of fatigue, anorexia, weight loss, and abdominal discomfort. Others may suffer from hepatic encephalopathy, ascites, splenomegaly, gastroesophageal varices, and coagulopathies. Physically, the patient may present with spider angiomata, palmar erythema, and in men, gynecomastia as evidence of hormonal imbalance and increased estrogen levels in relation to male androgens. Once again, the extra-hepatic features of chronic alcoholism such as polyneuropathy, Wernicke's encephalopathy, and signs of vitamin and protein malnutrition may lead to a diagnosis of alcoholic liver disease.

Pathologically, the liver may show both micronodular and macronodular degeneration with pericellular and pericentral fibrosis causing disorganization of lobular architecture. As stated, these changes are irreversible and therapy is aimed at controlling the symptoms of hepatic failure and portal hypertension. Abstinence from alcohol has been shown to improve the 5-year survival rate (Borowsky et al., 1981). Therapy includes provision of a nutritious low salt diet, multivitamins, and folic acid. Currently, there are ongoing trials on the use of colchicine, which seems to inhibit collagen synthesis in vitro and may reduce hepatic fibrosis; the results remain preliminary at this time despite some favorable trends (Kershenobich et al., 1988). One group investigated the use of oral clonidine to reduce portal pressure in a group of alcoholics with cirrhosis. Although this study reported favorable results, long-term benefits have not been proven (Albillos et al., 1992). Finally, liver transplantation is a definitive and successful treatment that is currently employed for a small and select group of alcoholics (Kumar et al., 1989). Unfortunately, the elderly alcoholic may not have the physiologic reserve to undergo this invasive therapeutic intervention.

EFFECT OF CHRONIC ALCOHOL USE ON ENDOCRINE FUNCTION

Chronic and excessive alcohol consumption is well known to effect the endocrine system. The most commonly documented effect is hypogonadism and feminization in the male cirrhotic; the patient presents with testicular atrophy, impotence, and decreased hair growth. Signs of hyperestrogenism include gynecomastia, palmar erythema, and spider angiomata. Many of these effects are related to liver dysfunction associated with cirrhosis. Alcohol also has a direct effect on testicular function. One study reported decreased plasma testosterone related to decreased testosterone production and increased testosterone clearance in healthy men ingesting alcohol (Gordon et al., 1976). Newer studies have confirmed these findings and report an apparent direct effect on the hypothalamic-pituitary axis. Plasma levels of luteinizing hormone (LH) and follicle stimulating hormone (FSH) were not elevated despite the reduced testosterone levels in a group of cirrhotic men (Wang et al., 1991). These patients did respond, however, to exogenous gonadotropin-releasing hormone with an elevated LH and FSH level, indicating a central disturbance.

The etiology of feminization seen in alcoholic men remains somewhat unclear but appears to be related to alcoholic liver dysfunction. An increased rate of conversion of adrenocorticosteroid precursors into estrogens may be seen in addition to decreased hepatic clearance of estrogen (Edman & MacDonald, 1975).

Recent studies have also implicated alcohol as affecting the hypothalamic-pituitary-adrenal axis, resulting in a transient, reversible Cushing's syndrome (Gordon & Southren, 1982). These patients manifest the clinical and laboratory features of Cushing's syndrome and, with abstinence from ethanol consumption, return to their prior health status within 2 to 4 weeks. Although there has been no clearly established pathogenetic mechanism, it appears that alcohol may have a dose-related, stimulatory effect on cortisol secretion, which may be mediated through adrenocorticotropic hormone.

In alcoholic liver disease the conversion of thyroxine (T4) to tri-iodothyronine (T3) is decreased with a concomitant increase in reverse T3 (rT3) levels (Chopra et al., 1975). This effect, in addition to changes in thyroxine-binding protein metabolism, may lead to abnormalities in thyroid function studies but are usually of small importance clinically.

EFFECT OF CHRONIC ALCOHOL USE
ON HEMATOLOGIC STATUS

Excessive alcohol use can effect the hematologic system through a variety of mechanisms. First, there are the multitude of nutritional deficiencies associated with excessive alcohol consumption. The patient may experience iron deficiency secondary to gastrointestinal blood loss. There is also a significant proportion of malnourished alcoholics who have a folate deficiency with megaloblastic anemia. The chronically malnourished alcoholic also has impaired jejunal absorption of folate (Cowan, 1980), and alcohol intake suppresses the hematologic response to folate (Sullivan & Herbert, 1964).

The chronic alcoholic may also develop a sideroblastic anemia associated with the megaloblastic changes seen with folate deficiency. Serum iron may be elevated in this condition, and pyridoxine deficiency is an essential characteristic. A smear of the patient's blood will show macrocytes, hypochromia, and microcytes (Larkin & Watson-Williams, 1984).

Alcoholics may also develop hemolytic anemia. This results largely from liver damage and the resulting portal hypertension and splenomegaly. The mean corpuscular volume (MCV) of the red cells may increase, and a pathologic target cell may be seen. These cells may then be sequestered and destroyed in the spleen. The alcoholic may also develop a severe hypophosphatemia capable of accelerating the hemolytic process (Jacobs & Amsden, 1971).

Alcohol has been shown to cause thrombocytopenia both by suppressing production and reducing survival of platelets (Cowan, 1980). This may result in a prolongation of bleeding time. Although under normal conditions this may not be clinically important, in a traumatic injury, such as a fall, or in association with gastrointestinal hemorrhage, it may be critical.

Immune function may also be suppressed in the alcoholic. There is a leukopenia associated with alcoholism, particularly with hypersplenism secondary to cirrhosis and portal hypertension. Granulocyte function may also be affected. Several studies have noted defective chemotaxis in chronic alcoholics (MacGregor et al., 1978). Cell-mediated immunity may be affected in patients with severe protein-energy malnutrition. Newer studies are investigating the effects of malnutrition and cirrhosis on the production of cytokines. The elderly alcoholic who has already experienced immune senescence as a physiologic process is at significantly increased risk of developing infection.

SUMMARY

Alcoholism is a significant cause of increased morbidity and mortality in the elderly. While a greater number of persons who have been drinking to excess are living longer than ever before, new cases of alcoholism remain a major problem. Alcohol is capable of affecting almost every cell, organ, and tissue of the body. For the elderly person, who already has reduced physiologic, emotional, and physical reserve due to a composite of normal aging and disease, the consequences are of paramount importance. Early recognition, attempts to reduce alcohol intake, and comprehensive management are all necessary to keep the older person as healthy as possible.

References

Albillos, A., Banares, R., Barrios, C., et al. (1992). Oral administration of clonidine in patients with alcoholic cirrhosis. *Gastroenterology, 102*, 248–254.

Anderson, A. J., Barboriak, J. J., & Rimm, A. A. (1978). Risk factors and angiographically determined coronary occlusion. *American Journal of Epidemiology, 107*, 8–14.

Arria, A. M., Tarter, R. E., Kabene, S. B., et al. (1991). The role of cirrhosis in memory functioning of alcoholics. *Alcoholism: Clinical and Experimental Research, 15*, 932–937.

Atkinson, R. M. (Ed). (1984). *Alcohol and drug abuse in old age*, (pp. 1–21). Washington DC. American Psychiatric Press.

Bilodeau, M., Rioux, L., Willems, B., & Pomier-Layrargues, G. (1992). Transjujular intrahepatic portacaval stent shunt as a rescue treatment for life-threatening variceal bleeding in a cirrhotic patient with severe liver failure. *American Journal of Gastroenterology, 87*, 369–371.

Borowsky, S. A., Strome, S., & Lott, E. (1981). Continued heavy drinking and survival in alcoholic cirrhotics. *Gastroenterology, 80*, 1405–1409.

Cala, L. A., Jones, B., Wiley, B., & Mastaglia, F. L. (1980). A computerized axial tomography (CAT) study of alcohol induced cerebral atrophy in conjunction with other correlates. *Acta Psychiatrica Scandinavica, 62*, 531–540.

Cello, J. P., et al. (1984). Endoscopic sclerotherapy versus portacaval shunt in patients with severe cirrhosis and variceal hemorrhage. *New England Journal of Medicine, 311*, 1589–1594.

Chopra, I. J., Chopra, U., Smith, S. R., et al. (1975). Reciprocal changes in serum concentrations of 3,3,5 triiodothyronine (reverse T) and 3,3,5 triiodothyronine (T) in systemic illnesses. *Journal of Clinical Endocrinology and Metabolism, 41,* 1043–1049.

Cowan, D. H. (1980). Effect of alcoholism on hemostasis. *Semin Hematology, 17,* 147–177.

Criqui, M. H. (1986). Alcohol consumption, blood pressure, lipids, and CV mortality. *Alcoholism: Clinical and Experimental Research, 10,* 564.

Criqui, M. H. (1987). The roles of alcohol in the epidemiology of cardiovascular diseases. *Acta Medica Scandinavica, 717,* 73–85.

Dufour, M. C., Archer, L., & Gordis, E. (1992). Alcohol and the elderly. *Clinics in Geriatric Medicine, 8,* 127–141.

Edman, C. D., & MacDonald, P. C. (1975). Extraglandular production of estrogen in subjects with liver disease. *Gastroenterology, 69,* A-19, 819.

Ettinger, P. O., Lyons, M., Oldewurtel, H. A., & Regan, T. J. (1976). Cardiac conduction abnormalities produced by chronic alcoholism. *American Heart Journal, 91,* 66–78.

Factor, S. M. (1976). Intramyocardial small vessel disease in chronic alcoholism. *American Heart Journal, 92,* 561–575.

Food and Nutrition Board, National Research Council. (1980). *Recommended dietary allowances* (4th ed. rev.). Washington, DC. National Academy of Sciences.

Friedman, G. D., Siegelaub, A. B., & Seltzer, C. C. (1974). Cigarettes, alcohol, coffee, and peptic ulcer. *New England Journal of Medicine, 290,* 469–473.

Fromm, D., & Robertson, R. (1976). Effects of alcohol on transport by isolated gastric and esophageal mucosa. *Gastroenterology, 70,* 220–225.

Gambert, S. R., Newton, M., & Duthie, E. H. (1984). Medical issues in alcoholism in the elderly. In J. T. Hartford & T. Samorajski, (Eds.), *Alcoholism in the elderly* (pp. 175–191). New York: Raven Press.

Gambert, S. R. (1992). Substance abuse in the elderly. In J. H. Lowinson, P. Ruiz, & R. B. Millman (Eds.), *Substance abuse: A comprehensive textbook* (2nd ed.) (pp. 843–851). Baltimore: Williams and Wilkens.

Gordon, G. G., Altman, K., Southren, A. L., et al. (1976). Effect of alcohol (ethanol) administration on sex-hormone metabolism in normal men. *New England Journal of Medicine, 295,* 793–797.

Gordon, G. G., & Southren, A. L. (1982). The effects of alcohol and alcoholic liver disease on the endocrine system and intermediary metabolism. In C. S. Lieber (Ed), *Medical disorders of alcoholism* (pp. 65–140). Philadelphia: W. B. Saunders.

Hartford, J. T., & Thienhaus, O. J. (1984). Psychiatric aspects of alcoholism in geriatric patients. *Aging, 25,* 253–262.

Hogan, W. J., Viegas de Androdi, S. R., & Winship, D. H. (1972). Ethanol induced acute esophageal motor dysfunction. *Journal of Applied Physiology, 32,* 755–760.

Hurt, R. D., Finlayson, R. E., Morse, R. M., & Davis, I. J. (1988). Alcoholism and prognosis of 216 inpatients. *Mayo Clinic Proceedings, 63,* 573–760.

Jacobs, H. S., & Amsden, T. (1971). Acute hemolytic anemia with red cells in hypophosphatemia. *New England Journal of Medicine, 285,* 1446–1450.

Kershenobich, D., Vargas, F., Garcia-Tsao, G., et al. (1988). ???? in the treatment of cirrhosis of the liver. *New England Journal of Medicine, 318,* 1709–1713.

Kumar, S., Batista, R. E., Stauber, J. S., et al. (1989). Orthototic liver-transplantation for alcoholic liver disease. *Gastroenterology, 96,* A616.

Larkin, E. C., & Watson-Williams, E. J. (1984). Alcohol and the blood. *Medical Clinics of North America, 68,* 105–120.

Lieber, C. S. (1982). General nutritional status in the alcoholic including disorders of minerals and vitamins. In C. S. Lieber (Ed), *Medical disorders of alcoholism* (pp. 551–569). Philadelphia: W. B. Saunders.

Linnoila, M., Stapleton, J. M., Lister, R., et al. (1986). Effects of alcohol on accident risk: Epidemiology and laboratory studies. *Pathologist, 40,* 36–41.

MacGregor, R. R., Gluckman, S. J., & Senior, J. R. (1978). Granulocyte function and levels of immunoglobulin and complement in patients admitted for withdrawal from alcohol. *Journal of Infectious Diseases, 138,* 747–758.

Monson, R. R., & Lyon, J. L. (1975). Proportional mortality among alcoholics. *Cancer, 36,* 1077–1079.

O'Caroll, R. E., Hayes, P. C., Ebmeir, K. P., et al. (1991). Regional cerebral blood flow and cognitive function in patients with chronic liver disease. *Lancet, 337,* 1251–1253.

Robins, L. N., Helzer, J. E., Weisman, M. M., et al. (1984). Lifetime prevalence of specific pschiatric disorders in three sites. *Archives of General Psychiatry, 41,* 949–958.

Roth, T., Roehrs, T., Zorick, F., et al. (1985). Pharmacologic effects of sedative-hypnotics, narcotic analgesics, and alcohol during sleep. Symposium on Sleep Apnea Disorders. *Medical Clinics of North America, 69,* 1281–1288.

Rothman, K., & Keller, A. (1972). The effect of joint exposure to alcohol and tobacco on risk of cancer of the mouth and pharynx. *Journal of Chronic Disease, 25,* 711–716.

Sherlock, S. (1981). *Diseases of the liver and biliary system.* Oxford, Great Britain: Blackwell Scientific Publications.

Sullivan, L. W., & Herbert, V. (1964). Suppression of hematopoiesis by ethanol. *Journal of Clinical Investigations, 43,* 2048–2062.

Torvik, A., Lindboe, C. F., & Rogde, S. (1982). Brain lesions in alcoholics: A neuropathologic study with clinical correlations. *Journal of Neurological Science, 56,* 233–248.

Torvik, A., & Torp, S. (1986). The prevalence of alcoholic cerebellar atrophy. A morphometric and histological study of an autopsy material. *Journal of Neurological Science, 75,* 43–51.

Tuyms, A. J. (1979). Epidemiology of alcohol and cancer. *Cancer Research, 39,* 2840–2843.

Urbano-Marquez, A., Estruch, R., Navarro-Lopez, F., et al. (1989). The effects of alcholism on skeletal and cardiac muscle. *New England Journal of Medicine, 320,* 409–415.

Victor, M. (1975). Polyneuropathy due to nutritional deficiency and alcoholism. In P. J. Dyke, P. K. Thomas, & E. H. Lambert (Eds.), *Peripheral neuropathy.* (pp. 1030–1066). Philadelphia: W. B. Saunders Co.

Victor, M. (1976). The Wernicke-Korsakcoff Syndrome. In P. J. Vinken & G. W. Bruyn (Eds.), *Handbook of clinical neurology,* Amsterdam: Elsevier-North Holland Press. pp. 243–270.

Wang, Y. J., Wu, J. C., Lee, S. D., et al. (1991). Gonadal dysfunction and changes in sex hormones in postnecrotic cirrhotic men in matched study with alcoholic cirrhotic men. *Hepatogastroenterology, 38,* 531–534.

Winship, D. H., Catlisch, C. R., Zboralske, F. E., et al. (1968). Deterioration of esophageal peristalsis in patients with alcoholic neuropathy. *Gastroenterology, 55,* 173–178.

Yano, K., Rhoads, G. G., & Kagan, A. (1977). Coffee, alcohol and risk of coronary heart disease among Japanese men living in Hawaii. *New England Journal of Medicine, 297,* 405–409.

Zimberg, S. (1978). Treatment of the elderly alcoholic in the community and in an institutional setting. *Addictive Diseases, 3,* 417–427.

6

Cognition, Aging, and Alcohol

RALPH E. TARTER

At the turn of this century, individuals over 65 years old comprised 4% of the U.S. population. By 1988, this proportion rose to 12.4%. It is estimated that in the year 2030 the elderly will comprise 22% of the population (Institute of Medicine, 1990). As the mean age of the general population escalates, the incidence of medical, psychiatric, and psychosocial problems associated with aging accordingly increases. It is against this backdrop that alcohol consumption, because of its high prevalence in the general population, and its numerous adverse impacts, is an especially important factor for understanding and preventing mortality and morbidity in the elderly. Alcohol consumption exacerbates the risk for injury, illness, and socioeconomic decline in the segment of the population that is already prone to these outcomes.

The results from the Epidemiological Catchment Area Study of the general population conducted in six U.S. cities indicate that among Euro-American men and women over 65 years of age, the lifetime prevalence of alcohol dependence is 12.5% and 1.46% respectively (Helzer et al., 1991). The prevalence of alcohol dependence among African-American males and females is 43% and 33% higher than Euro-Americans. Hispanic males exceed the lifetime prevalence of Euro-Americans by 31%, whereas the lifetime prevalence of alcohol dependence among Hispanic women is slightly more than half that of Euro-American women. Thus, differences between ethnic groups in the lifetime prevalence of alcohol problems need to be recognized in research directed at elucidating the biomedical consequences of alcohol consumption as well as by policymakers and legislators responsible for providing access to and funding for health services for this segment of the population.

Besides ethnic factors, it is noteworthy that the topography of drinking behavior sharply differs between males and females. The preferred beverage, quantity of alcohol consumed per drinking occasion, and the social context of alcohol consumption differs between genders within ethnic group (Bloom, 1983; Adams et al., 1990; Busby, Campbell, & Borrie, 1988).

In addition to ethnic and gender variation in pattern of alcohol intake, it is noteworthy that habitual excessive alcohol consumption predisposes to organ-system injury, culminating in an array of overlapping chronic and acute illnesses. However, the risk for adverse biomedical consequences is not equally distributed in the general population. For example, females are more vulnerable to cirrhosis than males (Gavaler, 1982). There is also suggestive evidence that Afro-Americans are at higher risk for developing this irreversible liver disease than Euro-Americans (Galambos, 1979). Significantly, cirrhosis in middle-aged persons is the primary cause of a chronic hepatic encephalopathy (Conn & Lieberthal, 1978) which underlies, in part, the cortical atrophy and cognitive deficits observed in alcoholics (Barthauer et al., 1992; Tarter, Van Thiel, & Moss, 1988).

Advancing age interacts with gender, ethnicity, drinking pattern, and organ-system susceptibility to produce biological injury. This presents unique circumstances for the elderly with respect to the effects of alcohol on the brain and ultimately cognition. For example, sedative use is prevalent in the elderly, particularly in females. Habitual use of these medications can induce a dementia (American Psychiatric Association, 1993). Furthermore, prolonged sedative use results in tolerance which generalizes to alcohol. The resulting cross-tolerance requires an increasingly larger quantity of alcohol to be consumed to achieve the desired subjective effect, and concomitantly magnifies the risk for organ-system pathology and accidental injury.

The risk for depression and its clinical manifestation is also greater with advancing age. Because of the major life changes that commonly occur with aging (retirement, widowhood, declining functional capacity, etc.), the likelihood for depression is high. Alcohol consumption is thus commonly an effort to medicate a negative affective state. In its severe manifestations, an affective disorder in late life, unlike major depression in middle age, has a debilitating effect on cognitive capacity. The magnitude of disruption can be so severe as to produce a pseudodementia. Among depressed individuals who also habitually consume alcoholic beverages, cognitive disturbances may, therefore, be augmented due to alcohol-induced dementia. The point to be made is that certain of the common etiological factors underlying cognitive disturbances in alcohol abusers are especially salient in the elderly population.

The changing demographics of the general population, combined with the particular circumstances of the elderly, underscores the need for research on the association between the effects of chronic alcohol consumption and the medical and psychosocial problems of aging. To date, however, a substantive empirical literature has yet to emerge. To illustrate this point, in 1993, the two premiere specialty journals, *Alcoholism: Clinical and Experimental Research* and *Journal of Studies on Alcohol*, together published less than a dozen research articles on the relation between aging and alcohol use. On the topic of cognition, there were no articles. The paucity of research focusing on the association between aging and alcohol consumption and the dearth of research directed at delineating the effects of alcoholism on cognition in the elderly prohibits drawing definitive conclusions. Recognizing this limitation, the ensuing discussion provides a conceptual framework for research, reviews the sparse empirical literature, and addresses the clinical issues pertinent to understanding the relation between alcohol consumption and cognition in the elderly population.

FRAMEWORK FOR RESEARCH ON COGNITION

Two general strategies have guided research directed at elucidating cognitive processes. First, cognition has been investigated from a psychometric perspective. This research is aimed at identifying the range of cognitive processes that together comprise the cognitive architecture. The emphasis is on measuring cognitive ability. Within this framework, manifold theories have been advanced of which the most influential have been proposed by Spearman (1904), Thurstone (1936), Guilford (1967), and Cattell (1963). And second, cognition has been investigated from an information processing perspective. The focus is on cognitive operations, which are investigated by decomposing complex tasks into their components. The information-processing perspective, having its origins in the cybernetic model first proposed by Miller, Galanter, & Pribram (1960), emphasizes the operations involved in performing cognitive tasks rather than quantifying abilities. This research strategy has been most effectively championed by Sternberg (1977) and Baddeley (1986).

Neuropsychology is concerned with understanding cognition within the context of brain-behavior relationships. Both psychometric (Reitan, 1955) and information processing (Kaplan et al., 1991) approaches are employed. An understanding of the representation and organization of cognitive processes in the brain, derived from the field of behavioral neurology, has fostered the development of psychological tests sensitive to detecting and localizing cerebral lesions. Application of psychometric tests for neurodiagnostic purposes essentially defines the specialty practice of clinical neuropsychology. Thus, pathology to the brain, either directly or indirectly, consequential to excessive habitual alcohol consumption, is amenable to investigation employing neuropsychological methods.

Initially, neuropsychological investigations into the study of alcoholism were concerned with the issue of lesion localization. Hypotheses were proposed based on the manifest pattern of cognitive deficits. Three general hypotheses guiding much of the early research were directed at testing whether alcoholism differentially affected the prefrontal cortex, right cerebral hemisphere, or produced lateralized pathology in the cerebral lesion. A synthesis of the neuropsychological literature, in conjunction with neuroradiological findings, implicates diffuse cerebral atrophy with proportionately greater pathology in the prefrontal region (Tarter & Edwards, 1986).

The focus of research has since shifted to correlating brain morphology with cognitive capacity (Wilkinson, 1987; Bernthal et al., 1987) and explorations into the etiology of cognitive impairment (Tarter & Edwards, 1986). During the past two decades, a large literature has emerged pertaining to young and middle-aged alcoholics. In contrast, research on the synergism among aging, alcohol consumption, and cognition has remained nascent. Consequently, in drawing conclusions about the cognitive status of elderly alcoholics, it is necessary to extrapolate from the research findings accrued from middle-aged individuals.

AGING AND MODELS OF COGNITIVE IMPAIRMENT IN ALCOHOLISM

The main issue that has engaged researchers for the past three decades pertains to whether habitual excessive alcohol consumption interacts with the normal aging process. In effect, do alcoholics manifest premature brain aging?

Figure 6.1 depicts two causal pathways linking alcohol consumption, aging and cognitive impairment. In pathway 1, alcohol neurotoxicity is presumed to disrupt putative biochemical and physiological mechanisms that regulate brain aging. Hence, it would follow that the lifetime quantity of alcohol consumed would covary in a dose-response

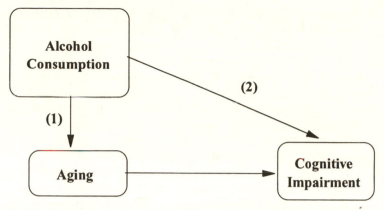

Figure 6.1. Causal pathways linking alcohol consumption and cognitive impairment.

relationship with biological aging of the brain. From the neuropsychological perspective, this would be manifest as a pattern of cognitive performance in alcoholics that is comparable to older nonalcoholics. The amount of alcohol-induced aging is presumably determined by the cumulative lifetime quantity of ethanol consumed. To date, studies have not been published demonstrating an association between total lifetime quantity of alcohol consumed and magnitude of deviation from normal performance on neuropsychological tests. However, it is noteworthy that duration of alcohol use and duration of alcoholism have been found to be either not correlated with cognitive capacity or correlated only modestly. To date, no study has shown that alcohol consumption history can explain more than 20% of variance on neuropsychological tests.

From a descriptive standpoint, the premature aging hypothesis has received confirmation. For example, alcoholics perform similarly to older normal controls on tests measuring vocational aptitude (Kish & Cheney, 1969), learning and memory capacity (Ryan & Butters, 1980), problem solving ability (Klisz & Parsons, 1977) and intelligence (Blusewicz et al., 1977). The performance of alcoholics on standardized neuropsychological tests (Fitzhugh, Fitzhugh, & Reitan, 1965), pattern of evoked cortical potentials (Porjesz & Begleiter, 1982), and morphological changes observed using magnetic resonance imaging (Chick et al., 1989) also reveal that alcoholics are comparable to older nonalcoholics.

It is important to emphasize that the evidence supporting the premature aging hypothesis is based entirely on the observation that there is similarity between alcoholics and a comparison group of older normal controls on a particular dependent variable. Although it is arguably heuristic to conceptualize the cumulative effects of alcohol on the brain in the context of brain aging, there is, however, no empirical evidence demonstrating that the mechanisms of alcohol action influence the endogenous aging process. Even though the topography of morphological, electrophysiological and cognitive disturbances may parallel the changes observed in normal aging, the causal mechanisms may be entirely different. To verify the premature aging hypothesis, it is necessary first to elucidate the factors regulating the normal aging process and then to determine whether acute alcohol consumption impacts directly on these processes.

In pathway 2, habitual excessive alcohol consumption is hypothesized to produce direct impairment in cognitive capacity. Alcohol is a potent neurotoxin, hence impaired cognitive capacity is conjectured to reflect the culmination of neuronal necrosis. The magnitude of cognitive impairment is determined conjointly, but independently, by the person's age and the total lifetime amount of alcohol consumed. Evidence demonstrating a direct neurotoxic effect of alcohol on cognitive processes is derived from controlled studies of rodents. In these studies, learning and memory capacities were found to be diminished following a period of alcohol consumption (Riley & Walker, 1978; Walker, Hunter, & Abraham, 1981; Freund & Walker, 1978; Freund, 1970). Research on humans has not supported these findings, at least with respect to performance on routine clinical neuropsychological tests. Alcoholics who are healthy and have no significant neuromedical history of trauma or disease perform comparably to normal controls (Grant, Adams, & Reed, 1979; Grant, Adams, & Reed, 1984). This finding is important because it demonstrates that where only an alcohol abuse history is present, and other factors that could potentially also induce neuropsychological impairment are not present, no cognitive deficits are manifest. Thus, even though the neurotoxic properties of alcohol are well established, the available evidence suggests that the neuropsychological impairments manifest by alcoholics are not due solely, or even substantively, to the direct effects of alcohol on the brain.

Figure 6.2 depicts a general model to account for the neuropsychological deficits in alcoholism consequent to multiple etiological factors. Although ethanol by itself potentially has a deleterious impact on neurological integrity and concomitantly also cognitive capacity, the major cause of the cognitive impairment is not considered to be ethanol neurotoxicity. Referring to the study by Grant et al. (1984), the association between alcoholism and cognitive capacity disappeared when neuromedical factors were controlled. In other words, neuromedical risk factors mediated the relationship between alcoholism and cognitive impairment. In another line of research, Tarter and colleagues (Tarter et al., 1988; Arria, Tarter, & Van Thiel, 1991) have shown that a subclinical hepatic encephalopathy, a consequence of cirrhosis, underlies to large extent the neuropsychological impairment observed in alcoholics. Controlling for cirrhosis, it has been shown that on most aspects of neuropsychological functioning, alcoholics are not distinguishable from persons with nonalcoholic cirrhosis (Tarter et al., 1988). Hence, among alcoholics with cirrhosis, the neuropsychological deficits are largely mediated by a subclinical hepatic encephalopathy. Numerous other factors could potentially also mediate the association between habitual excessive alcohol consumption

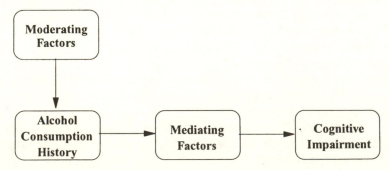

Figure 6.2. Causal pathways linking alcohol consumption and cognitive impairment, taking into account moderating and mediating influences.

and cognitive impairment. These factors include comorbid psychopathology, other drug use history, cerebral trauma, nutritional deficiency, and organ-system disease.

Moderating factors also influence the magnitude of association between alcohol consumption history and cognitive abilities. By definition, moderating factors interact with the independent variable which, in this case, is alcohol consumption history. Factors that are known to affect the pattern and severity of alcohol consumption include family history of alcoholism, gender, ethnicity, socioeconomic status, and age. With respect to the focus of this discussion, age of onset and period of peak alcohol consumption are particularly important. Significantly, susceptibility to neurological disruption from acute and chronic alcohol consumption increases with age (Abel & York, 1978; Linnoila et al., 1980; Vogel-Sprott & Barrett, 1984; Pfefferbaum et al., 1992). It is noteworthy that approximately one-third of elderly heavy alcohol consumers began their heavy drinking later in life, while about two-thirds have had a long standing history persisting from middle adulthood onward (Glatt, 1978). To date, neuropsychological studies have not, however, been conducted correlating neuropsychological test performance with natural history of drinking behavior in the elderly population.

Conceptualizing the association between alcohol consumption and cognitive impairment within a multivariate framework readily reveals the reasons for the substantial variation in level and type of cognitive impairment among the population of alcohol consumers and alcoholics. To date, multivariate modeling, incorporating moderating and mediating variables, has not been undertaken either to identify homogeneous subgroups or to detect specific subtypes based on particular etiological pathways. In practice, this task would be a daunting undertaking replete with numerous sampling and methodological problems. For example, because alcoholism in the elderly is a relatively low-prevalence disorder, combined with the fact that there are manifold moderators and mediators, it is very difficult to ascertain sufficiently large samples to incorporate the known salient variables for multivariate analyses.

FACTORS MODERATING AND MEDIATING THE ASSOCIATION BETWEEN CHRONIC ALCOHOL ABUSE AND COGNITIVE IMPAIRMENT

Dementia

Dementia concomitant to primary organic pathology (e.g., Alzheimer's disease, Pick's disease) affects approximately 8% of the population under 79 years of age (Kay & Bergman, 1980). Whether alcohol consumption promotes or catalyzes progression of the dementia in nonalcoholic individuals has only recently been investigated. Rosen et al. (1993) found no differences in cognitive capacity in a sample of putative Alzheimer patients stratified according to history of alcohol consumption. Further research is clearly required on this important topic.

It is difficult to establish the extent to which the cognitive deficits manifest by elderly consumers of alcohol beverages reflect an alcoholic dementia. This is due to the fact that the cognitive deficits presumed to be caused by the alcohol may be due to the conjoint presence of a primary dementing disease. This task is complicated by the fact that a definite diagnosis of primary dementia (e.g., Alzheimer) can only be made post mortem. Because of this limitation, inferences about the likelihood of a primary de-mentia can only be drawn by prospectively monitoring cognitive changes and by doc-umentation of noncognitive symptoms (e.g., affect, behavior).

Acute Alcohol Effects

The pharmacokinetic actions of alcohol are not constant across the lifespan. Tolerance to alcohol decreases with advancing age. Thus, a given dose of alcohol has greater pharmacological impact in older than younger individuals. The efficiency of the liver for metabolizing alcohol is lower in older people, and this is likely accompanied by greater neurological sensitivity to alcohol metabolities (e.g., acetaldehyde) (Galambos, 1979). Indirectly, drinking in the elderly also augments the risk for traumatic neuro-logical injury concomitant to the more severely experienced acute effects.

A related issue pertains to the intake of sedatives because habitual use of these compounds produce tolerance to alcohol, which in turn leads to consumption of an unsafe quantity of alcohol. Quantity of alcohol consumption per occasion has been reported to be significantly, albeit modestly, related to cognitive status (Parker et al., 1980) and superficially to resemble the pattern of deficits concomitant to aging (Parker et al., 1982). In effect, lower tolerance combined with greater neurological sensitivity to alcohol, sedative drug use, and increased risk for trauma interact to predispose to cognitive impairment in the elderly.

Lifestyle

As society progresses toward increasingly greater technological complexity, the cog-nitive requirements for optimal social adjustment will accordingly increase. Hence, even subtle cognitive deficits potentially can exert pronounced limitations on adjustment. Among nonalcoholics, cognitive capacity is correlated with quality of social adjustment and capacity to perform the activities of daily living (Heaton, Chelune, & Lehman, 1978; Heaton & Pendleton, 1981).

The extent to which particular patterns of alcohol consumption interact with quality of life in the elderly has not been investigated. These relationships need to be delineated within a framework of reciprocal person-environment interactions. For example, the elderly commonly experience downward social mobility which, not uncommonly, re-sults in poverty. The poor quality of life associated with economic disadvantage inter-acts with alcohol consumption to augment the risk for disease and traumatic injury. In addition, declining sensorimotor capacity increases the risk for accidents but also has the effect of fostering a passive lifestyle in which alcohol consumption is a dominant activity. Retirement, and concomitantly the cessation of habitual routines and goal-directed activities, in conjunction with boredom, predisposes to alcohol consumption. Thus, not only does alcohol consumption potentially impact adversely on life quality, mediated in part by cognitive processes, but also lifestyle interacts with the pattern of alcohol consumption to augment the risk for cognitive impairment.

Disease

The prevalence of chronic diseases increases with aging. Because the brain is dependent totally on other organ systems to satisfy its metabolic needs (oxygen, nutrients, etc.), pathology can disrupt neurological integrity and ultimately produce cognitive impairments. Deficits on neuropsychological tests have been reported to be manifest in association with a variety of diseases affecting the cardiovascular, pulmonary, digestive, and endocrine systems as well as consequent to diseases of specific organs such as the heart, liver, and pancreas (see Tarter, Van Thiel, & Edwards, 1988, for review).

Habitual excessive alcohol consumption commonly results in organ-system disease. Whether or not the elderly are more susceptible than middle-aged persons to organ-system injury from a specific dose of alcohol is, however, not known. Nonetheless, because chronic diseases are more prevalent in the elderly, it is plausible to conclude that the impaired cognitive capacity observed in older alcoholics may be due in part to organ-system injury and disease, conditions that may be both independent of, as well as caused by, alcohol consumption.

Pattern of Alcohol Consumption

Approximately 16% of the elderly population can be characterized as heavy drinkers (Bloom, 1983). Different drinking patterns have yet to be systematically studied with respect to their unique or particular association with cognition. The extent to which the parameters of quantity, frequency, beverage type, quantity consumed per drinking occasion, and duration of drinking history predict or account for performance on tests of cognitive capacity remains to be determined. Compared to younger individuals, there is greater cognitive and psychomotor impairment in older social drinkers following a fixed dose of alcohol (Vogel-Sprott & Barrett, 1984; Linnoila et al., 1980); however, whether these age differences parallel cognitive functioning following long-term alcohol consumption is not known. To date, the association between drinking topography and cognitive abilities has not been investigated in the elderly population.

Heterogeneity of Cognitive Impairment in Alcoholics

The population of alcoholics is very heterogeneous with respect to the magnitude and pattern of cognitive deficits. On tests of motor regulation and control, it appears, for example, that younger alcoholics are more impaired than older alcoholics (Alterman et al., 1984). These findings suggest perhaps that the impairments either presage the onset of alcoholism or emanate from an interaction between alcohol and aging in some individuals. Also, abstracting deficits have been frequently observed in alcoholics (Tarter & Ryan, 1983). With the exception of one study, the investigations conducted so far have been based on subjects recruited from psychiatric facilities. However, a recent study of alcoholics with Laennec's cirrhosis recruited from a gastroenterology service failed to reveal an abstracting deficit (Tarter et al., in press). These findings underscore the heterogeneity of deficit according to age and ascertainment source as well as illustrate the multifactorial etiology of neuropsychological deficits manifest by alcoholics.

Investigations focusing specifically on cognitive capacities among elderly alcoholics (over 60 years of age) have not yet been conducted. It is likely that heterogeneity is even greater in this segment of the population because of the larger number of risk factors (disease, injury, other drug use, etc.).

Studies of middle-aged alcoholics are, however, informative. Specifically, it has been shown that there are two broad types of neuropsychological profiles. One pattern is characteristic of the Wernicke-Korsakoff syndrome. This disorder has been comprehensively described with respect to etiology, natural history, and clinical phenomenology. The most salient disturbances are in short-term memory and semantic encoding. The second general category of disorder is dementia. This is the more common outcome of chronic alcohol abuse and is manifest in manifold patterns of cognitive disturbances.

Dementia in the elderly has been documented since ancient times. Maudsley (1879) was first to hypothesize that alcohol excess was a cause of dementia. Currently, dementia is consensually accepted to comprise one outcome of chronic alcoholism (American Psychiatric Association, 1993). Although dementia concomitant to alcoholism is well documented, an unresolved question concerns whether there is a primary alcoholic dementia; that is, whether the dementia is caused specifically by the long-term actions of ethanol on the brain.

There is sound reason to suspect that older drinkers would be particularly susceptible to developing a primary dementia. The breakdown of the blood-brain barrier with aging, coupled with a reduction in total water in proportion to body mass, produces higher blood alcohol concentrations in older persons following a fixed dose of ethanol compared to younger individuals. Because the aging brain is more susceptible to the neuropharmacological effects of ethanol, it follows that neuronal necrosis would be more insidious. Empirical evidence directly addressing this question is limited, however, to the finding by Pfefferbaum et al. (1992) who observed significant gray and white matter loss after correcting for age. This study demonstrates that the aging brain may be more vulnerable to the effects of alcohol. The available evidence also indicates, however, that among middle-aged alcoholics, ethanol neurotoxicity is not the sole or even major determinant of neuropsychological deficit (Grant et al., 1979). It is not known whether the same holds true for elderly alcoholics; that is, no cognitive deficits are observed in persons who are healthy or without significant neurological history or medical complications.

In DSM-IV, the diagnosis of *substance-induced persisting dementia* is applied if the following three criteria are satisfied:

1. Anterograde and retrograde amnesia
2. Cognitive disturbance involving at least one of the following:
   a. Aphasia
   b. Apraxia
   c. Agnosia
   d. Impairment in executive cognitive processes
3. Social or occupational decline caused by the cognitive deficits

Dementia within the DSM-IV framework is thus a rather broad category consisting of a diverse set of complex symptoms. For example, an impairment in executive cognitive processes, as one defining feature of dementia, consists of several distinct processes such as planning, self-monitoring, and regulating behavior, and each process is subserved by basic mechanisms such as attentional control, abstracting ability, and language. The point to be made is that there are manifold constellations of disturbances that could qualify a person for a dementia diagnosis. And, these disturbances most likely have a multifactorial etiology. In the elderly alcoholic, this is particularly salient because of the prevalence of Parkinson's disease, cerebrovascular disease, and medical disorders. These latter conditions independently as well as in combination with excessive habitual alcohol consumption can induce dementia. Furthermore, because alcohol and sedatives are commonly used conjointly, the risk for dementia is exacerbated. Thus, while it is relatively easy to diagnose dementia, it is difficult to identify the etiological mechanisms.

NEUROPSYCHOLOGICAL CAPACITY
IN ELDERLY ALCOHOLICS

Investigations have not been conducted that specifically examined alcoholic subjects over 60 years of age. Almost all of the research conducted to date has employed advancing age as an exclusionary criterion. Several studies have, however, been carried out in which an older comparison group was accrued for comparison to Korsakoff subjects (Oscar-Berman & Bonner, 1989; Oscar-Berman & Bonner, 1985). The results indicated that older alcoholics did not perform more poorly than age-matched normal controls on various components of a matching to sample task. The results are, however, difficult to interpret because only response time (which reflects efficiency and not capacity) was measured, and the results are based on only seven subjects. Thus, the possibility of a type II error cannot be discounted. In another study, 12 elderly alcoholics performed on average more poorly than age-matched normal controls under conditions requiring short but not long delay of a response (Oscar-Berman, Hunter, & Bonner, 1992). Because the longer response delay condition is more difficult, this finding is contrary to expectation. Employing more traditional measures, Kramer, Blusewicz, & Preston (1989) compared old and young alcoholics and age-matched normal controls on·the California Verbal Learning Test. Immediate and delayed recall capacity was associated with both aging and alcoholism. However, alcoholism was associated with a differential pattern of mistakes (intrusions, false positive errors) and more impaired recognition memory. These findings suggest that older alcoholics manifest certain cognitive impairments that are not due to aging alone. Further research on larger samples is clearly needed.

The paucity of research notwithstanding, it appears that elderly alcoholics are not invariably impaired relative to age-matched normal controls. This conclusion is buttressed by the observation that there are no observable differences between Alzheimer patients who either have abused alcohol in the past or had no significant alcohol involvement. However, it is important to emphasize that elderly alcoholics and nonalcoholics have not been directly compared across a broad spectrum of cognitive processes, including those processes that are commonly impaired in middle-aged alcoholics. Furthermore, prospective studies have not been conducted to determine whether cognitive decline covaries with advancing age among the subpopulation of alcoholics who manifest cognitive disturbances. Finally, whereas the neurotoxic properties of ethanol are well established, there is no convincing evidence that alcohol toxicity significantly contributes to the deterioration in cognitive capacities or directly causes dementia in alcoholics. Cerebral trauma, cerebrovascular pathology, sedative drug use, and chronic disease are prevalent in the elderly and may account for the manifest cognitive deficits in alcohol abusers. The point to be made is that a large number of general risk factors as well as certain risk factors that are particular to the elderly population underlie the cognitive deficits in the elderly.

RAMIFICATIONS OF COGNITIVE IMPAIRMENT

Reversibility

Abstinence from alcohol in middle-aged alcoholics is associated with substantial improvement in cognitive capacities. However, complete reversibility does not occur. Long-term memory, for example, remains impaired even after a period of 7 years of continuous sobriety (Brandt et al., 1983). In contrast, short-term memory and psychomotor capacity improve substantially with abstinence. Research has not yet been directed at determining whether the potential for cognitive recovery covaries with age. It is plausible to hypothesize that elderly alcoholics would experience less recovery compared to young or middle-aged alcoholics because of diminished neurological plasticity. This important issue remains to be examined empirically.

Cognitive Rehabilitation

Providing middle-aged alcoholics with the opportunity to practice on cognitive tests results in improvement on other tests of cognitive capacity (Goldman, 1987; Goldman, Williams, & Klisz, 1983). With increasing availability of computer interactive software for cognitive rehabilitation, it would appear that the application of these procedures would be effective for maximizing recovery of cognitive capacities. Research has yet to be conducted on the elderly alcoholic population.

Medical Management

Organ-system pathology, having diverse etiologies, has not been generally considered to be a major factor underlying impaired cognitive functioning in alcoholics. Yet there is abundant evidence demonstrating that cognitive deficits emanate from a variety of diseases that are commonly present in alcoholics. Consequently, it is reasonable to theorize that aggressive medical management of disease in alcoholics would have a beneficial effect on cognitive functioning. Apart from research on cirrhosis, little is known about the disease-related origins of the cognitive deficits in alcoholics. Recently, some attention has been directed at delineating the association between cerebral hypoxia, sleep apnea, and alcoholism in the elderly (Vitiello et al., 1990). However, it is not known whether oxygen perfusion in apneic alcoholics can reverse the cognitive deficits. In summary, research needs to address the question of whether or not cognitive recovery can be facilitated by more intensive medical intervention than is currently practiced.

Treatment Prognosis

Several studies on middle-aged alcoholics have been conducted to determine the extent to which cognitive capacity predicts treatment prognosis. In one study it was found that cognitively limited alcoholics responded best to structured or directive intervention such as pharmacotherapy, whereas more cognitively sophisticated alcoholics responded better to didactic interventions (Kissin, Platz, & Su, 1970). This finding raises the important issue of designing interventions that are tailored to the specific psychological characteristics and needs of the individual. Within the framework of patient-treatment matching, the benefits, if any, of incorporating cognitive capacity in the matching criteria to augment prognosis remain to be determined.

Several studies have examined the extent to which neuropsychological test scores can predict treatment outcome. Because there is great disparity across studies with respect to the characteristics of the sample, the cognitive processes measured, and type of treatments provided, it is to be expected that inconsistency in the findings across studies would occur. Several investigations have found that cognitive capacity is unrelated to treatment outcome (Donovan, Kivlahan, & Walker, 1984; Eckardt et al., 1988; Price et al., 1988), while other studies observed only a modest relationship between cognitive capacity and treatment prognosis (Abbott & Gregson, 1981; Berglund, Leijonquist, & Harlen, 1977; McCrady & Smith, 1986). In one study of middle-aged alcoholics, Parsons, Schaeffer, and Glenn (1990) found that a combined summary score derived from a battery of neuropsychological tests accurately classified 66% of individuals who either relapsed or remained abstinent from alcohol for 8 to 14 months posttreatment. In a follow-up study, Glenn, Sinha, and Parsons (1993) found that the N1 and P3 components of the event-related potential successfully predicted 65.6% of alcoholics who either sustained sobriety or relapsed. These ERP waveform components are the neurophysiological substrate of attentional and short-term memory processes, respectively. Overall, however, the results of the available studies indicate that cognitive capacity is only modestly predictive of treatment outcome.

Quality of Life

Cognitive capacity, measured by neuropsychological tests, is associated with social and vocational adjustment among psychiatric patients (Heaton, Chelune, & Lehman, 1978; Heaton & Pendleton, 1981). In addition, it has been found that neuropsychological test scores of individuals with dementia are correlated with the instrumental aspects of daily living (e.g., balancing a checkbook) but not physical capacity (Saxton et al., 1986). In this latter study, no specific aspect of neuropsychological capacity was related to instrumental abilities, suggesting that general level of cognitive functioning is the salient factor. Whether cognitive capacity covaries with quality of life in elderly alcoholics has not yet been investigated.

NEUROPSYCHOLOGICAL ASSESSMENT

Tarter, Ott, and Mezzich (1991) have proposed a three-stage procedure for conducting a cost-efficient neuropsychological evaluation. The first stage, a screening process, is directed at detecting cognitive deficits using tests having high sensitivity but low specificity. Tests serving this purpose include the Trailmaking Test and Symbol Digit Modalities Test. If a deficit is observed, a comprehensive assessment is then conducted using standard batteries such as the Halstead-Reitan or Luria-Nebraska instruments. These batteries survey a broad range of cognitive processes and afford the opportunity to lateralize and localize cerebral lesions. The third stage of the evaluation process entails a modality-specific assessment. In this phase of the assessment, disturbances detected in the second stage are fully delineated to characterize the nature and severity of deficit in particular domains of cognition.

The neuropsychological evaluation should not only yield a profile of an individual's cognitive strengths and weaknesses but also should attempt to identify the causes of impairment. This is arduous and not always possible for alcoholics because of the large number of factors that could induce cognitive impairment. Toward this end, the neuropsychological evaluation should be viewed as one aspect of the comprehensive examination directed at clarifying both current clinical status and etiology.

The ultimate aim is to tailor interventions to identified problems. Toward this end, the Drug Use Screening Inventory (DUSI) was developed originally for adolescents and modified subsequently for adults to facilitate the thorough description of medical, neuropsychiatric, and psychosocial problems concomitant to alcohol and drug use (Tarter, 1990). This 149-item self-report questionnaire quantifies severity of disturbance in ten domains: (1) substance use, (2) behavior disorder, (3) psychiatric illness, (4) health status, (5) family adjustment, (6) work, (7) social competence, (8) peer relationships, (9) school adjustment (if applicable), and (10) leisure and recreation. Severity of disorder is ranked across the 10 domains on a common scale ranging from 0 to 100% to prioritize intervention needs. In this manner, treatment modality can be targeted to identified areas of disturbance and resources provided that are commensurate to the severity of disturbance.

SUMMARY

Although the proportion of elderly is rising in the general population, little is known about the effects, if any, of alcohol consumption on cognitive functioning. Available evidence indicates that the same factors underlying cognitive impairment in middle-aged individuals also apply to the elderly. However, additional factors that are more prevalent in the elderly, such as diseases related to aging along with increased sedative and other drug use, likely contribute to the manifest cognitive disturbances. Thus, there is reason to believe that the factors underlying cognitive disturbances in older alcoholics differ somewhat from those of younger alcoholics. Nonetheless, in the absence of systematic research, this conclusion is necessarily tentative.

References

Abbott, M., & Gregson, R. (1981). Cognitive dysfunction in the prediction of relapse in alcoholics. *Journal of Studies on Alcohol, 42*, 230–243.

Abel, E., & York, J. (1978). Age-related differences in the response to ethanol in the rat. *Physiological Psychology, 7*, 391–395.

Adams, W., Garry, P., Rhyme, R., Hunt, W., & Goodwin, J. (1990). Alcohol intake in the healthy elderly: Changes with age in a cross-sectional and longitudinal study. *Journal of the American Geriatrics Society, 38*, 211–216.

Alterman, A., Tarter, R., Petrarulo, E., & Baughman, T. (1984). Evidence for impersistence in young male alcoholics. *Alcoholism: Clinical and Experimental Research, 8*, 448–450.

American Psychiatric Association. (1993). *DSM-IV Draft Criteria*. Washington, D.C.

Arria, A., Tarter, R., & Van Thiel, D. (1991). Improvement in cognitive functioning of alcoholics following orthotopic liver transplantation. *Alcoholism: Clinical and Experimental Research, 15*, 956–962.

Baddeley, A. (1986). *Working Memory.* Oxford, England: Oxford University Press.

Barthauer, L., Tarter, R., Hirsch, W., & Van Thiel, D. (1992). Brain morphology characteristics of cirrhotic alcoholics and nonalcoholics: An MRI study. *Alcoholism: Clinical and Experimental Research, 16*, 982–985.

Berglund, M., Leijonquist, H., & Harlen, M. (1977). Prognostic significance and reversibility of cerebral dysfunction in alcoholics. *Journal of Studies on Alcohol, 38*, 1761–1770.

Bernthal, P., Hays, A., Tarter, R., Lecky, J., Hegedus, A., & Van Thiel, D. (1987). Cerebral CT scan abnormalities in cholestatic and hepatocellular disease and their relationship to psychometric indices of encephalopathy. *Hepatology, 7*, 107–114.

Bloom, P. (1983). Alcoholism after sixty. *American Family Physician, 28*, 111–113.

Blusewicz, J., Justman, R., Schenkenberg, T., & Beck, E. (1977). Neuropsychological correlates of chronic alcoholism and aging. *Journal of Nervous and Mental Disease, 165*, 348–355.

Brandt, J., Butters, N., Ryan, C., & Bayog, R. (1983). Cognitive loss and recovery in long-term alcohol abusers. *Archives of General Psychology, 40*, 435–442.

Busby, W., Campbell, A., & Borrie, M. (1988). Alcohol use in a community based sample of subjects aged 70 years or older. *Journal of the American Geriatrics Society, 36*, 301–305.

Cattell, R. (1963). Theory of fluid and crystallized intelligence. A critical experiment. *Journal of Educational Psychology, 54*, 1–22.

Chick, J., Smith, M., Engleman, H., Kean, D., Mander, A., Douglas, R., & Best, J. (1989). Magnetic resonance imaging of the brain in alcoholics: Cerebral atrophy, lifetime alcohol consumption, and cognitive deficits. *Alcoholism: Clinical and Experimental Research, 13*, 512–518.

Conn, H., & Lieberthal, M. (1978). *The hepatic coma syndrome and lactulose* (pp. 1–419). Baltimore: Williams & Wilkins.

Donovan, D., Kivlahan, D., & Walker, D. (1984). Clinical limitations of neuropsychological testing in predicting treatment outcome among alcoholics. *Alcoholism: Clinical and Experimental Research, 8*, 470–475.

Eckardt, M., Rawlings, R., Graubard, B., Faden, V., Martin, R., & Gottschalk, L. (1988). Neuropsychological performance and treatment outcome in male alcoholics. *Alcoholism: Clinical and Experimental Research, 12*, 88–93.

Fitzhugh, L., Fitzhugh, K., & Reitan, R. (1965). Adaptive abilities and intellectual functioning of hospitalized alcoholics. Further considerations. *Quarterly Journal of Studies on Alcohol, 26*, 402–411.

Freund, G. (1970). Impairment of shock avoidance learning after long-term alcohol ingestion in mice. *Science, 168*, 1599–1601.

Freund, G., & Walker, D. (1978). Impairment of avoidance learning by prolonged ethanol consumption in mice. *Journal of Pharmacology and Experimental Therapeutics, 197*, 284–292.

Galambos, J. (1979). Cirrhosis: epidemiology. In L. Smith (Ed.), *Major problems in internal medicine* (pp. 97–121). Philadelphia: W. B. Saunders.

Guilford, J. (1956). The structure of intellect. *Psychology Bulletin, 53*, 267–293.

Gavaler, J. (1982). Sex-related differences in alcohol-induced liver disease. Artificial or real? *Alcoholism: Clinical and Experimental Research, 6*, 186–196.

Glatt, M. (1978). Experience with elderly alcoholics in England. *Alcoholism: Clinical and Experimental Research, 2*, 23.

Glenn, S., Sinha, R., & Parsons, O. (1993). Electrophysiological indices predict resumption of drinking in sober alcoholics. *Alcohol, 10*, 89–95.

Goldman, M. (1987). The role of time and practice in recovery of function in alcoholics. In O.

Parsons, N. Butters, & P. Nathan (Eds.), *Neuropsychology of alcoholism: Implications for diagnosis and treatment.* New York: Guilford.

Goldman, M., Williams, D., & Klisz, D. (1983). Recoverability of psychological functioning following alcohol abuse: Prolonged visual-spatial dysfunction in older alcoholics. *Journal of Consulting and Clinical Psychology, 51,* 370–378.

Guilford, J. (1967). *Nature of human intelligence.* New York: McGraw-Hill.

Grant, I., Adams, K., & Reed, R. (1979). Normal neuropsychological abilities of alcoholic men in their late thirties. *American Journal of Psychology, 136,* 1263–1269.

Grant, I., Adams, K., & Reed, R. (1984). Aging, abstinence, and medical risk factors in the prediction of neuropsychological deficits amongst chronic alcoholics. *Archives of General Psychology, 41,* 710–718.

Heaton, R., Chelune, G., & Lehman, R. (1978). Using neuropsychological and personality tests to assess the likelihood of patient employment. *Journal of Nervous and Mental Disease, 166,* 408–416.

Heaton, R., & Pendleton, M. (1981). Use of neuropsychological tests to predict adult patients' everyday functioning. *Journal of Consulting and Clinical Psychology, 49,* 807–821.

Helzer, J., Burman, A., & McEvoy, L. (1991). Alcohol abuse and dependence. In L. Robins & D. Regier (Eds.), *Psychiatric disorders in America. The Epidemiological Catchment Area Study.* New York: Free Press.

Institute of Medicine (1990). *The second fifty years: Promoting health and preventing disability.* Washington, DC: National Academy Press.

Kaplan, E., Fein, D., Morris, R., & Delis, D. (1991). *WAIS-R as a neuropsychological Instrument* (manual). San Antonio, TX: Psychological Corporation.

Kay, D., & Bergman, K. (1980). Epidemiology of mental disorders among the aged in the community. In J. Birren and R. Sloane (Eds.), *handbook of mental health and aging.* Englewood Cliffs, NJ: Prentice Hall.

Kish, G., & Cheney, T. (1969). Impaired abilities in alcoholism measured by the General Aptitude Test Battery. *Quarterly Journal of Studies on Alcohol, 30,* 384–388.

Kissin, B., Platz, A., & Su, W. (1970). Social and psychological factors in the treatment of chronic alcoholism. *Journal of Psychatric Research, 8,* 13–27.

Klisz, D., & Parsons, O. (1977). Hypothesis testing in younger and older alcoholics. *Journal of Studies on Alcohol, 38,* 1718–1729.

Kramer, J., Blusewicz, J., & Preston, K. (1989). The premature aging hypothesis: Old before its time? *Journal of Consulting and Clinical Psychology, 37,* 257–262.

Linnoila, M., Erwin, C., Ramon, D., & Cleveland, W. (1980). Effects of age and alcohol on psychomotor performance of men. *Journal of Studies on Alcohol, 41,* 488–495.

Maudsley, H. (1879). *The pathology of the mind.* London: MacMillan.

McCrady, B., & Smith, D. (1986). Implications of cognitive impairment for the treatment of alcoholism. *Alcoholism: Clinical and Experimental Research, 10,* 145–149.

Miller, G., Galanter, E., & Pribram, K. (1960). *Plans and the structure of behavior.* New York: Holt, Rinehart, & Winston.

Monteiro, M. (1990). DSM-III-R diagnostic criteria for dementia associated with alcoholism—a critical review. *Annals of Clinical Psychiatry, 2,* 263–275.

Oscar-Berman, M., & Bonner, R. (1985). Matching- and delayed matching-to-sample performance as measures of visual processing, selective attention, and memory in aging and alcoholic individuals. *Neuropsychologia, 23,* 635–651.

Oscar-Berman, M., & Bonner, R. (1989). Nonmatching- (oddity) and delayed nonmatching-to-sample performance in aging, alcoholic, and alcoholic Korsakoff individuals. *Psychobiology, 17,* 424–430.

Oscar-Berman, M., Hunter, N., & Bonner, R. (1992). Visual and auditory spatial and nonspatial delayed-response performance by Korsakoff and non-Korsakoff alcoholic and aging individuals. *Behavioral Neuroscience, 106,* 613–622.

Parker, E., Birnbaum, I., Boyd, B., & Noble, E. (1980). Neuropsychological decrement as a function of alcohol intake in male students. *Alcoholism: Clinical and Experimental Research, 4,* 330–334.

Parker, E., Parker, D., Brody, J., & Schoenberg, R. (1982). Cognitive patterns resembling premature aging in male social drinkers. *Alcoholism: Clinical and Experimental Research, 6,* 46–52.

Parsons, O., Schaeffer, K., & Glenn (1990). Does neuropsychological test performance predict resumption of drinking in post-treatment alcoholics? *Addictive Behaviors, 15,* 297–307.

Pfefferbaum, A., Linn, K., Zipursky, R., Mathalon, D., Rosenbloom, M., Lane, B., Ha, C., & Sullivan, C. (1992). Brain gray and white matter volume accelerates with aging in chronic alcoholics: A quantative MRI study. *Alcoholism: Clinical and Experimental Research, 16,* 1078–1089.

Porjesz, B., & Begleiter, H. (1982). Evoked brain potential deficits in alcoholism and aging. *Alcoholism: Clinical and Experimental Research, 6,* 53–63.

Price, J., Mitchell, S., Willshire, B., Graham, J., & Williams, G. (1988). A follow-up study of patients with alcohol-related brain damage in the community. *Australian Drug and Alcohol Review, 7,* 83–87.

Reitan, R. (1955). Investigation of the validity of Halstead's measures of biological intelligence. *Archives of Neurological Psychiatry, 73,* 28–35.

Riley, J., & Walker, D. (1978) Morphological alterations in hippocampus after long-term alcohol consumption in mice. *Science, 201,* 646–648.

Rosen, J., Colantonio, A., Becker, J., DeKosky, S., & Moss, H. (1993). Effects of a history of heavy alcohol consumption on Alzheimer's disease. *British Journal of Psychiatry, 163,* 358–363.

Ryan, C., & Butters, N. (1980). Learning and memory impairment in young and old alcoholics: Evidence for the premature aging hypothesis. *Alcoholism: Clinical and Experimental Research, 4,* 288–293.

Saxton, J., Housley, S., Becker, J., & Boller, F. (1986). Cognitive function and activities of daily living in Alzheimer's disease. *Clinical Neuropsychologist, 1,* 97.

Spearman, C. (1904). "General Intelligence," objectively determined and measured. *American Journal of Psychology, 15,* 201–293.

Sternberg, R. (1977). *Intelligence, information processing, and analytical reasoning. The componential analysis of human abilities.* Hillsdale, NJ: Erlbaum.

Tarter, R. (1990). Evaluation and treatment of adolescent substance abuse: A decision tree method. *American Journal of Drug and Alcohol Abuse, 16,* 1–46.

Tarter, R., & Edwards, K. (1986). Multifactorial etiology of neuropsychological impairment in alcoholics. *Alcoholism: Clinical and Experimental Research, 10,* 128–135.

Tarter, R., Ott, P., & Mezzich, A. (1991). Psychometric assessment in drug abuse. In R. Frances & S. Miller (Eds.), *The clinical textbook of addictive disorders.* New York: Guilford Press.

Tarter, R., & Ryan, C. (1983). Neuropsychology of alcoholism: Etiology, phenomenology, process and outcome. In M. Galanter (Ed.), *Recent developments in alcoholism* (pp. 449–469). New York: Plenum.

Tarter, R., Switala, J., Lu, S., & Van Thiel, D. (in press). Abstracting capacity in cirrhotic alcoholics. *Journal of Studies on Alcohol.*

Tarter, R., Van Thiel, D., & Edwards, K. (Eds.). (1988). *Medical neuropsychology: The impact of disease on behavior.* New York: Plenum.

Tarter, R., Van Thiel, D., & Moss, H. (1988). Impact of cirrhosis on the neuropsychologic test performance of alcoholics. *Alcoholism: Clinical and Experimental Research, 12*, 619–621.

Thurstone, L. (1936). The factorial isolation of primary abilities. *Psychometrika, 1*, 175–182.

Vitiello, M., Prinz, P., Personius, J., Nuccio, M., Koerker, R., & Scurfield, R. (1990). Nighttime hypoxemia is increased in abstaining chronic alcoholic men. *Alcoholism: Clinical and Experimental Research, 14*, 38–41.

Vogel-Sprott, M., & Barrett, P. (1984). Age, drinking habits and the effects of alcohol. *Journal of Studies on Alcohol, 45*, 517–521.

Walker, D., Hunter, B., & Abraham, W. (1981). Neuroanatomical and functional deficits subsequent to chronic ethanol administration in animals. *Alcoholism: Clinical and Experimental Research, 5*, 267–282.

Wilkinson, D. (1987). CT scans and neuropsychological assessments of alcoholism. In O. Parsons, N. Butters, P. Nathan (Eds.), *Neuropsychology of alcoholism* (pp. 76–102). New York: Plenum.

7

Alcohol, Aging, and Genetics

DEBRA A. HELLER AND GERALD E. McCLERN

Studies spanning several decades have left little doubt that genetic factors play at least some role in alcohol-related behaviors, and the heredity of human alcoholism has been the subject of intensive research (for reviews, see Cotton, 1979; Devor & Cloninger, 1989). Much of this research has involved twin, family, and adoption studies. For example, adoption studies have found that biological first-degree relatives of alcoholics have a fourfold increased risk of developing alcoholism themselves (Goodwin, 1986). Other lines of evidence have been provided by researchers such as Schuckit (1988, 1991), who has demonstrated that many sons of alcoholics experience decreased reactions to ethanol as compared to controls. Investigations into the heterogeneity in the severity of alcoholism have also implicated genetic factors. Studies of adopted men in the 1970s and 1980s by Cloninger and his colleagues led them to postulate two broad types of alcoholism, which varied in severity, sensitivity to environmental factors, and genetic transmissibility (Cloninger et al., 1981). More recently, research efforts into the genetics of alcoholism have focused on the identification of biochemical pathways and markers, such as the dopamine D_2 receptor, which may be involved in the development of some types of alcoholism (Cloninger, 1991). Although still somewhat controversial, such findings nevertheless provide plausible evidence for potential genetic mechanisms in the development of alcoholism.

Fewer studies have examined genetic contributions to alcohol use in the normal range, as distinct from alcohol abuse and alcoholism. A shift in focus from abuse to use, however, has several important merits. The study of alcohol ingestion, a necessary though insufficient condition for alcoholism, should illuminate at least some aspects of this complex problem. From a methodological standpoint, greater power may be achieved with studies of variation in drinking behavior in the general population, due to the much larger sample sizes that can be attained. Perhaps most important, however, is the increasing interest in the role of alcohol as a cofactor in disease and health, even at low to moderate levels of intake.

A central theme of this book is the consideration of alcohol issues that may be unique to the elderly. Some of these considerations include alterations in pharmacokinetics, pharmacodynamics, and increased health consequences that may accompany alcohol use in the elderly. Although alcohol use and abuse in elderly groups have been examined epidemiologically and clinically, very few investigations have looked at genetic factors.

Consideration of developmental processes may yield a useful orientation from which to examine issues relating to genetics, alcohol, and aging. Alcoholism itself is a clear example of a developmental condition, and much research has concerned the factors that operate before and during the period of peak risk to determine or influence its onset. Developmental forces in the broad sense, meaning forces that influence change from one age to another, are not, of course, restricted to early life, but can operate throughout the lifespan. A developmental view of this sort may be valuable in exploring variability in alcohol-related issues in advanced age.

The goals of this chapter are:

1. To provide a theoretical framework from which to examine genetic and environmental influences on alcohol-related behaviors, problems, and processes from a developmental perspective
2. To summarize briefly research done to date in this area
3. To present some of our own recent findings from the Swedish Adoption/Twin Study of Aging (SATSA)

A THEORETICAL FRAMEWORK

A basic, although oversimplified, representation of the causal matrix through which genes act upon complex phenotypes is given in Figure 7.1. Genes are denoted by pairs of double helices, representing stretches of DNA, at the left of the figure. The genetic information encoded by the nucleotide sequences in the DNA molecules is transcribed

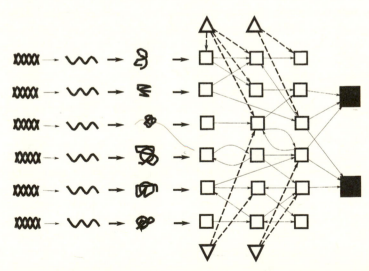

Figure 7.1. Representation of a causal matrix through which genetic and environmental factors may act upon complex phenotypes. DNA is transcribed into RNA, which is translated into polypeptides and proteins. Actions and interactions involving polypeptides give rise to physiological functions and structures, shown as open boxes. Interrelationships among these functions and structures lead to complex phenotypes, represented as black boxes at the right of the figure. Environmental factors, shown as triangles, also enter into the causal nexus, and complex control mechanisms may be present at any level.

into corresponding segments of ribonucleic acid (RNA). The RNA is in turn translated, by complex cellular mechanisms, into amino acids which, when joined together, form polypeptides and proteins, shown in Figure 7.1 as globular, coiled structures. The sequence of events (DNA–RNA–protein) was designated by Francis Crick (1970) as the "Central Dogma" of molecular biology and is in fact the foundation for all life processes.

The polypeptides formed by transcription and translation constitute the array of structural, transport, and catalytic proteins of the body. Their actions and interactions give rise to the anatomical, biochemical, and physiological properties (represented by open boxes in Figure 7.1) of the organism. The interrelationships among these structures and functions may be extremely complicated, with such control features of complex systems as feedback inhibition, feedback activation, etc. Ultimately, this intricate causal nexus gives rise to complex phenotypes, here represented by the black boxes at the right of the figure.

Several points may be drawn from this representation. First, a given gene may have widespread effects, through processes in which its primary products, the polypeptides, participate. This phenomenon is termed *pleiotropy*. Second, a given phenotype may be influenced by many genes; this phenomenon may be labeled *polygeny*, or *multigenic inheritance*. Third, there are no genes "for" a complex trait; genes code for polypeptides that enter into the processes of the organism; these processes eventually culminate in the phenotype of interest. Fourth, the complexities of the causal nexus will lead to correlations of varying magnitude among the differing phenotypes, due to shared pathways of influence originating at the level of the genes. Finally, it will be apparent that what is called a phenotype is an arbitrary matter. Each of the elements of Figure 7.1 may constitute a phenotype of interest, depending on the purpose of the study. For example, a molecular geneticist could be interested in the polypeptide as the phenotype, a physiologist may be interested in metabolic products or organ functions, and a quantitative geneticist may focus on a complex, continuously distributed phenotype quite distant from the effects of any of its contributory genes.

The model may also be extended to include the effects of environmental factors, designated by triangles in Figure 7.1. These environmental variables may impinge on the same causal pathways that mediate the influence of the genes. The term *environment* has a sweeping definition in this context: Environment is anything that is not coded in the DNA. Everything from the cytoplasmic gradients of the fertilized egg to peer group influences is included in the environmental domain. There are also environmental analogs of pleiotropy and polygeny: Multiple effects may arise from a single environmental factor, and multiple environment factors may work together to influence a single phenotype.

Figure 7.1 is essentially a cross-sectional depiction of genetic and environmental influences occurring at one point of time. In this sense, it is only a "snapshot" of the complex pathways influencing a phenotype. Of course, genetic and environmental factors are not static forces, but rather may be expected to change over time. Figure 7.2 attempts to put such a dynamic network into perspective.

It is undeniable that environmental forces come and go throughout our lives; the case is not so obvious, however, with respect to genetic factors. After all, one's full complement of genes is present at conception. However, while the full genomic complement may be present in all cells, only a limited subset will be operational. Both liver cells

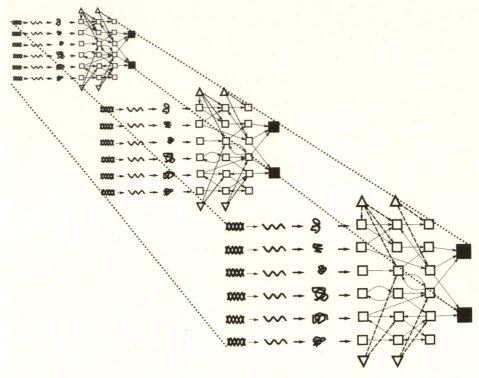

Figure 7.2. Extension of the causal matrix shown in Figure 7.1 to a dynamic perspective, illustrating that genetic and environmental influences may change over time.

and brain cells, for example, may share a number of active genes in common (the "housekeeping" genes required for all cellular function), but will differ in subsets of active genes pertinent to the specific organ functions of liver and brain. Furthermore, different genes may function in a particular organ or system at different times. Hence the effective genotype of the same individual's liver cells may be different at different times. Genes may be turned on or off and may interact in changing ways with environmental influences. Similarly, environmental factors may have differing onsets and offsets. It is probably most useful to think of differing onsets and differing durations, because both genetic and environmental factors may have a brief presence but lasting influence through structures or functions that persist once established.

QUANTITATIVE GENETIC THEORY

Figures 7.1 and 7.2 illustrate that genetic and environmental factors both contribute to phenotypes. Quantitative genetic methods can be used to estimate the relative importance of various genetic and environmental influences. Quantitative genetic theory may be regarded as an extension of the laws of Mendelian inheritance to the polygenic case. The theoretical basis for quantitative genetic analysis was established by geneticists such as Ronald Fisher, Sewall Wright, and J.B.S. Haldane in the 1920s and 1930s. A primary contemporary source is provided by Falconer (1989). Although space does not permit an extensive elaboration of quantitative genetic theory, a brief summary of quantitative genetic terminology is presented.

Using notation described in Falconer (1989), an individual's phenotype, P, is determined by the effects of both genotype, G, and the environment, E, which includes all nongenetic effects (Equation 1).

$$P = G + E \qquad \text{[Equation 1]}$$

It is only by considering population variability, however, that the relative magnitude of these components may be estimated. Quantitative genetic analyses, then, have as their goal the decomposition of phenotypic variance into genetic and environmental sources (Equation 2).

$$V_P = V_G + V_E \qquad \text{[Equation 2]}$$

The genetic portion of the phenotypic variance can be divided into two types of genetic variance: additive and nonadditive. Additive genetic variance, V_A, is the portion of variance due to many genes that act together additively. Nonadditive genetic variance, V_D, reflects the effects of dominance (interactions within gene loci) and epistasis (interactions between loci). For many purposes, however, we shall not differentiate between V_A and V_D, but shall instead consider them together as V_G.

The environmental variance, V_E, can also be partitioned further, into common, or shared environmental effects (environmental influences shared by individuals, such as relatives), and nonshared environmental effects, which are unique to individuals.

The relative importance of genetic contributions to a phenotype is expressed as *heritability* (often abbreviated as h^2), which can be broadly defined as the proportion of population variation attributable to genetic variance (V_G/V_P). It is important to note that heritability is a feature of populations, not individuals. For example, if the heritability for some trait, such as alcohol consumption, is reported as 0.40, we may conclude that 40% of the population variability for that trait is due to genetic variation. We cannot, however, conclude that 40% of an individual's consumption is due to his or her genotype, and the remainder due to the environment!

The genetic and environmental components of variance are estimated by examining familial resemblance for relatives differing in their degree of relatedness. For example, first-degree relatives, such as parents and offspring or siblings, share on average 50% of their additive genetic variance, V_A. Second-degree relatives, such as half-siblings, aunt-uncle/niece-nephew relations, and grandparents with grandchildren, share only 25% of V_A, and so on. Environmental effects may also contribute substantially to familial resemblance.

Twins are of special interest. Monozygotic (MZ), or identical, twins are genetically identical and share all of their genetic variance. Dizygotic (DZ), or fraternal twins, in contrast, are genetically no more alike than siblings and therefore share on average only 50% of their segregating genes. The twin intraclass correlation, t, reflects the degree to which co-twins resemble one another. A traditional method of estimating heritability is to compare intraclass correlations between MZ and DZ twins. Doubling the difference between t_{MZ} and t_{DZ} yields a classic estimate of heritability.

Keeping the theoretical framework of quantitative genetic theory in mind, we can now turn our attention to some of the previous research that has examined genetic influences on alcohol-related behaviors.

PREVIOUS INVESTIGATIONS OF ALCOHOL-RELATED PHENOTYPES

Although many studies over the last half-century or so have attempted to clarify the role of familial components in alcoholism, fewer studies have examined the genetic and environmental contributions to normal drinking variability. Some of these studies are listed in Table 7.1 and will be discussed briefly here. For a more extensive review, see Heath (1994).

Table 7.1. Heritability for Alcohol Use in Selected Twin and Family Studies

Reference	Study Sample	Estimated Heritability
Partanen et al., 1966	Finnish twins Age: 28–37	0.27–0.39
Medlund et al., 1977 (reanalyzed by Heath, 1994)	Swedish Twin Registry Age: 16–47	0.34
Clifford et al., 1981, 1984	London Twin-Family Survey Age: 18–70+	0.27–0.40
Swan et al., 1990	NAS-NRC Veteran Twin Registry Age: 52–66	0.43–0.60
Carmelli et al., 1993	NAS-NRC Veteran Twin Registry 1st Survey 1967–69 16-year followup in 1983–85	Baseline 0.21–0.33 Followup 0.23–0.48
de Castro, 1993	Minnesota Twin Registry Average age: 38	0.50
Kaprio et al., 1981	Finnish Twin Registry Age: 18–60+	0.51
Kaprio et al., 1981	Finnish Twin Registry, 1975 Survey 1932–50 cohort = age 25–43 1951–57 cohort = 18–24	Men 0.28, women 0.41 Men 0.57, women 0.42
Kaprio et al., 1987, 1991	Finnish Twin Registry, 1981 Survey 1932–50 cohort = age 31–49 1951–57 cohort = age 24–30	Men 0.20, women 0.17 Men 0.71, women 0.72
Jardine & Martin, 1984	Australian National Health and Medical Research Council Twin Survey Age: 18–88	Males 0.36 Females 0.55
Tambs & Vaglum, 1990	Norwegian spouses and their children aged 18 and older	Upper limit 0.44

An Important Resource—The Nordic Twin Registries

Inspection of Table 7.1 reveals that many of the studies examining genetic influence on alcohol use have come from Sweden, Norway, and Finland. A primary reason is the existence of large population-based twin registries in these countries. The Nordic countries have a long tradition, dating back several centuries, of population registration. Historically, births, marriages, and deaths were registered in local parishes and reported to the authorities (Kaprio et al., 1990). Beginning in the 1960s, these records were used to form national twin registries in Sweden, Norway, Denmark, and Finland. Although there is variation from country to country, the registries generally include information on all twins born in the late 1800s up to today (Schwartz et al., 1986).

These databases have great value for research purposes, for several reasons. One is sheer size—each national registry contains information on many thousands of twin pairs, so far greater statistical power and flexibility in research design are possible than for other types of studies. Another key feature is the representativeness of these samples, which are population-based, in contrast to twin panels, which are often volunteer-based and may not be representative of the general population.

Although their analyses predated the actual formation of the Finnish Twin Registry, the work by Partanen et al. (1966) was a major contribution to the study of genetic variability in alcohol use. They examined 902 male twins, aged 28 to 37, and found that alcohol consumption in the normal range, as well as abstinence and heavy use, showed significant heritability. Overall heritability estimates for quantity and frequency of alcohol consumed were in the range of 0.36 to 0.39, indicating that 36 to 39 percent of the population variability was due to genetic variability. Similarly, an investigation of the Swedish Twin Registry by Medlund et al. (1977) (reanalyzed by Heath, 1994) estimated h^2 to be 0.34. More recently, a great deal of work has been done by Kaprio and his colleagues using data from the Finnish Twin Registry (Kaprio et al., 1981, 1987, 1991). Some of their findings are summarized in Table 7.1; overall estimates of h^2 for alcohol quantity and frequency range from 0.20 to 0.51.

Other Twin Studies

In addition to investigations using the Nordic registries, other twin studies have found evidence for substantial genetic influence on alcohol consumption (see Table 7.1).

In England, Clifford et al. (1981) conducted the London Twin-Family Survey, which included twins, siblings, and parents from 572 families, and found $h^2 = 0.37$. Further analysis (Clifford et al., 1984) revealed that cohabitation affected the twin correlations: Twins living together were more similar than twins living apart. Another major twin study was the Australian National Health and Medical Research Council Twin Surveys (Jardine & Martin, 1984; Heath & Martin, 1988; Heath et al., 1991; Heath, 1994). These studies have found substantial heritability for alcohol abstinence and alcohol consumption, with heritability estimates as high as 61%, depending on the subsample examined.

Most twin and family studies of alcohol use have been conducted on relatively young subjects, often in their twenties and thirties. Exceptions, however, include several studies of U.S. veterans using the NAS-NRC Twin Registry of male veteran twins (Carmelli et al., 1990, 1993; Swan et al., 1990). Although the subjects in these studies were significantly older than some of the others listed in Table 7.1, heritability estimates were still substantial. For example, Swan et al. (1990), using data from the second exam of the NHLBI Twin Study, found heritability for alcohol use in the range of 43 to 60%.

The general consensus of the studies summarized in Table 7.1 is that there is substantial genetic influence on drinking behaviors, and that genetic variability accounts for one- to two-thirds of the total population variation in alcohol consumption.

Age Differences in Genetic Factors Affecting Alcohol Use

Investigations into the genetics of alcoholism have suggested age-related heterogeneity in inheritance. Prima facie evidence for age-related heterogeneity in genetic factors has been provided by studies such as that by Atkinson et al. (1990), who found that alcoholics who experienced onset late in life (over age 60) as a group reported much less family alcoholism. Other reports have shown that familial alcoholism tends to have an early onset and a severe course (Cloninger et al., 1981). A twin study by McGue et al. (1992), using DSM-III criteria for alcohol abuse and dependence, found that, for men, heritability was higher for early-onset versus late-onset alcoholism. They concluded that genetic influences may be most substantial for early-onset male alcoholism. Results from other studies of alcoholism have not been as clear. One study found that although twin correlations in males decreased with age of onset, these decreases were equal in MZ and DZ twins, suggesting that genetic factors were not associated with the age differences (Pickens et al., 1991).

Most studies of alcohol use, such as those listed in Table 7.1, have not considered age differences in heritability. A few studies have included age comparisons, though, and these will be briefly discussed here. Tentative evidence for age heterogeneity was provided by Partanen et al. (1966), although this Finnish sample was relatively young, including only male twins aged 28 to 37. Within this age range, however, the authors found consistently higher heritability in younger than older twins when 1-year increments were used. The Finnish twin sample of Kaprio et al. (1981) had a greater age range (18 to 60+). When these investigators evaluated heritability for alcohol use by decade, they found relatively constant heritabilities for age groups from 18 to 59 (ranging from 0.48 to 0.65), but in the oldest group (over age 60), heritability was near zero. In a later study, Kaprio et al. (1991) found apparent differences in heritability between those under and over age 30. Similarly, in their Australian sample, Jardine and Martin (1984) found that for males, heritability was much higher in the group aged 18 to 30 than in the group over age 30.

It is difficult to reconcile and draw conclusions from these studies, which differ in their measures of alcohol use, statistical treatment of abstainers, and age range of subjects. A further confounding variable is that it is difficult to disentangle cohort effects from developmental effects. Many studies have demonstrated that sociocultural factors have an impact on alcohol use. Some of these factors can also affect familial similarity, as well as age differences, for drinking behaviors. For example, Reich et al. (1988) have demonstrated that significant secular trends in the familial transmission of alcoholism have occurred in the United States in recent decades. They found that younger cohorts have earlier ages of onset than older cohorts, and that familial transmissibility is greater in younger cohorts. Cultural as well as genetic modes of inheritance are included in the familial parameters in these models. It is clear that the increases in familial transmissibility seen are due to cultural, environmental factors, rather than to genetic factors, since the trends have occurred too rapidly to be associated with genetic changes. However, these findings suggest that cohort differences associated with cultural factors must be taken into consideration when evaluating age differences in genetic studies of alcohol use or abuse.

The Role of Common Environment

In the classic twin method, the difference between intraclass correlations for MZ and DZ twins is doubled to estimate heritability. The remaining population variation can then be attributed to environmental factors. These factors may include cultural factors, factors shared by relatives living together, or factors that are unique to individuals. Path-modeling approaches facilitate the division of total phenotypic variance into genetic, shared environmental, and nonshared environmental components. The importance of shared family environment is often indicated when familial similarity is greater than that expected based on biological relatedness alone. For example, path modeling of alcoholism data by Allgulander et al. (1991) estimated heritability to be 0.16, and common environment to be 0.32. Some studies of alcohol use have also quantified the relative importance of common environment. Clifford et al. (1984) found that common environment accounted for 42% of the variation in alcohol use; this was greater than the heritability estimate of 37%. However, other studies, such as an adoption study conducted by Gabrielli and Plomin (1985), found that shared family environment did not contribute significantly to variability in drinking behaviors. More recently, Kaprio et al. (1991) and de Castro (1993) found no evidence for a role of shared family environment in alcohol intake.

A separate line of evidence regarding the importance of family environment was provided by Kaprio et al. (1990), who found that MZ twin similarity increased as a function of cohabitation. Social contact may affect twin similarity for alcohol use in more than one way. For example, both twins may be exposed to similar environmental factors, resulting in similarity for alcohol use. Alternatively, sibling interactions may occur in which one twin's use of alcohol has a direct influence on the drinking behavior of his or her co-twin.

Studies of Twins Reared Apart

One criticism of twin and family studies is that they may overestimate heritability by confounding genetic and environmental factors, in that relatives living together share environments as well as genes. One research design that helps resolve these issues is the study of twins who were separated early in life and reared apart from each other. Although the occurrence and identification of such separations are relatively infrequent, several genetic studies of twins reared apart have been conducted. In the United States, the Minnesota Study of Twins Reared Apart (see Bouchard et al., 1981) has examined alcohol abuse in MZ twins (Grove et al., 1990). Although study designs using DZ as well as MZ twins have greater power than studies of only monozygotic twins, if MZ twins reared apart share no common environment then their correlation may estimate heritability directly. Initial analyses have suggested zero heritability for alcohol-related problems; however, the relatively small sample lacks sufficient statistical power to draw strong conclusions.

Using twins identified through the Finnish Twin Registry, Kaprio et al. (1984) compared 307 pairs of MZ and DZ twins who had been separated before the age of ten. Analyzing men and women separately, they estimated heritability for alcohol consumption to be 0.36 for men and 0.52 for women, while common environment accounted for 33 to 45% of the variance (see Table 7.1).

The Swedish Adoption/Twin Study of Aging (SATSA)

The largest sample of twins reared apart to date is that of the Swedish Adoption/Twin Study of Aging (SATSA). This sample of twins separated early in life was identified through the Swedish Twin Registry and contacted by questionnaire in 1984, along with a sample of matched control twin pairs who had been reared together (Pedersen et al., 1984). The SATSA subregistry is made up of 346 pairs of twins reared apart and 404 pairs of twins reared together. The initial questionnaire included measures of self-reported health, personality, family and work environments, and alcohol, tobacco, and drug use. Longitudinal follow-ups of the sample have been conducted at 3-year intervals (Pedersen et al., 1991).

Because the primary goal of SATSA is to examine individual differences in aging, it provides a unique opportunity to look at issues relating to alcohol, genetics, and aging. For the present analyses, we focused on alcohol quantity-frequency measures from the 1984 questionnaire. This contained a series of questions about quantity and frequency of beer, wine, and liquor consumption. Total monthly ethanol consumption was computed based on these responses, and was log-transformed and corrected for relative body weight.

The mean age of the 1984 questionnaire sample was 58.7 years; the entire age range was 26 to 87, although only about 10% of the sample was under age 40. In order to look at broad group differences here, we divided the sample roughly at the median to form two age groups: those under and over age 60. The median split allows us to consider broad age-group differences while maximizing sample size.

The left portion of Table 7.2 presents the intraclass correlations for the two age groups, by rearing and zygosity group. Both age groups show a pattern of correlations in which MZ twins reared together (MZT) have much higher correlations than MZ

Table 7.2. Analyses of Monthly Ethanol Consumption[a] from the Swedish/Adoption Twin Study of Aging (SATSA) Intraclass Correlations and Modeling Results, by Age Group

	Intraclass Correlations (Controlling for Sex and Age in Years Within Age Group)[b]				Percent Variance Accounted for by Age in Years	Genetic and Environmental Components of Variance (Independent of Age Effects within Group)[c]			
	MZA	MZT	DZA	DZT		Ga	Es	Ec	Ens
Younger (< 60)	0.16	0.47	0.20	0.31	3.2%	18.7%	17.8%	8.3%	55.1%
Older (60+)	0.24	0.50	0.33	0.37	6.0%	11.2%	11.2%	25.4%	52.1%

[a]Log-transformed and corrected for relative weight.

[b]For comparison of intraclass correlations, the mean effects of sex, age in years, and the sex by age interaction were removed in a prior multiple regression analysis.

[c]In the structural equation modeling, the mean effects of sex were first removed in a prior linear regression analysis. The effects of age were directly controlled for within the model after Neale and Martin (1989).

twins reared apart (MZA). DZ twins reared together (DZT) have somewhat higher correlations than DZ twins reared apart (DZA), but the difference is not as great as that seen with the MZ twins. If we were to average across rearing group, it is apparent that the overall MZ correlations would be somewhat higher than the DZ correlations, but this is due largely to the MZT effect.

Path Modeling of Twin Covariances

In order to test the genetic and environmental effects on alcohol consumption, variances and covariances among the twins were subjected to structural-equation modeling with the LISREL 7 program (Jöreskog & Sörbom, 1989). The use of structural-equation models has become standard in twin research (Boomsma et al., 1989, Neale & Cardon, 1992). To control for the effects of age-in-years which may be present within age group, a model that included age effects (Neale & Martin, 1989) was used.

The study of twins reared apart provides a unique opportunity to decompose environmental variance, V_E, into shared and nonshared components, which we designate as V_{ES} and V_{ENS}. The shared rearing environment, E_S, contributes to similarity in twins reared together, but not twins reared apart. Evidence for E_S is obtained if twins reared together are more similar than those reared apart. Nonshared environment, E_{NS}, is by definition the environmental parameter contributing to individual, intrapair differences. Regardless of rearing status or zygosity, members of twin pairs have no covariance for E_{NS}. It is important to note that E_{NS} encompasses anything that is not shared by co-twins: It can include subtle differences in parental treatment and different experiences within the home, as well as unique experiences away from the rearing environment. Some investigators have used Hamlet's famous words ''the slings and arrows of outrageous fortune'' to describe the effects of nonshared environmental effects (Neale & Cardon, 1992). Any residual error variance is also contained within the E_{NS} component.

In some cases twin similarity cannot be explained by either zygosity or rearing status. A third environmental parameter, which we term *correlated environment*, E_C, is defined to absorb this covariance. One potential source of E_C is prenatal influences—before birth, both members of a twin pair may be affected by maternal factors such as nutrition, toxins, and stress. E_C may also be due to similarities in adult life style, such as dietary habits. In twins reared apart, E_C may also reflect similarity of rearing environments due to selective placement.

For these analyses, we did not break down the sample by sex. Since estimates of heritability in twins of the same sex may be biased unless the effects of sex are controlled for (McGue & Bouchard, 1984), multiple regression was used to assess the linear effects of sex, and the residuals were then used for subsequent analyses. The right portion of Table 7.2 summarizes the estimates for the components of variance that were obtained with LISREL modeling. For both age groups, heritability estimates are low in comparison to some other studies: 18.7% for those under age 60, and 11.2% for those over age 60. Shared environmental effects are higher in the younger group (17.8% versus 11.2%), while the effects of correlated environment are higher in the older group (25.4% versus 8.3%). For both age groups, the largest component of variance is that of nonshared environment, which accounts for 52 to 55% of the variance.

In some respects, it is unsatisfying to limit age comparisons to two age groups. Additional age groups would be preferable, but due to sample size considerations, the number of age groups that can be defined in the present study is limited. Therefore, for descriptive purposes, alternative analyses that used moving intervals as a sampling technique were also employed. Moving averages are commonly used in econometric time-series applications to study temporal trends and to correct for seasonal variations. Borrowing this concept, the SATSA sample was divided into overlapping age bands in order to study multiple age groups while preserving sample size. Structural equation modeling was performed for each age band. The significance of parameter estimates across the age bands cannot be evaluated since the age bands are not independent; however, the moving interval analyses are useful for descriptive purposes as a means of examining age trends.

Figures 7.3 and 7.4 illustrate the moving-interval analysis results for men and women separately.

A somewhat different picture emerges from that seen in Table 7.2. Figures 7.3 and 7.4 suggest that the components of variance across the age range are different in men and women. Genetic factors appear to be most salient for women, with no clear age gradient in heritability. For men, genetic factors appear sporadically (around age 55 and again around age 79); given the sample sizes involved, these should not be overinterpreted. For both women and men, shared environmental factors in the form of E_S and E_C appear to be present over the entire age range, although at some ages, especially for women, E_C appears to be greater than E_S.

Many other studies have suggested that there are large sex differences in alcohol-related behaviors. Although most genetic studies of alcoholism have been on men, several studies have suggested that genetic factors are less important in the development

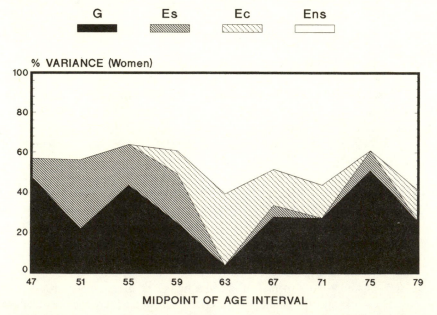

Figure 7.3. Genetic and environmental components of variance for alcohol consumption, based on moving-interval analyses across age, for women. G = genetic variance, Es = shared environmental effects, Ec = correlated environmental effects, Ens = nonshared environmental effects. (Source: The Swedish Adoption/Twin Study of Aging.)

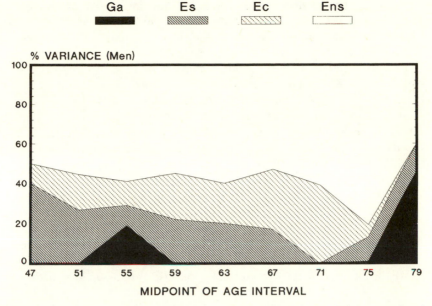

Figure 7.4. Genetic and environmental components of variance for alcohol consumption, based on moving-interval analyses across age, for men. G = genetic variance, Es = shared environmental effects, Ec = correlated environmental effects, Ens = nonshared environmental effects. (Source: The Swedish Adoption/Twin Study of Aging.)

of alcoholism for women than men (Pickens et al., 1991). However, Kendler et al. (1992) recently conducted a population-based twin study of alcoholism in women and concluded that genetic factors play a major factor in the development of alcoholism in women as well as in men.

Other Factors Affecting Heritability Estimates

The heritability estimates from SATSA reported here are somewhat lower than those found in most other studies (see Table 7.1). Several factors should be taken into consideration. One is that this sample is older than those of many other genetic studies. When Kaprio et al. (1981) evaluated heritability in different age groups, they found that heritability was near zero in the age group over age 60. Although some other studies have included adults in their fifties and sixties (e.g., Carmelli et al., 1990, 1993; Swan et al., 1990), the SATSA age range is greater, with significant numbers of individuals in their seventies and eighties. It is possible that heritability for alcohol use declines with age. However, it is important to keep in mind that the findings reported here are cross-sectional and may reflect cohort differences rather than age-related changes. Without longitudinal data, it is impossible to make inferences regarding changes in heritability. Other studies have suggested that there are strong sociocultural and cohort effects on genetic studies for drinking behaviors. There may be cultural effects specific to this Swedish cohort that are reflected in the heritability estimates.

The pattern of correlations apparent in Table 7.2 suggests that there may be sibling interactions present, as well. Gurling et al. (1985), for example, have discussed ''mutual effects" that may be operative within twin pairs. These interactions may include conforming effects in MZ twins reared together, making them more similar, and competition effects in DZ twins reared together, making them dissimilar. Our observed pattern of correlations suggests that such influences may have affected the SATSA sample. An important assumption of the twin method is that MZ and DZ twins experience equal environments. If MZ co-twins interact with each other differently than do DZ co-twins, this constitutes a violation of the equal environments assumption.

Assortative mating can also have an impact on familial correlations and estimates of heritability. It has been suggested that heritability estimates from twin studies may be deflated if the effects of assortative mating for alcohol use are not considered (Tambs et al., 1990). Several studies (Price & Vandenberg, 1980; Tambs et al., 1990) have found that spouse correlations for alcohol consumption increase with years of marriage, suggesting that spouses become similar to each other over time. Other researchers, however, have found that spouse correlations are due more to assortative mating than to convergence of habits after marriage (Hall et al., 1983). It is clear that assortative mating, if present, can influence estimates of both genetic and shared environmental transmission. Research designs that include information on family members, as well as twins, may help to resolve problems related to the effects of assortative mating.

CONCLUSIONS

The results of the studies reviewed in this chapter suggest that genetic factors are important in variation in levels of alcohol consumption, as well as in the development of alcoholism itself. Relatively few studies, however, have evaluated age-related differences or changes in the genetic and environmental framework involved in drinking behaviors. Some studies, such as those from the Finnish Twin Registry and the Swedish Adoption/Twin Study of Aging, have reported much lower heritability estimates in the elderly, in comparison with many other studies of younger individuals. However, it is difficult to disentangle sociocultural and cohort differences from true aging and developmental effects. It is likely that further research efforts focusing on longitudinal follow-ups of twin and family samples across different cultural settings will help to clarify these issues.

References

Allgulander, C., Nowak, J. & Rice, J. P. (1991). Psychopathology and treatment of 30,344 twins in Sweden. II. Heritability estimates of psychiatric diagnosis and treatment in 12,884 twin pairs. *Acta Psychiatric Scandinavica, 83*, 12–15.

Atkinson, R. M., Tolson, R. L. & Turner, J. A. (1990). Late versus early onset problem drinking in older men. *Alcoholism: Clinical and Experimental Research, 14*, 574–579.

Boomsma, D. I., Martin, N. G., & Neale, M. C., (Eds.). (1989). Genetic analysis of twin and family data: Structural modeling using LISREL. *Behavior Genetics*, (special issue), *19(1)*.

Bouchard, T. J., Heston, L., Eckert, E., Keyes, M., & Resnick, S. (1981). The Minnesota study of twins reared apart: Project description and sample results in the developmental domain. *Progress in Clinical and Biological Research, 69* Part B, 227–233.

Carmelli, D., Swan, G. E., Robinette, D., & Fabsitz, R. R. (1990). Heritability of substance use in the NAS-NRC twin registry. *Acta Geneticae Medicae et Gemellologiae, 39*, 91–98.

Carmelli, D., Heath, A. C., & Robinette, D. (1993). Genetic analysis of drinking behavior in World War II veteran twins. *Genetic Epidemiology, 10*, 201–213.

Clifford, C. A., Fulker, D. W., Gurling, H. M. D., & Murray, R. M. (1981). Preliminary findings from a twin study of alcohol use. In L. Gedda, P. Parisi, & W. E. Nance (Eds.) *Twin research 3: Epidemiological and clinical studies* (pp. 47–52). Alan R. Liss: New York.

Clifford, C. A., Hopper, J. L., Fulker, D. W., & Murray, R. M. (1984). A genetic and environmental analysis of a twin family study of alcohol use, anxiety, and depression. *Genetic Epidemiology, 1*, 63–79.

Cloninger, C. R., Bohman, M., & Sigvardsson, S. (1981). Inheritance of alcohol abuse: Cross-fostering analysis of adopted men. *Archives of General Psychiatry, 38*, 861–868.

Cloninger, C. R. (1991). D_2 dopamine receptor gene is associated but not linked with alcoholism. *Journal of the American Medical Association, 266*, 1833–1834.

Cotton, N. S. (1979). The familial incidence of alcoholism: A review. *Journal of Studies on Alcohol, 40*(1), 89–116.

Crick, F. (1970). Central dogma of molecular biology. *Nature, 227*(258), 561–563.

de Castro, J. M. (1993). Genetic influences on daily intake and meal patterns of humans. *Physiology and Behavior, 53*, 777–782.

Devor, E. J., & Cloninger, C. R. (1989). Genetics of alcoholism. *Annual Review of Genetics, 23*, 19–36.

Falconer, D. S. (1989). *Introduction to quantitative genetics* (3rd ed.). Essex: Longman Scientific and Technical.

Gabrielli, W. F., & Plomin, R. (1985). Drinking behavior in the Colorado Adoptee and Twin Sample. *Journal of Studies on Alcohol, 46*, 24–31.

Goodwin, D. W. (1986). Genetic factors in the development of alcoholism. *Psychiatric Clinics of North America, 9*, 427–433.

Grove, W. M., Eckert, E. D., Heston, L., Bouchard, T. J., Segal, N., & Lykken, D. T. (1990). Heritability of substance abuse and antisocial behavior: A study of monozygotic twins reared apart. *Biological Psychiatry, 27*, 1293–1304.

Gurling, H. M. D., Grant, S., & Dangl, J. (1985). The genetic and cultural transmission of alcohol use, alcoholism, cigarette smoking and coffee drinking: A review and an example using a log linear cultural transmission model. *British Journal of Addiction, 80*, 269–279.

Hall, R. L., Hesselbrock, V. M., & Stabenau, J. R. (1983). Familial distribution of alcohol use: II. Assortative mating of alcoholic probands. *Behavior Genetics, 13*, 373–382.

Heath, A. C., & Martin, N. G. (1988). Teenage alcohol use in the Australian Twin Register: Genetic and social determinants of starting to drink. *Alcoholism: Clinical and Experimental Research, 12*, 735–741.

Heath, A. C., Meyer, J., Jardine, R., & Martin, N. G. (1991). The inheritance of alcohol consumption patterns in a general population twin sample: II. Determinants of consumption frequency and quantity consumed. *Journal of Studies on Alcohol, 52*, 425–433.

Heath, A. C. (1994). Genetic influences on drinking behavior in humans. In H. Begleiter, & B. Kissin (Eds.). *Alcohol and alcoholism. Vol. 1, Genetic factors and alcoholism.* Oxford: Oxford University Press.

Jardine, R., & Martin, N. G. (1984). Causes of variation in drinking habits in a large twin sample. *Acta Geneticae Medicae et Gemellologiae, 33*, 435–450.

Jöreskog, K. G., & Sörbom, D. (1989). *LISREL 7: A guide to the program and applications* (2nd ed.). Chicago: SP55.

Kaprio, J., Koskenvuo, M., & Sarna, S. (1981). Cigarette smoking, use of alcohol, and leisure-time physical activity among same-sexed adult male twins. In *Twin research 3: Epidemiological and clinical studies* (pp. 37–46). New York, Alan R. Liss.

Kaprio, J., Koskenvuo, M., & Langinvainio, H. (1984). Finnish twins reared apart. IV: Smoking and drinking habits. A preliminary analysis of the effect of heredity and environment. *Acta Geneticae Medicae et Gemellologiae, 33*, 425–433.

Kaprio, J. K., Koskenvuo, M., Langinvainio, H., Romanov, K., Sarna, S. & Rose, R. J. (1987). Genetic influences on use and abuse of alcohol: A study of 5638 adult Finnish twin brothers. *Alcoholism: Clinical and Experimental Research, 11*, 349–356.

Kaprio, J., Koskenvuo, M., & Rose, R. J. (1990). Change in cohabitation and intrapair similarity of monozygotic (MZ) cotwins for alcohol use, extraversion, and neuroticism. *Behavior Genetics, 20*, 265–276.

Kaprio, J., Rose, R. J., Romanov, K., & Koskenvuo, M. (1991). Genetic and environmental determinants of use and abuse of alcohol: The Finnish Twin Cohort Studies. *Alcohol and Alcoholism*, Suppl 1, 131–136.

Kendler, K. S., Heath, A. C., Neale, M. C., Kessler, R. C., & Eaves, L. J. (1992). A population-based twin study of alcoholism in women. *Journal of the American Medical Association, 268*, 1877–1882.

Medlund, P., Cederlöf, R., Floderus-Myrhed, B., Friberg, L., & Sörensen, S. (1977). A new Swedish twin registry. *Acta Medica Scandinavica*, Suppl. 600.

McGue, M., & Bouchard, T. J. (1984). Adjustment of twin data for the effects of age and sex. *Behavior Genetics, 14*, 325–343.

McGue, M., Pickens, R. W., & Svikis, D. S. (1992). Sex and age effects on the inheritance of alcohol problems: A twin study. *Journal of Abnormal Psychology, 101*, 3–17.

Neale, M. C., & Cardon, L. R. (1992). *Methodology for genetic studies of twins and families*. Dordrecht, the Netherlands: Kluwer Academic Publishers.

Neale, M. C., & Martin, N. G. (1989). The effects of age, sex, and genotype on self-report drunkenness following a challenge dose of alcohol. *Behavior Genetics, 19*, 63–78.

Partanen, J., Bruun, K., & Markkanen, T. (1966). Inheritance of drinking behavior: A study of intelligence, personality, and use of alcohol of adult twins. Helsinki: Finnish Foundation for Alcoholic Studies.

Pedersen, N. L., Friberg, L., Floderus-Myrhed, B., McClearn, G. E., & Plomin, R. (1984). Swedish early separated twins: Identification and characterization. *Acta Geneticae Medicae et Gemellologiae, 33*, 243–250.

Pedersen, N. L., McClearn, G. E., Plomin, R., Nesselroade, J. R., Berg, S., & de Faire, U. (1991). The Swedish Adoption/Twin Study of Aging: An update. *Acta Geneticae Medicae et Gemellologiae, 40*, 7–20.

Pickens, R. W., Svikis, D. S., McGue, M., Lykken, D. T., Heston, L. L., & Clayton, P. J. (1991). Heterogeneity in the inheritance of alcoholism. *Archives of General Psychiatry, 48*, 19–28.

Price, R. A., & Vandenberg, S. G. (1980). Spouse similarity in American and Swedish couples. *Behavior Genetics, 10*, 59–71.

Reich, T., Cloninger, C. R., Van Eerdewegh, P., Rice, J. P., & Mullaney, J. (1988). Secular trends in the familial transmission of alcoholism. *Alcoholism: Clinical and Experimental Research, 12*, 458–464.

Schuckit, M. A. (1988). Reactions to alcohol in sons of alcoholics and controls. *Alcoholism: Clinical and Experimental Research, 12*, 465–469.

Schuckit, M. A. (1991). A 10-year followup of sons of alcoholics: Preliminary results. *Alcohol and Alcoholism*, Suppl. 1, 147–149.

Schwartz, R. M., Keith, L. G., & Keith, D. M. (1986). The Nordic contribution to the English language twin literature. *Acta Obstetrica et Gynecologica Scandinavica, 65*, 599–604.

Swan, G. E., Carmelli, D., Rosenman, R. H., Fabsitz, R. R., & Christian, J. C. (1990). Smoking and alcohol consumption in adult male twins: Genetic heritability and shared environmental influences. *Journal of Substance Abuse, 2*, 39–50.

Tambs, K., & Vaglum, P. (1990). Alcohol consumption of parents and offspring: A study of the family correlation structure in a general population. *Acta Psychiatrica Scandinavica, 82*, 145–151.

II

BIOLOGY AND BIOCHEMISTRY

8

Ethanol Metabolism and Intoxication in the Elderly

THOMAS P. BERESFORD
AND MICHAEL R. LUCEY

There is increasing evidence to suggest that the pharmacokinetic and pharmacodynamic effects of ethanol may differ among elderly as compared to younger persons. Epidemiological surveys, for example, note that absolute amounts of alcohol drunk decrease with age for light and moderate as well as for heavy drinkers (Mishara & Kastenbaum, 1980; Nordstrom & Berglund, 1987). At the same time, however, other studies note that significant numbers of elderly begin abusive drinking after age 60 and that the absolute numbers of abusive and dependent drinkers will continue to increase in this fastest growing segment of the U.S. population (Atkinson, 1990). The two existing studies of the differential effects of a standard ethanol dose among persons of different age indicate that elderly persons may be more sensitive to ethanol that their younger counterparts (Vogel-Sprott & Barrett, 1984; Jones & Neri, 1985). Another more recent study found that older subjects performed significantly worse in driving simulation than did younger subjects at the same alcohol dose (Roehrs et al., 1992).

Yet, despite the convergence of two large public health problems—alcohol use and aging—little research has been done to elucidate the metabolic and pharmacodynamic effects of ethanol among elderly subjects. Vestal and colleagues (1977) first studied the relationship of aging with the distribution and elimination of ethanol in a group of 50 healthy nonalcoholic subjects, ranging in age from 21 to 81 years, who were given a continuous 1-hour infusion of ethanol in a dose of 0.57 gm/kg body weight. Serial blood ethanol levels were taken and the values were plotted in standard metabolic curves. These data were then assessed using tests of statistical correlation against the age spectrum of their study subjects. While age had no effect on observed rates of ethanol elimination, peak ethanol concentration in blood at the end of the infusion period correlated directly with age ($r = 0.55$, $p < .001$). From this, they concluded that a smaller volume of distribution, associated with characteristically decreased lean body mass among their elderly subjects, explained the higher peak ethanol concentrations. They did not report intoxication testing in their study nor did they investigate the effects of feeding.

Vogel-Sprott and Barrett (1984) studied a sample of 41 male social drinkers aged 19 to 63. Their subjects performed balance beam and bead-stringing tasks after receiving a single dose of 0.57 g/kg of ethanol served in divided doses 20 minutes apart and taken after a 4-hour fast. All subjects were given the same dose without adjustment for age. On average, this dose resulted in a peak level of 0.69 ± 6.8 mg/dL for all 41 subjects; the data were not reported by age except to say, echoing Vestal, that older subjects had proportionately less body water and therefore obtained higher blood alcohol levels. When individual differences in peak blood alcohol level were controlled statistically, alcohol-induced impairment in task performance increased during peak exposure in association with age in this nonstratified sample. From these data the authors concluded that a reduction in the volume of distribution for alcohol and "an intensified behavioral effect" of alcohol, that is, a postulated increase in sensitivity to ethanol, may operate jointly to cause older nonalcoholic persons to reduce the doses of alcohol drunk on social occasions. Interestingly, however, they noted that an index used to estimate the proportion of body water accounted for only 25% of the variance in peak blood ethanol levels. There was no analysis of area under the metabolic curve (AUC) and, since peak blood alcohol levels may not reflect the actual magnitude of difference in ethanol exposure between the young and the elderly, these data must be regarded as preliminary. At the same time, there was no age stratification and therefore the sample size was inadequate to allow analysis of stratified age cohorts.

Jones and Neri (1985) studied four groups of healthy men in their twenties, thirties, forties, and fifties (N = 12 per group). After a 12-hour fast, each of the subjects drank 0.68 g/kg ethanol within 20 minutes and each was asked to estimate feelings of intoxication on a 10-point scale. In their sample, the distribution volume of ethanol per kg body weight decreased by only 8%, comparing subjects in their twenties with those in their fifties. They concluded that age was associated with increased feelings of intoxication at the set dose. They did not administer performance tasks, nor did they investigate the effects of feeding on ethanol kinetics. They did not include subjects over 60, nor did they adjust the ethanol dose in relation to age.

While these early studies piqued interest in metabolic and pharmacodynamic issues related to age, they raised more questions than they answered. Contrasting data from Vestal and colleagues against that from Jones and Neri raises questions of the clinical importance of distribution volume and ethanol dilution, for example. Since ethanol must be absorbed through the gastrointestinal tract, putative differences in absorption might have accounted for some of the peak level differences between young and old subjects. Data published subsequently on young subjects (Frezza et al. 1990) suggested possible gender differences in which nonalcoholic women were thought to absorb more alcohol than nonalcoholic men given the same dose. This study introduced administration route as a variable when it compared areas under the metabolic curve (AUC) in intravenous (IV) and oral (PO) doses of ethanol given to the same subject. Finally, with respect to intoxication effects, each of the three previous studies gave doses of alcohol that might be considered substantial for elderly but not for youthful subjects.

AGE AND ETHANOL METABOLISM

With these concerns in mind, we studied the combined effect of age and gender on blood ethanol given orally and intravenously to healthy nonalcoholic volunteers. We used a stratified sample of young and old subjects representing both genders. All of the subjects were screened for illness or surgical conditions that might affect absorption through slowed gastric motility or inadequate gastric acid secretion. Achlorhydria among the elderly was excluded on the basis of response to pentagastrin challenge during the screening period. A total of 57 subjects (28 male, 29 female) were studied, 28 in the young (21 to 40 years) and 29 in the old (> 60 years) cohort; there were 14 to 17 subjects in each of the four resulting subject groups. All subjects received a low dose of ethanol (0.3 g/kg) on three occasions: (1) orally after an overnight fast (PONF), (2) orally after a standard breakfast (POF), and (3) IV after a standard breakfast (IV Fed). The blood ethanol response (mEq/l) was represented by AUC over 240 minutes.

The metabolic curves for each of the four subject groups are depicted in Figures 8.1 to 8.4. In all cohorts, there was a hierarchy of blood ethanol AUC responses: oral fasted > IV fed > oral fed.

Viewed by age and gender, blood ethanol AUCs among males were significantly greater in older subjects than younger subjects in the oral fasted ($p < 0.04$, Figure 8.5) and IV fed ($p < 0.05$) states *but not* in the oral fed state. Among female subjects, the old-young difference was striking in the oral fasted state alone ($p < 0.001$, Figure 8.6) with no significant age difference seen in either the oral or IV fed states. These data are presented numerically in Table 8.1.

The average magnitude of the AUC difference between the elderly and young male groups exposed to PO alcohol in a fasted state was 13%; the like figure was three times greater, 39%, for elderly versus young females. Average peak levels for elderly males were 10.8 mEq/L as compared to 8.5 mEq/L for younger males, and 12.8 mEq/L versus 9.0 mEq/L for older and younger females, in the oral fasted state. There were no ethanol AUC gender differences among the cohorts. Controlling for gastric motility differences,

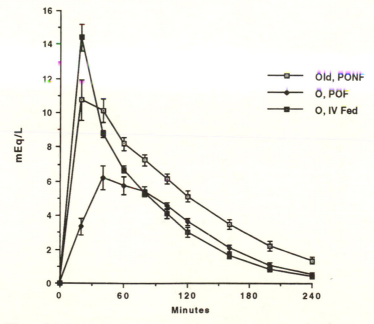

Figure 8.1. Blood ethanol concentrations, elderly men (N = 14), 0.3 g/kg.

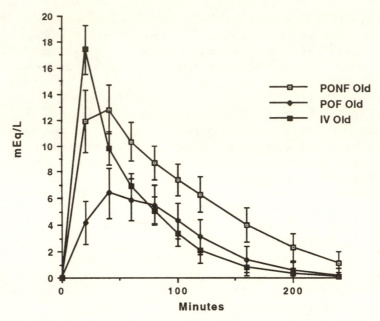

Figure 8.2. Blood ethanol concentrations, elderly women (N = 17), 0.3 g/kg.

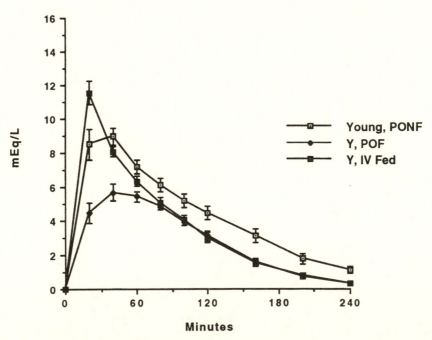

Figure 8.3. Blood ethanol concentrations, young men (N = 15), 0.3 g/kg.

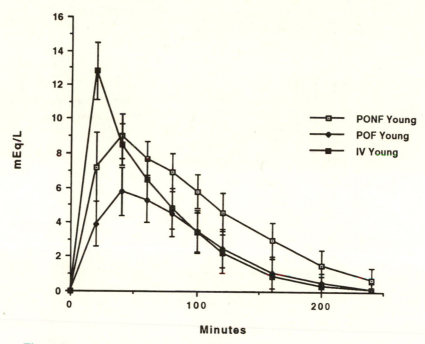

Figure 8.4. Blood ethanol concentrations, young women (N = 15), 0.3 g/kg.

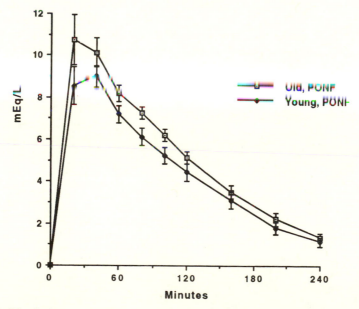

Figure 8.5. Blood ethanol concentration; oral fasted, 0.3 gm/kg, old (N = 14) and young (N = 15) men.

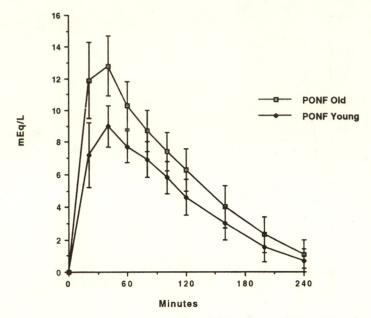

Figure 8.6. Blood ethanol concentration; oral fasted, 0.3 gm/kg, old (N = 17) and young (N = 15) women.

we found no age or gender differences in gastric emptying rates studied by radionuclide emptying techniques, negating emptying time as a confounding variable.

These data further elucidate an influence of age on ethanol metabolism, especially in the fasting state, for both genders. They also show that the mechanism underlying the age effect that appears to lessen ethanol metabolism is unlikely to be related to gastric metabolism or motility since average AUC was greater in the fasting state than in the fed state *irrespective* of IV or PO administration. This age-related difference, seen most clearly in the oral fasted state and not at all in the oral fed state, suggests an involvement of one or more mechanisms responsible for rapid ethanol metabolism within the first hour after ingestion.

Table 8.1. Area under the Curve (AUC) for Ethanol (0.3 g/kg single dose)

Condition	Older Males	Younger Males	Older Females	Younger Females
	(N = 15)	(N = 14)	(N = 16)	(N = 14)
Oral, fasted	1317 ± 176[a]	1168 ± 192	1504 ± 387[b]	1081 ± 200
IV, fed	942 ± 150[c]	829 ± 145	960 ± 185	842 ± 194
Oral, fed	745 ± 227	690 ± 113	706 ± 335	602 ± 230

[a]Older males > younger males, $p < .04$

[b]Older females > younger females, $p < .001$

[c]Older males > younger males, $p < .05$

Note: Older males and older females do not differ statistically. Younger males and younger females do not differ statistically. When gender data is pooled, average AUCs for old subjects are greater than those for young, both oral fasted ($p < .0001$) and IV fed ($p < .01$). When age data is pooled, no differences by gender exist.

AGE-RELATED CHARACTERISTICS OF INTOXICATION

Route of administration and feeding status appear to be important factors not only in metabolism but in the intoxication that follows exposure to alcohol by persons of different ages. In one part of the study noted above, subjects were asked (1) to rate their subjective sense of intoxication (Cognitive Sensations) and fatigue resulting from ingestion of alcohol (Fatigue Score), (2) to perform pencil and paper tasks of perceptual motor functioning (Line Tracing, Rotatable Letters, Identical Pictures), and (3) to perform a test of reaction time. This was done after the standard dose of 0.3 g/kg given IV after a standard breakfast. Ratings were done at baseline, at 30 minutes near the peak ethanol concentration, and at 100 minutes in the decay phase of the ethanol metabolism curve.

The results, noted in Table 8.2, described no baseline differences between the age groups on subjective intoxication measures but a clear subjective sense of intoxication for both groups that was independent of age. There was a clear age difference in performing perceptual motor tests at baseline that continued over the course of the ingestion. Only the Identical Pictures test demonstrated a significant differential effect caused by the *interaction* of age and ethanol intoxication ($p < .02$), suggesting that the ethanol worsened the performance of the elderly group on this task beyond the expected difference caused by the subject's age alone. There were no significant alterations in reaction time between groups at this dose. These data suggested that, at this low dose and in this unusual route of administration, some of the toxic effects of ethyl alcohol among elderly subjects, when compared to their baseline performance, are no greater that those seen among younger persons in comparison to their baseline.

To pursue these findings further, we administered the same measures of intoxication to split groups of subjects who had ingested the same dose of alcohol orally either after a 12-hour overnight fast or after a standard breakfast. In addition to the tests noted above, we added two clinical tests of balance and gait. Figure 8.7 presents subjective intoxication data from this experiment. Elderly subjects of both genders achieved greater degrees of subjective intoxication over baseline at the ethanol peak in the fasted state when compared to the same perceptions at the same time after ingesting ethanol in a fed state. The increased perception of intoxication in the fasted state was still significantly higher than baseline when assessed again at 100 minutes. The data portrayed in Figures 8.8 and 8.9 demonstrate that, within gender groups, elderly subjects were significantly less likely than their younger counterparts to recover from an intoxicated state when ingesting alcohol in fasted, but not in fed, states.

Table 8.2. Age/Trial Effects during Ethanol Exposure, 0.3 g/kg, IV, Fed, for Elderly ($N = 29$) and Young ($N = 28$) Subjects

Test	Age Effect	Trial Effect	Age/Trial Interaction
Cognitive Sensations	n.s.	$p < .0001$	n.s.
Fatigue Score (POMS)	n.s.	$p < .01$	n.s.
Line Tracing	$p < .0001$	$p < .05$	n.s.
Rotatable Letters	$p < .0002$	n.s.	n.s.
Identical Pictures	$p < .0001$	$p < .0001$	$p < .02$
Reaction Time	n.s.	n.s.	n.s.

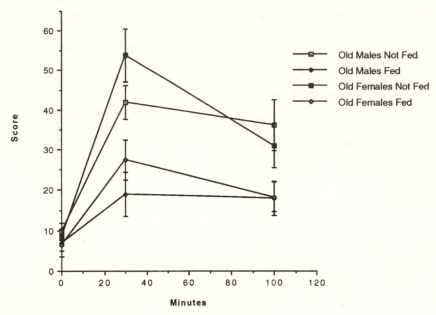

Figure 8.7. Cognitive sensations, 0.3 g/kg EtOH PO. Old males, not fed (N = 7) and fed (N = 7); old females, not fed (N = 9) and fed (N = 8).

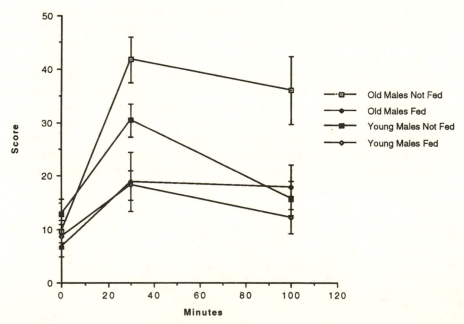

Figure 8.8. Cognitive sensations, 0.3 g/kg EtOH, PO. Old males, not fed (N = 7) and fed (N = 7); young males, not fed (N = 8) and fed (N = 7).

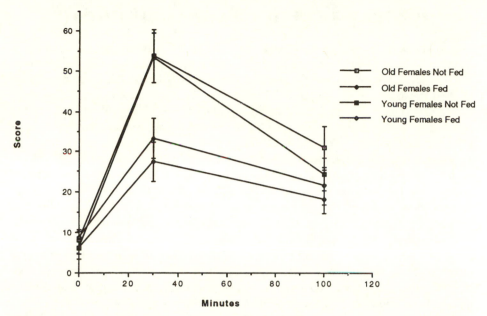

Figure 8.9. Cognitive sensations, 0.3 g/kg EtOH PO. Old females, not fed (N = 9) and fed (N = 8); young females, not fed (N = 8) and fed (N = 7).

Since the earlier metabolic data noted a significantly greater AUC for ethanol among the fasted elderly, these data suggest that the differential response to alcohol and the lengthened subjective recovery after acute ingestion among the elderly may be a dose-related phenomenon. This supposition can only be confirmed by further testing with a higher dose of ethanol as compared to placebo, however. Interestingly, the more objective tasks and measures of intoxication demonstrated a lessening functional capability that declined in parallel fashion among subjects of both age groups in both fed and fasted states. This suggests too that the low dose used in this study might not have been sufficient to bring out age-specific, objectively measurable intoxication.

In summary, this line of research has shown (1) that elderly persons absorb significantly more alcohol than do young persons when drinking in a fasted, but not in a fed, state. A corollary finding is that younger male subjects require a dose of ethanol approximately 15% greater and younger females a dose as much as 30% greater than their elderly counterparts to reach similar peak levels and to maintain approximately equal AUCs after a single ingestion in the fasted state. (2) Feeding lessens the blood ethanol concentration through an unknown mechanism independent of the route of administration. And (3), at this low dose, elderly subjects show differentially increased subjective but not objective intoxication effects relative to younger persons. These findings offer further evidence of probable differences related to age and to gender that may serve to explain in part the nature of changes in alcohol use and dependence among elderly persons and may suggest a physiologic basis for other phenomena reputedly affected by age. They make it clear that age comparisons of intoxication must include age adjustment of ethanol dosage, gender related differences among older persons, and careful attention to fasting state and administration route.

POSSIBLE CHARACTERISTICS OF AGE-RELATED DIFFERENCES

This study suggests that mechanisms more complicated than differential volumes of distribution may be at work. Unlike previous investigators, we assessed differential metabolism and intoxication characteristics among elderly ($>$ 60 years) versus younger (21 to 40 years) nonalcoholic persons in three different metabolic settings. Elderly male and female subjects, given a single administration of a small dose of ethanol, yielded areas under the metabolic curve that were significantly greater than younger subjects in an oral fasted ($p < .0001$) and an IV fed ($p < .01$) state *but not* in an oral fed state. Previous knowledge would have predicted differing AUCs in *all three* states if volume of distribution had been the only or the primary critical variable. AUC differences did not separate the two genders in our study but, on average, the age differences in absorption were significantly greater between young and old women ($p < .001$) than that between young and old men ($p < .04$) given oral ethanol in a fasting state.

While exposure to ethanol in the blood was greater among elderly subject groups as judged by AUC, most but not all measures of impaired functioning were worse among the elderly both at baseline and after alcohol ingestion. By contrast, subjective perceptions of intoxication compared in oral fasted versus oral fed states appeared to separate elderly from younger subjects, especially during the recovery phase of the ethanol metabolic curve. The subjective sense of intoxication appears due to an effect of alcohol that may be unique to the elderly subjects (age-alcohol interaction), whereas differences in measures of function between age groups, such as in gait and balance testing, appear to be functions of age alone at this dose. Whether this is true at higher doses is unknown. Previous work by other investigators suggests that higher doses of alcohol than the dose used in this study are usually required to achieve intoxication in younger nonalcoholic subjects (Schuckit, 1991). But there are no research data establishing appropriate intoxicating doses or blood alcohol levels for elderly nonalcoholic persons. Data from young subjects mentioned above (Frezza et al., 1990) also suggested apparent gender differences in which nonalcoholic women were thought to absorb more alcohol than nonalcoholic men given the same dose; we could not replicate this controversial finding.

CLINICAL IMPLICATIONS

Perhaps the first conclusion that can be drawn from this study is that, from a metabolic point of view, a ''standard drink'' for an elderly person contains about 20% less ethanol than that for a younger person, based on average AUC determinations. Similarly, a ''standard drink'' for an elderly female may contain less alcohol than that for an elderly male.

Second, the dose of ethanol used in our study was approximately half that given by previous investigators. It is the rough equivalent of one standard drink for most elderly people. In our experience this amount of ethanol resulted in considerable subjective feelings of intoxication among the elderly subjects of either gender, and these effects were longer lasting among the elderly than they were in the younger subject groups. Alcohol ingestion rather than age seemed to be the primary cause of these responses.

Third, considering only the objective intoxication data of the young and old subjects, the nonalcoholic elderly began with lessened perceptual motor capability at baseline, experienced a greater degree of impairment after ethanol because of their age than did their younger colleagues, and took longer to return to baseline functioning on some measures. This suggests that at this commonly used dose, age rather than alcohol accounts for most of the differences in the kinds of neural functions that come into play in activities such as walking, driving, or writing. Results from the one previous study that considered objectively measurable intoxication effects at a higher dose (Vogel-Sprott & Barrett, 1984) suggest that age and alcohol may have more of an interactive effect on functioning as the dose increases, although this is difficult to determine because of the previous study's design.

Fourth, the ethanol dose used in this study is approximately that commonly prescribed for or taken by elderly persons as an aid to sleep. While both alcohol and age are known to lessen sleep, in our study the extended recovery time among the aged subjects after a dose of ethanol suggests that alcohol may exert a more potent toxic effect on an aged central nervous system than previously appreciated. The initial tranquilizing effect, often thought to induce sleep, may be superseded by a more profound rebound effect in elderly than in younger persons. While folklore and some clinicians may suggest a glass of wine or other standard amount of an alcoholic beverage as a sleep aid for elderly individuals, few sleep researchers make such a recommendation. Our data, suggesting an increased neural sensitivity to alcohol among the elderly, joins with the great preponderance of sleep data in suggesting that bedtime alcohol be avoided as a sleep-inducing drug, and especially so among the elderly.

Finally, our study suggests that both subjective and objective measures of intoxication were worsened by fasting. While ethanol absorption was markedly increased when subjects of any age had not eaten, the age difference between young and old women was especially striking and may account for the drop in ethanol consumption reported among elderly women in large population surveys. While the metabolic mechanism for this is unclear at present, its elucidation may afford us some useful insight into the biology of ethanol metabolism that might be applicable to old and young alike.

References

Atkinson, R. M. (1990). Aging and alcohol use disorders. Diagnostic issues in the elderly. International Psychogeriatrics, 2, 55–72.

Frezza, M., diPadova, C., Pozatto, G., et al. (1990). High blood alcohol levels in women: The role of decreased gastric alcohol dehydrogenase activity in first-pass metabolism. New England Journal of Medicine, 322, 95–99.

Jones, A. W., Neri, A. (1985). Age-related differences in blood ethanol parameters and subjective feelings of intoxication in healthy men. Alcohol and Alcoholism, 20, 45–52.

Mishara, B. L., & Kastenbaum, R. (1980). Alcohol and old age. New York: Grune and Stratton.

Nordstrom, G., & Berglund, M. (1987). Ageing and recovery from alcoholism. British Journal of Psychiatry, 151, 382–388.

Roehrs, T. A., Beare, D. J., Roth, T. (1992). Sleepiness and ethanol effects on simulated driving performance. Alcoholism: Clinical and Experimental Research, 16, 371.

Schuckit, M. A. (1991). Drug and alcohol abuse, a clinical guide to diagnosis and treatment. New York: Plenum.

Vogel-Sprott, M., Barrett, P. (1984). Age, drinking habits and the effects of alcohol. Journal of Studies on Alcohol, 45, 517–521.

Vestal, R. E., McGuire, E. A., Tobin, J. D., et al. (1977). Aging and ethanol metabolism. Clinical Pharmacology and Therapeutics, 21, 343–354.

9

Alcohol, Aging, Infections, and Immunity

MADHAVAN NAIR, STANLEY A. SCHWARTZ, AND ZIAD A. KRONFOL

A number of studies gathered mostly during the last decade have shown that alcohol exerts a significant regulatory effect on hosts' immune response against various infections and tumors. Although the mechanisms of alcohol-induced immunomodulations are multifactorial and incompletely understood, the main effects of alcohol-induced abnormalities are associated with humoral (Drew et al., 1984; Delacroix et al., 1982; Morgan et al., 1980; Chang et al., 1990) and cellular immunity (Chang et al., 1990; Jerrels et al., 1990; Meadows et al., 1989, 1992; Ericsson et al., 1980; Watson et al., 1984), including dysfunctions of suppression (Watson et al., 1984; Hodgson et al., 1978; Woltjen & Zelterman, 1981; Kawanishi et al., 1981), helper (McKeever et al., 1988), and cytotoxic activities (Abdallah et al., 1983; Saxena et al., 1980; Stacey, 1984; Charpentier et al., 1984; Meadows et al., 1989).

Natural killer (NK) cell activity is believed to be the early immune surveillance response against nascent tumors and viral infection (Welsh, 1981; Herberman & Holden, 1978). The body's ability to mount an antigen-specific immune response is directly dependent on the production of multiple immunoregulatory proteins called cytokines. Cytokines are also known to exert significant regulatory effects on various immune functions of lymphocytes (Henderson & Blake, 1992; Cairo, 1991). Cytokines, therefore, are important mediators that protect the host against microbial invasion, injury, or other inflammatory insults by restoring normal homeostasis (Moore, 1991; Rees, 1992). Previous studies showed that alcoholics are characterized by disturbance in the production and functions of various cytokines (Nelson et al., 1990; Chadha et al., 1990; Rees, 1992), potentially predisposing them to various infections.

There is also a substantial body of evidence suggesting a decline in various immunological functions with age (Miller, 1991). Previous studies have shown that all four antigen-responsive immune cells—T cells, B cells, monocytes, and killer cells—are affected by aging and that T cells are particularly vulnerable to aging (Makinoden et al., 1987; Dogget et al., 1981). More recently there has been growing interest in the effects of aging on cytokine gene expression. The production of interferon (IFN) has been reported to be decreased (Abb et al., 1984), unchanged (Rytel et al., 1986) or increased (Chopra et al., 1989) with aging. Similarly, IFN messenger RNA (mRNA) has been reported to be increased (Chopra et al., 1989) or decreased (Gauchat et al., 1988). Diminished IL-2 mRNA production by lymphocytes of aged donors has also been reported (Wu et al., 1986).

Studies on a combined effect of aging and alcohol on various immune functions have been limited. In mouse models, ethanol produced significantly more suppressive effects on young splenic T cell proliferative response to mitogen than on splenic cells from old mice (Chang et al., 1990). Similar age-related changes in alcohol-induced immune suppression were reported by other investigators (Roselle et al., 1989; Domiate-Saad & Jerrels, 1990). Recently Chang and Norman (1991) showed a decrease in T cell proliferation and T cell dependent antibody response in both young and old mice subjected to extended alcohol intake. The effects of alcohol and aging on hosts' immune responses and the mechanisms of immunomodulations are not clear.

EFFECTS OF AGE AND ALCOHOL ON NK AND ADCC ACTIVITIES

We recently examined the effects of alcohol and age on NK and antibody-dependent cellular cytotoxic (ADCC) activities to further elucidate the mechanisms of alcohol-induced immunosuppression seen in alcoholic patients. Early studies of the effects of aging on NK and ADCC activities were contradictory. Some showed an increase of NK activity (Rabatic et al., 1988) while others showed either a decrease (Fernandes & Gupta, 1981) or no change (Penschow & Mackay, 1980) during aging. Since chronic alcoholism was known to be associated with various immune dysfunctions and since

Table 9.1. NK and ADCC Activities of Cord and Adult Peripheral Blood Lymphocytes[a]

Targets	Effector Source	Effector: target cell ratio	
		10:1	5:1
		Cytotoxicity (%)[b]	
K562[c]	a-PBL[e]	19.6 ± 5.0	12.6 ± 2.3
		(p < .025)	(p < .005)
	CBL[f]	6.2 ± 3.3	3.6 ± 2.1
SB[d]	a-PBL	23.6 ± 5.6	8.5 ± 1.9
		(p < .025)	(p < .025)
	CBL	7.7 ± 3.2	2.6 ± 1.7

[a]Effector cells were mixed with targets at varying E:T cell ratios in a 4-hr ^{51}Cr release assay. The results are means ± SD of 15 different cord blood lymphocyte samples and 10 unrelated adult (mean age 27.5 years) peripheral blood lymphocyte samples.

[b]Percentage cytotoxicity was calculated as described (Nair et al., 1986.) used as targets in the NK assay.

[c]Erythroleukemia cell line (k562) used as targets in the NK assay.

[d]B-Leukemia cell line sensitized with anti-SB antibody used as target in the ADCC assay.

[e]Adult peripheral blood lymphocytes (a-PBL) depleted of adherent cells.

[f]Cord blood lymphocytes (CBL) depleted of adherent cells.

Note: Differences in values between CBL and a-PBL were statistically significant at both E:T ratios in both NK and ADCC assays using Student's 't' test.

certain immunological impairments were often manifested with aging, we studied the effect of aging and alcohol on NK and ADCC reactions.

Lymphocytes depleted of adherent cells from 15 cord blood and 10 adult (mean age 25.7 ± 3.5 years) peripheral blood samples were tested for their NK and ADCC activity against tumor target cells. Data presented in Table 9.1 show that cord blood lymphocytes (CBL) depleted of adherent cells demonstrated significantly lower NK and ADCC activities, respectively, against K562 and antibody-coated SB target cells compared to normal adult lymphocytes at 10:1 and 5:1 E:T cell ratios. E:T cell ratios higher than 10:1 also produced similar differences (data not shown).

In a separate set of experiments we also studied the NK and ADCC activities of two different age groups, young (mean age 20.54 ± 3.34 years) and old (mean age 67.46 ± 4.75 years) individuals. Data presented in Figure 9.1 show that both NK (48%, $p <$ .05) and ADCC (46%, $p <$ .02) activities of elderly individuals manifested significant increases in cytotoxicity at 100:1 E:T cell ratio compared to that of young adults (35% and 25% cytotoxicity, respectively). However, statistically significant increases in cytotoxic activities were not demonstrated at lower E:T cell ratios (50:1, 25:1, and 12.5:1), although the cytotoxic response was marginally higher at lower E:T cell ratios.

Since earlier studies showed that the immune system of the newborn is deficient in several aspects of humoral and cellular immunity that include NK activity, we examined whether alcohol can have a selective inhibitory effect on NK activity of lymphocytes from neonates. Data presented in Figure 9.2 demonstrate that direct addition of EtOH at 0.1%, 0.2%, and 0.3% to culture of peripheral blood lymphocytes from normal adult

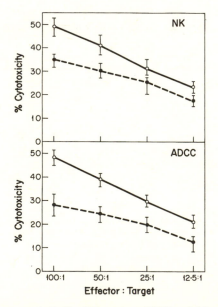

Figure 9.1. Twenty-eight young individuals (mean age 20.54 ± 3.34 years) and forty-one elderly individuals (mean age 67.46 ± 4.75) were included in this study. All participants were free from drinking or smoking habits. Lymphocytes were isolated from freshly drawn blood using lymphocyte separation medium (Organon Teknika Corp., Durham, NC). NK activity was determined using ^{51}Cr-labelled human erythroleukemia (K-562) cells. ADCC assays were carried out using ^{51}Cr-labelled Raji cells treated with Lym-1 antibody. ○———○, elderly ○---○, young adults.

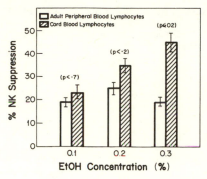

Figure 9.2. EtOH at final concentrations of 0.1, 0.2 and 0.3% (v/v) was added directly to a mixture of effector cells and target cells and incubated for 4 hours and the NK activity was measured against K562 target cells at 25:1 E:T cell ratios. The percent NK suppression calculated on the basis of NK activity produced by untreated control culture. Values represent mean % NK blood samples and five adult peripheral blood samples. Statistical significance of differences in the mean values was determined by Student's 't' test.

donors (mean age 25.7 ± 3.5 years) did not produce any significant suppression of NK activities. However, EtOH at higher concentrations (0.3%, v/v) significantly ($p < .02$) suppressed the NK activity of lymphocytes from cord blood. These studies suggest that alcohol can have a selective inhibitory effect on NK activities of cord blood lymphocytes; such inhibitory effects were not observed in adult peripheral blood lymphocytes.

EFFECTS OF ALCOHOL ON INTERFERON PRODUCTION

Since chronic alcoholics manifest dysregulations of various immune functions that are influenced by various cytokines including interferons, we examined the ability of lymphocytes to produce interferons α and γ in response to Sendai virus and *Staphylococcal* enterotoxin B (Sigma Chemical Co., St. Louis, MO), respectively (Table 9.2). Significant differences were seen in the ability of peripheral blood lymphocytes to produce both interferons α and γ when healthy individuals were compared to chronic alcoholics. Lymphocytes from chronic alcoholics (MAST score > 17.15) produced significantly lower levels of both interferon α and γ. However, chronic alcoholism did not signifi-

Table 9.2. Interferons and Natural Killer Cell Activity in Controls and Alcoholic Patients

Variables	Healthy Controls ($N = 40$)	Alcoholic Patients ($N = 40$)
Interferon-α[a]	5483	1168 ($p < .001$)
Interferon-γ[a]	556	143 ($p < .001$)
NK Cytotoxicity (%)	49	46 ($p > .05$)
MAST[b] Score	0.97	17.15 ($p < .001$)

Note: Lymphocytes were isolated from freshly drawn blood, induced with 150 HAU of Sendai virus (IFN-α) or 1.0 ug/ml of Staphylococcal enterotoxin-B (IFN-γ). Interferon antiviral activity was determined on human foreskin fibroblast cells. NK activity was determined using ^{51}Cr labeled human erythroleukemia (K-562) cells as target.

[a]Interferon titers are expressed as units calculated on the basis of a standard reference curve.

[b]Michigan Alcohol Screen Test. Statistical significance of the difference were calculated by Student's 't' test.

Table 9.3. Lymphocyte Subsets in Normal Controls and Alcoholic Patients

Lymphocyte Marker	Normal Controls	Alcoholic Patients	Significance
CD_2 (total T)	63.3 ± 13.9	61. ± 14.8	NS
CD_4 (T-helper/inducer)	40.9 ± 12.1	41.1 ± 13.6	NS
CD_8 (T-suppressor/cytotoxic)	24.2 ± 9.4	20.2 ± 8.8	.063
CD_4/CD_8	1.9 ± 0.9	2.6 ± 1.8	.0545
CD_{20} (total B)	6.3 ± 4.1	7.6 ± 5.9	NS
CD_{56} (NK Cells)	12.3 ± 10.0	11.8 ± 7.6	NS
IL_2R_1 (interleukin-2 receptor)	5.5 ± 3.0	9.0 ± 4.5	.022
I_2 (HLA-D/DR related)	9.6 ± 4.1	15.6 ± 4.8	.005

Note: Results are expressed in percentages (mean ± SD) of lymphocyte subsets as quantitated by flow cytometry analysis using specific monoclonal antibodies.

cantly alter the level of NK activity as compared to healthy controls. It is conceivable that chronic alcoholics have some potential subclinical infection(s) that triggers the low-level interferon production that, in turn, enhances NK activity, thus masking NK suppression induced by alcoholism.

LYMPHOCYTE SUBSETS IN NORMAL AND ALCOHOLIC PATIENTS

Since we did not find a significant difference in NK activity in chronic alcoholics compared to that of age- and sex-matched normal controls, and because of significant suppression of IFN production in chronic alcoholics in response to various stimuli, studies were undertaken to investigate whether chronic alcohol consumption results in any phenotypic alteration of lymphocyte subsets. Results presented in Table 9.3 demonstrate a trend and a lowered percentage of CD8 lymphocytes and an increase in CD4/CD8 ratio in alcoholic patients compared to matched controls. We also found a significant increase in the percentage of lymphocytes with the activation markers IL-2R1 and I2 in the alcoholic group. There was a trend ($p < .06$) for a negative association between CD8 lymphocytes and age in alcoholic patients, but not in the control group. The significant increase in the percentage of lymphocytes bearing activation markers in alcoholics may be attributed to possible subclinical infections that are often present in alcoholics more than in normal subjects.

CONCLUDING REMARKS

Previous studies have shown that chronic alcoholism is associated with various immune dysfunctions. A decline of various immunological functions is also known to be associated with the aging process. The present study was undertaken to study the role of alcohol and aging on lymphocyte cytotoxicity and on interferon production. Our studies reported herein demonstrate that neonatal lymphocytes produced significantly lower levels of NK and ADCC activities compared to that of adult peripheral blood lymphocytes. We also have shown that alcohol selectively suppresses NK activity of cord blood lymphocytes, whereas no suppression was demonstrable with adult peripheral blood lymphocytes at similar concentrations of alcohol. Chronic alcoholics demonstrated significantly decreased levels of both α and γ interferon production compared to that of age- and sex-matched normal controls, although both groups demonstrated comparable levels of NK activity. Chronic alcoholism also seems to induce certain activation markers on lymphocytes. These studies suggest that alcohol causes a selective inhibitory effect on NK activity of cord blood lymphocytes and exerts a significant immunomodulatory effect on interferon production that may be of clinical significance. While age and chronic alcohol use exert independent effects on immune function, a synergy between these two factors remains unproven to this point.

Acknowledgments

The authors wish to express since appreciation for Carol Sperry and Gerry Sobkowiak for their expert secretarial assistance.

This work was supported in part by NIH grant No. 51R01 42988, 2 R01 CA 35922, 1R01 MH 47225, 1P50 AA 07378, 1P50MH, 43564, and grants from the Robert Cameron and Margaret Duffy Troup Memorial Fund of the Buffalo General Hospital, 229865 and 229879.

References

Abb, J., Abb, H., & Deinhardt, F. (1984). Age-related decline of human interferon alpha and interferon gamma production. *Blut, 48,* 285.

Abdallah, R. M., Starkey, J. R., & Meadows, G. (1983). Alcohol and related dietary effects on mouse natural killer cell activity. *Immunology, 50,* 131.

Cairo, M. S. (1991). Cytokines: a new immunotherapy. *Clinical Perinatology, 18,* 343–359.

Chadha, K. C., Whitney, R. B., Cummings, M. K., Norman, M., Windle, M., & Stadler, I. (1990). Evaluation of interferon system among chronic alcoholics. In D. Seminara, R. R. Watson, & A. Pawlowski (Eds.), *Alcohol immunomodulation and AIDS* New York: Alan R. Liss. (pp. 123–133).

Chang, M. P., & Norman, D. E. (1991). Immunotoxicity of alcohol in young and old mice. II. Impaired T cell proliferation and T cell-dependent antibody responses of young and old mice fed ethanol-containing liquid diet. *Mechanisms of Aging and Development, 57,* 175–186.

Chang, M. P., Norman, D. C., & Makinodan, T. (1990). Immunotoxicity of alcohol in young and old mice. I. In vitro suppressive effects of ethanol on the activities of T and B immune cells of aging mice. *Alcoholism, 14,* 210–215.

Charpentier, B., Franco, D., Paci, L., Charra, M., Martin, B., & Friss, V. D. (1984). Deficient natural killer cell activity in alcohol cirrhosis. *Clinical Experimental Immunology, 58,* 107.

Chopra, R. K., Holbrook, N. I., Powers, D. C., et al. (1989). Interleukin 2 receptors and interferon-gamma synthesis and mRNA expression in phorbol myristate acetate and calcium ionophore A23187-stimulated T cells from elderly humans. *Clinical Immunology and Immunopathology, 53,* 297.

Delacroix, D. L., Elkon, K. B., Genbel, A. R., Hedgson, H. E., Dive, C., & Verman, J. F. (1982). Changes in size, subclass and metabolic properties of serum immunoglobulin A. *American Journal of Clinical Investigation, 71,* 358–367.

Dogget, D. L., Chang, M. P., Makinodan, T., et al. (1981). Cellular and molecular aspects of immune system aging. *Molecular Cell Biochemistry, 37,* 137.

Domiati-Saad, R., & Jerrells, T. R. (1993). The influence of age on blood alcohol levels and ethanol-associated immunosuppression in a murine model of ethanol consumption. *Alcoholism, 17,* 382–388.

Drew, P. A., Clifton, P. M., Labrooy, J. T., & Shearman, D. J. C. (1984). Polyclonal B cell activation in alcoholic patients with no evidence of liver dysfunction. *Clinical Experimental Immunology, 51,* 479–486.

Ericsson, D. C., Kohl, S., Pickering, L. K., Davis, G. S., & Faillace, L. A. (1980). Mechanisms of host defense in well nourished patients with chronic alcoholism. *Alcoholism, 4,* 261.

Fernandes, G., & Gupta, S. (1981). Natural killing and antibody-dependent cytotoxicity by lymphocyte subpopulations in young and aging humans. *Journal of Clinical Immunology, 1,* 141–148.

Gauchat, J. F., Deweck, A. L., & Stadler, B. M. (1988). Decreased cytokine messenger RNA levels in the elderly. *Aging: Immunity, Infectious Disease, 1,* 191.

Herberman, R. B., & Holden, J. (1978). Natural cell mediated immunity. *Advanced Cancer Research, 27,* 305.

Henderson, B., & Blake, S. (1992). Therapeutic potential of cytokine manipulation. *Trends in Pharmacological Science, 13,* 1145.

Hodgson, H. J. K., Wands, J. R., & Isselbaeber, K. J. (1978). Alteration in suppressor cell activity in chronic active hepatitis. *Proceedings of the National Academy of Science USA, 75,* 1549.

Jerrels, T. R., Peritt, D., Marietta, C., & Eckardt, M. J. (1990). Mechanisms of suppression of cellular immunity induced by ethanol. *Alcoholism: Clinical and Experimental Research, 13,* 490.

Kawanishi, H., Tavassoli, H., MacDermott, R. P., & Sheagren, J. N. (1981). Impaired concanacalin-A inducible suppressor T cell activity in active alcoholic disease. *Gastroenterology, 80,* 510.

Makinodan, T., Lubinski, J., & Fong, T. C. (1987). Cellular biochemical and molecular basis of T-cell senescence. *Archives Pathology Laboratory Medicine, 111,* 910–914.

McKeever, Y., Mahoney, C. O., Whelan, C. A., Weir, D. G., & Feighery, C. (1988). Helper and suppressor T lymphocyte function in severe alcoholic liver disease. *Clinical and Experimental Immunology, 60,* 39.

Meadows, G. G., Wallendal, W., Kosngi, A., Weinderlich, J., & Singer, D. S. (1992). Ethanol induced marked changes in lymphocyte population and natural killer cell activity in mice. *Alcoholism: Clinical and Experimental Research, 16,* 474.

Meadows, G. G., Blank, S. E., & Duncad, D. D. (1989). Influence of ethanol consumption on natural killer cell activity in mice. *Alcoholism: Clinical and Experimental Research, 13,* 476.

Miller, R. A. (1991). Aging and immune function. *International Review of Cytology, 124,* 187.

Moore, M. A. (1991). The future of cytokine combination therapy. *Cancer, 67,* 2718–2726.

Morgan, M. Y., Ross, M. G., Ng CM, Adams, D. M., Thomas, H. C., & Sherlock, S. (1980). HLA-B8, immunoglobulins and antibody response in alcohol related liver disease. *Journal of Clinical Pathology, 33,* 488–492.

Nair, M. P. N., Laing, T. J., & Schwartz, S. S. (1986). Decreased natural and antibody-dependent cellular cytotoxic activities in intravenous drug abusers. *Clinical Immunology and Immunopathology, 38,* 68–78.

Nelson, S., Bagby, G. J., & Summer, W. R. (1990). Alcohol-induced suppression of tumor necrosis factor—a potential risk factor for secondary infection in the acquired immunodeficiency syndrome. *Progress in Clinical Biological Research, 325,* 211–220.

Penschow, J., & Mackay, J. (1980). NK and K cell activity of human blood; differences according to sex, age and disease. *Annals of Rheumatic Disease, 39,* 82.

Rabatic, S., Sabioncello, A., Dekaris, D., & Kardum, I. (1988). Age-related changes in functions of peripheral blood phagocytes. *Mechanics of Ageing and Development, 45,* 223–229.

Rees, R. C. (1992). Cytokines as biological response modifiers. *Journal of Clinical Pathology, 45*, 93–98.

Roselle, G. A., Mendenhall, C. L., & Grossman, C. J. (1989). Age dependent alteration of host immune responses in the ethanol-fed rat. *Journal of Clinical Immunology, 29*, 99.

Rytel, M. W., Larratt, K. S., Turner, P. A., et al. (1986). Interferon response to mitogens and viral antigens in elderly and young adult subjects. *Journal of Infectious Disease, 153*, 984.

Saad, A. J., & Jerrells, T. R. (1990). Flow cytometry and immunohistochemical evaluation of ethanol-induced changes in splenic and thymic lymphoid cell populations. *Alcoholism: Clinical and Experimental Research, 15*, 796.

Saxena, Q. B., Nezey, E., & Adler, W. H. (1980). Regulation of natural killer activity *in vivo*. II. The effect of alcohol consumption on human peripheral blood natural killer cell activity. *International Journal of Cancer, 26*, 413.

Stacey, N. H. (1984). Inhibition of antibody dependent cell mediated cytotoxicity by ethanol. *Immunopharmacology, 8*, 155.

Watson, R. R., Eskelson, C., & Hartman, B. R. (1984). Severe alcohol abuse and cellular immune functions. *Arizona Medicine, 10*, 665.

Welsh, R. M. (1981). Natural cell-mediated immunity during viral infections. *Current Topics in Microbiology and Immunology, 92*, 83.

Woltjen, J. A., & Zelterman, R. K. (1981). Suppressor cell activity in primary biliary cirrhosis. *Digestive Disease Science, 25*, 104.

Wu, W., Pahlavani, M., Cheung, H. T., et al. (1986). The effect of aging on the expression of interleukin 2 messenger ribonucleic acid. *Clinical Immunology, 100*, 224.

10

Age Differences in Effects of Alcohol on Brain Membrane Structure, Neurotransmitters, and Receptors

W. GIBSON WOOD

Age differences in effects of ethanol in animals have been reported for responses such as sleep-time, chronic intoxication, severity of withdrawal, and hypothermia and have been reviewed previously (Wood et al., 1984; Wood, 1976; Wood & Armbrecht, 1982b). For example, it can be seen in Table 10.1 that 28-month-old male C57BL/ 6Nnia mice lost the righting reflex for a longer time following an injection of ethanol than 8- and 18-month-old mice (Wood & Armbrecht, 1982a). The blood ethanol level was significantly lower when the righting response was regained in the 28-month-old group as compared to the 8-month group (Table 10.1). In the same study, it was observed that ethanol-induced changes in body temperature were significantly less in the 28-month age group as compared to the younger group (Figure 10.1). The younger mice showed the well-documented hypothermic effects of an ethanol injection. However, the body temperature of the older mice was less affected at loss of the righting reflex and when the righting reflex was regained (Figure 10.1).

Effects of chronic ethanol administration are also age-related. Severity of intoxication was significantly greater in 25-month-old mice administered an ethanol liquid diet over a 14-day period than effects in 3-month-old mice (Wood et al., 1982). The aged mice did not develop tolerance to ethanol. Blood ethanol levels did not differ significantly between age groups. Withdrawal was significantly more severe and of a longer duration in the 25-month-old group than the 3-month group.

The mechanism(s) to explain age differences in effects of acute and chronic ethanol administration have not been identified. Possible reasons that may explain the effects of ethanol in the aged organism include age differences in ethanol metabolism, body water content, and effects of ethanol on brain (Wood et al., 1984; Wood & Armbrecht, 1982b). Several studies have suggested that age differences in ethanol metabolism do not play a significant role in age effects of ethanol. An exception was a study that found that ethanol metabolism increased with age in Fischer 344 rats (Ott et al., 1985). Body water content has been reported to decrease with increasing age. When ethanol dose was based on estimated body water content, effects of ethanol in aged rats were reduced (York, 1982). Age differences in body water content may contribute in part to effects

Table 10.1. Effects of an Ethanol Injection on Sleep-Time and Blood Ethanol Levels in Different Age Groups of Mice

Age Group (months)	Sleep-Time (minutes)	Blood Ethanol Level (mg/dl)
8	66.37 ± 4.43	393 ± 19
18	72.37 ± 6.79	371 ± 11
28	87.50 ± 7.53[a]	338 ± 20[a]

Note: Mice were injected with ethanol (3g/kg, I.P.). Sleep-time was measured from loss of the righting reflex until the righting reflex was regained. Data are the means ± SE of 8 mice for each age group.

[a]$p < 0.03$ as compared to the 8-month-old group. Data are from Wood and Armbrecht (1982a).

of ethanol in aged brain. However, age differences in body water content do not account for the findings showing that old animals lose and regain the righting reflex at lower brain and blood ethanol levels as compared to younger animals (Ritzmann & Springer, 1980; Wood & Armbrecht, 1982a).

Effects of ethanol on responses involving brain function (sleep-time, intoxication, temperature regulation) differ in aged as compared to younger animals. As discussed earlier, aged animals sleep longer following an injection of ethanol and wake at a lower blood ethanol concentration. It has been reported that aged mice lose and regain the righting reflex at lower brain and blood ethanol levels than younger mice (Ritzmann & Springer, 1980). In Fischer rats, even though blood ethanol levels were lower in 30-month-old rats, sleep time between 3-month and 30-month-old rats did not differ, sug-

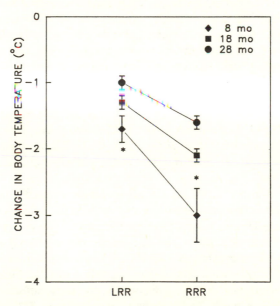

Figure 10.1. Age differences in effects of an injection of ethanol (3 g/kg, IP) on body temperature at loss (LRR) and regaining (RRR) of the righting reflex in C57BL mice. Data expressed as the mean ± SE of 8 animals for each age group. *$p < .001$ as compared to the 28-month-old group. Data are adapted from Wood and Armbrecht, 1982a.

gesting greater brain sensitivity to effects of ethanol in the aged animals (Ott et al., 1985).

Age differences in ethanol metabolism and body water content do not fully explain differences in effects of ethanol on sleep-time, righting reflex, intoxication, and severity of withdrawal. Results of the studies discussed above support the hypothesis that ethanol behaves differently in the aged brain as compared to effects on brain of younger organisms. Effects of ethanol and/or aging on brain can be examined at several different levels, ranging from neuropsychological function to neurochemical changes. A primary effect of ethanol and of aging has been seen in brain membrane structure and function (Wood et al., 1984; Wood & Armbrecht, 1982b; Deitrich et al., 1989; Rubin & Rottenberg, 1982; Hunt, 1985; Wood & Schroeder, 1992; Wood & Schroeder, 1988a; Wood et al., 1989a). The purpose of this chapter will be to review studies that have examined age differences in response to ethanol in vitro and chronically on brain membrane structure, neurotransmitters, and receptors.

MEMBRANE STRUCTURE AND EFFECTS OF ETHANOL

Membrane Fluidity

Fluidity will be used in this chapter in its most general application, describing the lateral motion of membrane lipids. Ethanol in vitro fluidizes membranes. The fluidizing effects of ethanol have been well documented using different types of membranes (e.g., synaptic plasma membranes, mitochondrial membranes, microsomes, erythrocytes) and techniques such as fluorescent probes, nuclear magnetic resonance, and electron spin resonance (Wood & Schroeder, 1988a; Deitrich et al., 1989; Wood et al., 1989a; Rubin & Rottenberg, 1982; Klemm, 1990; Hunt, 1985; Wood et al., 1991; Wood & Schroeder, 1992). A positive correlation between in vivo ethanol sensitivity and disordering of brain membranes by ethanol in vitro has been reported in genetic lines of mice (Goldstein et al., 1982). Long-sleep mice slept longer following an injection of ethanol than short-sleep mice, and the long-sleep mice showed greater ethanol-induced fluidization than the short-sleep mice. Membranes of ethanol-tolerant animals and alcoholic patients have been found to be fluidized less by ethanol in vitro as compared to membranes of controls (Beauge et al., 1985; Chin & Goldstein, 1977; Harris et al., 1984; Rottenberg et al., 1981; Taraschi et al., 1986; Taraschi et al., 1990; Wood et al., 1989b; Wood et al., 1987).

Both in vivo sensitivity and tolerance to ethanol are associated with effects of ethanol on membrane fluidity. We proposed that membranes of aged mice would be fluidizied more by ethanol in vitro as compared to membranes of younger mice (Armbrecht et al., 1983). That hypothesis was tested in synaptic plasma membranes (SPM), brain microsomes, and erythrocyte membranes of three different age groups of C57BL/6Nnia male mice using 5-doxyl stearic acid and electron spin resonance. Fluidity in the absence of ethanol in vitro did not differ significantly in the three different membrane types with respect to age (Table 10.2). It can be seen in Table 10.2 that brain microsomes were more fluid than SPM and that erythrocyte membranes were the least fluid. When ethanol was added to the membranes, effects on membrane fluidity were significantly less in membranes of the older animals than in membranes of the younger animals

Table 10.2. Baseline Membrane Order of Membranes Isolated from Three Age Groups of Mice

Age Group (mo)	Membrane Order (S)		
	SPM	BMM	RBC
3–5	0.591 ± 0.002	0.577 ± 0.001	0.607 ± 0.001
11–13	0.594 ± 0.001	0.578 ± 0.004	0.603 ± 0.002
22–24	0.593 ± 0.001	0.573 ± 0.002	0.604 ± 0.001

Note: Membrane order was measured using the 5-doxyl stearic acid spin label and electron spin resonance at 37°C. Data are the means ± SE of three preparations (Armbrecht et al., 1983).

(Figure 10.2). Data are presented in Figure 10.2 on SPM, but effects of ethanol on fluidity were similar in microsomes and erythrocyte membranes. The finding that membranes of aged animals were less affected by ethanol in vitro was surprising in view of data showing that aged animals were more sensitive to effects of ethanol on sleep time and effects of chronic ethanol consumption. The effects of ethanol on membranes of aged animals were similar to the resistance to ethanol-induced fluidization observed in membranes of short-sleep mice and ethanol-tolerant animals. Resistance to fluidization by ethanol in aged membranes, however, was consistent with the in vivo data that showed that ethanol had less of an effect on body temperature in aged as compared to younger mice.

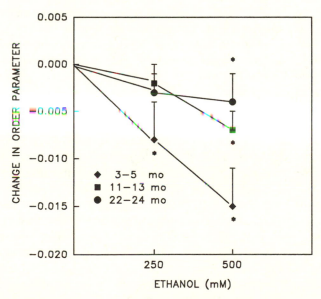

Figure 10.2. Effect of ethanol in vitro on the order parameters of synaptic plasma membranes from three different age groups of C57BL mice. Order parameters were determined using the 5-doxyl stearic acid spin label and electron spin resonance at 37°C. Data are the difference between order parameters in the presence of ethanol minus no ethanol and are expressed as the mean ± SE of three preparations for each age group. *$p < 0.05$ as compared to the age-related baseline control order parameter. Data are adapted from Armbrecht et al., 1983.

Membrane Lipid Composition

Lipids are a primary structural component of membranes and are involved in regulation of certain proteins (Yeagle, 1989). Effects of ethanol on membrane lipid composition have been examined in several different studies (Sun & Sun, 1985). In addition, lipid composition of membranes of different age groups has also been reported (Wood & Schroeder, 1988b; Strong et al., 1991). Changes in the lipid composition of the membrane can have an effect on membrane fluidity. Effects of chronic ethanol consumption on lipid composition of synaptosomes were examined in mice 6 months and 28 months of age. Cholesterol content and total lipid phosphorus content of synaptosomes were highest in the 28-month-old ethanol and control groups as compared to the 6-month-old ethanol and control groups. Chronic ethanol consumption did not alter total membrane cholesterol content and lipid phosphorus in either the 6-month-old or 28-month-old groups. Changes in the percentage of individual membrane phospholipids also did not differ with age or with chronic ethanol consumption.

Poly-phosphoinositides (Poly-PI) have been shown to play a major role in receptor-mediated signal transduction mechanisms (Berridge, 1987). Poly-PI are affected by chronic ethanol consumption. It has been reported that chronic ethanol consumption resulted in a threefold increase in Poly-PI level in 6-month-old mice but that Poly-PI level was not changed in synaptosomes of 28-month-old mice (Sun et al., 1987). In a recent study, it was reported that PIP_2 and PIP (Poly-PI) were increased in synaptosomes of chronic ethanol-treated 12-month-old mice but that both PIP_2 and PIP were reduced in chronic ethanol-treated 26-month-old mice (Sun et al., 1992). The increase in PIP_2 and PIP in synaptosomes of the 12-month-old ethanol-treated mice may be an adaptive response that was impaired in brain of aged mice.

Ethanol effects on membrane bulk (total changes in membrane structure and lipid content), fluidity, and lipid composition do not fully explain the increased sensitivity to ethanol observed in aged animals. The hypothesis that sensitivity and tolerance to ethanol can be explained by ethanol-induced changes in bulk membrane fluidity and lipid composition has been questioned (Wood & Schroeder, 1988a; Deitrich et al., 1989; Wood et al., 1989a; Klemm, 1990; Wood et al., 1991; Wood & Schroeder, 1992). We and other groups have proposed that ethanol has a specific effect on membrane lipid domains (Wood & Schroeder, 1992; Stout & Kreishman, 1992). Recent findings of our laboratory (Schroeder et al., 1988) have shown that ethanol in vitro had a greater effect on the fluidity of the exofacial leaflet as compared to the cytofacial leaflet. It can be seen in Figure 10.3 that the exofacial leaflet was significantly more fluid than the cytofacial leaflet and that ethanol had a significantly greater effect on the exofacial leaflet. Ethanol did not modify the fluidity of the cytofacial leaflet even at concentrations above 200 mM (data not shown). Chronic ethanol consumption was also observed to have a more pronounced effect on the fluidity of the exofacial leaflet (Figure 10.4) than the cytofacial leaflet (Wood et al., 1989b). The exofacial leaflet of the chronic ethanol-treated mice became more rigid and the cytofacial leaflet became more fluid as compared to the pair-fed control group. In a subsequent study (Wood et al., 1990), it was reported that chronic ethanol consumption modified the transbilayer distribution of membrane cholesterol in the exofacial and cytofacial leaflets of SPM (Figure 10.5). There was a twofold increase in cholesterol in the exofacial leaflet of chronic ethanol-treated mice and a reduction in cholesterol in the cytofacial leaflet. These data were consistent with the study that found that the fluidities of the two leaflets were altered

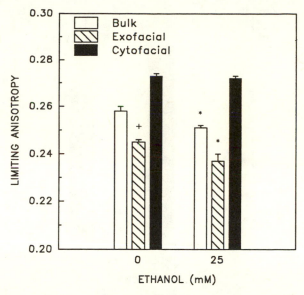

Figure 10.3. Limiting anisotropy of DPH in SPM leaflets in the presence and absence of ethanol. Data are the mean $\pm$ SE (N = 5). *$p <$ .01 as compared to the cytofacial leaflet and *$p <$ .05 as compared to the exofacial leaflet minus ethanol. Data are adapted from Schroeder et al., 1988.

differently by chronic ethanol consumption. It has also been reported that the movement of cholesterol between membranes was reduced by chronic ethanol consumption (Wood et al., 1992). An important finding of both studies was that chronic ethanol consumption altered specific properties of membrane cholesterol domains in the absence of changing the total amount of membrane cholesterol.

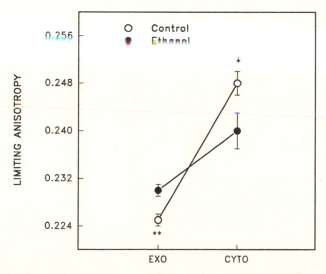

Figure 10.4. Limiting anisotropy of DPH in SPM of chronic ethanol-treated and pair-fed control groups. Individual values are the mean $\pm$ SE (N = 3–5). *$p <$ .05 as compared with the cytofacial leaflet of the chronic ethanol group; **$p <$ .02 compared with the exofacial leaflet of the chronic ethanol group. Data are from Wood et al. (1989b).

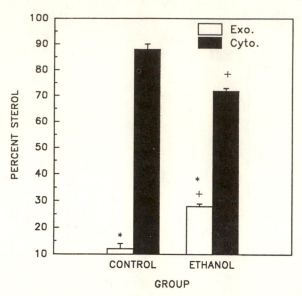

Figure 10.5. Transbilayer distribution of dehydroergosterol (a cholesterol analogue) in SPM of control and chronic ethanol groups. Data are the mean ± SE of the percent sterol (N = 4 membrane preparations per group). *$p < .01$ compared with the cytofacial leaflet and *$p < .01$ compared with the exofacial or cytofacial leaflet of the control group. Data are from Wood et al. (1990).

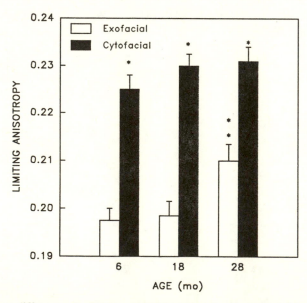

Figure 10.6. Age differences in fluidity of SPM exofacial and cytofacial leaflets of C57BL/6Nnia mice. Data are the mean ± SE of limiting anisotropy of DPH (N = 3 preparations of each age group). *$p < .01$ compared to the exofacial leaflet and **$p < .01$ as compared to the exofacial leaflets of the 6- and 18-month-old mice.

142

There have not been any studies on membrane lipid domains and effects of ethanol in membranes of aged animals. Previous studies have reported on changes in bulk lipid properties of membranes; that would not reveal alterations in membrane lipid domains. Addressing the effects of aging and membrane lipid domains, preliminary data showed that increasing age was associated with changes in the fluidity of the exofacial and cytofacial leaflets (Figure 10.6). Both the exofacial and cytofacial leaflets became less fluid with increasing age as compared to leaflets of the 6-month-old group (Figure 10.6). The largest change in the two leaflets occurred in the exofacial leaflet of the aged mice. Chronic ethanol consumption and increasing age affect leaflet fluidity. The exofacial leaflet of ethanol-treated animals becomes less fluid, whereas the cytofacial leaflet becomes more fluid. In SPM of aged mice, fluidity of both leaflets was reduced and would suggest that chronic ethanol consumption and aging have very different effects on membrane structure.

NEURONAL FUNCTION

There have been several studies on effects of ethanol both in vitro and chronically on neurotransmitters and receptors (Watson, 1992). We have reported, for example, that potassium chloride or veratridine increased the release of GABA from cortical synaptosomes of young mice two- to threefold above the unstimulated baseline conditions (Strong & Wood, 1984). Ethanol significantly depressed the release above baseline but had no effect on baseline release. Dose response curves were generated with a series of alcohols of increasing chain length. The concentration of alcohol required to inhibit GABA release by 50% (IC_{50}) was highly correlated with the membrane/buffer partition coefficients of different alcohols. Since the membrane/buffer partition coefficients of alcohols were correlated with the fluidity in electron spin resonance studies, the results suggested that alcohols inhibit GABA release by fluidizing the membrane.

Based on our finding that membranes of aged animals were fluidized less by ethanol in vitro than young animals, effects of ethanol in vitro on GABA release in cortical synaptosomes of different age groups of mice (4, 14, and 28 months) were determined (Strong & Wood, 1984). Baseline release did not differ among the three age groups. However, ethanol was significantly less effective in depressing the depolarization-induced GABA release in cortical synaptosomal preparations of aged mice as compared to younger mice. Age differences in effects of ethanol on GABA release could be further seen when comparisons were made among the three age groups for the IC_{50} of ethanol (Figure 10.7). The IC_{50} was twofold higher for the oldest group as compared to the youngest group. Synaptosomes of aged mice were resistant to perturbation by ethanol in vitro. The diminished response of aged synaptosomes to ethanol in vitro was consistent with the results showing that membranes of aged mice were fluidized less by ethanol in vitro as compared to membranes of young mice.

We next examined effects of chronic ethanol consumption on GABA release in synaptosomes of 4- and 28-month-old mice. Age-matched, pair-fed controls received a liquid control diet. Inhibition of potassium-stimulated GABA release in response to ethanol in vitro was greatest in the young control group as compared to any other group (Figure 10.8). Significant differences were observed between the young ethanol-treated

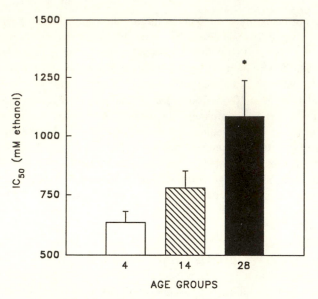

Figure 10.7. Comparison of the IC_{50} of ethanol among different age groups. The IC_{50} was the concentration of ethanol required to reduce net GABA release by 50%. Each value is the mean ± SE of four experiments using six ethanol concentrations (0, 125, 250, 500, 750, 1000 mM). *$p < .05$ compared with the 4-month group. Data are from Strong and Wood (1984).

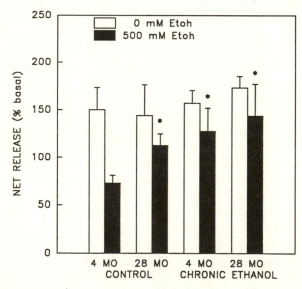

Figure 10.8. Effect of chronic ethanol consumption on GABA release. Each value is the mean ± SE of 4 experiments. *$p < .05$ as compared with the 4-month control group. Data are from Strong and Wood (1984).

group and the young pair-fed control group. The young ethanol-treated group was resistant to the effects of ethanol in vitro, which can be interpreted as cellular tolerance. On the other hand, potassium-stimulated GABA release did not differ between the old chronic group and the old control group when ethanol was added in vitro. Aged animals were impaired in the capacity to adapt to effects of chronic ethanol consumption as measured by depolarized GABA release.

It has been reported that the affinity of the GABA receptor was lower in ethanol-treated rats (12 to 15 months) as compared to rats 3 months of age (Komiskey et al., 1988). Significant differences in affinity of the GABA receptor were not observed, however, between the 3-month-old and 28-month-old rats. The maximum number of GABA binding sites was not affected by ethanol treatment or age. An interesting observation in that study was that the 28-month-old animals received a lower ethanol dose than the other two age groups, but the brain ethanol levels were equivalent.

Release of neurotransmitter amino acids was found to be associated with age and ethanol (Peinado et al., 1987). Glutamate and glutamine release was decreased in 24-month-old rats as compared to 3-month-old rats following an ethanol injection (1.5 g/kg). A 3.0 g/kg dose increased efflux of taurine in the old as compared to the younger animals. Release of aspartate and glycine was not affected by ethanol dose in the two age groups. It was concluded that age differences in effects of ethanol on these amino acid neurotransmitters may be associated with tolerance and dependence.

Ethanol in vitro had different effects on potassium conductance in hippocampal slices from 6- to 8-month-old versus 25- to 29-month-old Fischer 344 rats (Niesen et al., 1988). In young neurons, ethanol was found to have a hyperpolarizing effect, whereas ethanol depolarized old neurons. Ethanol enhanced potassium conductance in young neurons and decreased potassium conductance in old neurons.

In an interesting study that combined aging, genotype, and chronic ethanol consumption, effects were examined on somatostatin levels in hippocampus and striatum in C57BL/6J and Balb/cJ mice (Fuhrmann et al., 1986). The Balb/c strain showed a significant decrease in somatostatin levels with increasing age. Age differences in somatostatin levels were not observed until 27 months in the C57BL strain. Chronic ethanol consumption resulted in an increase in somatostatin levels in the older Balb/c mice, but no effects were observed in the C57BL strain. The ethanol-induced increase in somatostatin counteracted the decline observed with increasing age. The data very convincingly showed that chronic ethanol consumption did not result in accelerated or premature aging. That study also demonstrated the importance of using different strains when examining effects of ethanol in different age groups of animals. The use of selective lines and strains is an approach that has gained importance in alcohol studies (Crabbe et al., 1992).

Effects of aging and chronic ethanol consumption on brain muscarinic cholinergic receptors were recently examined (Pietrzak et al., 1990). Rats received ethanol as their only source of fluid for 25 months. Increasing age was found to be associated with a decrease in quinuclidinyl benzilate binding to muscarinic receptors in the hippocampus, cerebral cortex, and striatum. An association between ethanol consumption and aging was only observed in the cerebral cortex at 3 or 9 months. In another study on ethanol, muscarinic receptors, and aging, it was reported that rats receiving ethanol for 3 months beginning at 2 months and 21 months of age differed in muscarinic receptor density

(Pietrzak et al., 1989). There was approximately a 48% increase in cortical muscarinic receptor density in the young but not the old ethanol-treated groups. Brain muscarinic receptors did not adapt to the effects of chronic ethanol consumption in the old ethanol group.

CONCLUSION

Increasing age is a factor that is associated with effects of ethanol on brain membrane structure, neurotransmitters, and receptors. A general conclusion is that there is an altered capacity to respond to ethanol in aged brain as compared to brain of young organisms. For example, adaptation to the chronic effects of ethanol was not observed for depolarized GABA release or Poly-PI activity in aged animals. The impaired capacity to respond to ethanol was observed when ethanol was administered acutely or chronically. Whether the altered capacity of the aged brain to respond to ethanol is an explanation for age differences in sleep time, temperature regulation, and withdrawal is not known. Another conclusion that can be drawn from several of the studies reviewed in this chapter is that ethanol has a different effect on brain as compared to changes that normally occur with increasing age. The idea that chronic ethanol consumption accelerates aging has no substantive support.

Understanding the molecular mechanisms of age differences in response to ethanol is complicated by the fact that we do not know what mechanisms are involved in intoxication, tolerance, and dependence in young organisms. There has been a large increase in studies on ethanol and brain, but no one approach has unequivocally explained the cellular mechanisms of intoxication, tolerance, and dependence. Those ethanol phenomena may involve a cascade of effects such as specific effects of ethanol on membrane lipid domains that in turn modify membrane proteins, signal transduction, and intracellular events. It might be argued that before we can understand how aged individuals differ in response to ethanol, we will have to understand the effects of ethanol in organisms not complicated by changes associated with aging.

The data base on effects of ethanol in aged brain, particularly potential neurochemical mechanisms, has not grown appreciably over the past five years. A notable exception is recent work on chronic ethanol consumption and Purkinje dendritic morphology in different age groups of rats (Pentney & Quigley, 1987; Pentney et al., 1989; Pentney & Quackenbush, 1990; Pentney & Quackenbush, 1991). Future studies on the effects of ethanol on the aged brain could focus on areas of investigation such as cerebellar dendritic function, NMDA receptor, protein kinases, calcium homeostasis, and lipid domains.

Acknowledgments

This work was supported in part by NIH grants NIAAA 07292, NIA 11056 the Geriatric Research, Education, and Clinical Center, and the Medical Research Service of the Department of Veterans Affairs. Appreciation is extended to Drs. H. James Armbrecht, Friedhelm Schroeder, Randy Strong, Albert Sun, and Grace Sun, who collaborated previously with the author on several of the studies reviewed in this chapter.

References

Armbrecht, H. J., Wood, W. G., Wise, R. W., Walsh, J. B., Thomas, B. N., & Strong, R. (1983). Ethanol-induced disordering of membranes from different age groups of C57BL/6NNIA mice. *Journal of Pharmacology and Experimental Therapeutics, 226*, 387–391.

Beauge, F., Stibler, H., & Borg, S. (1985). Abnormal fluidity and surface carbohydrate content of erythrocyte membrane in alcoholic patients. *Alcoholism: Clinical and Experimental Research, 9*, 322–328.

Berridge, M. J. (1987). Inositol trisphosphate and diacylglycerol: two interacting second messengers. *Annual Review Biochemistry, 56*, 159–193.

Chin, J. H., & Goldstein, D. B. (1977). Drug tolerance in biomembranes: A spin label study of the effects of ethanol. *Science, 196*, 684–685.

Crabbe, J. C., Phillips, T. J., Cunningham, C. L., & Belknap, J. K. (1992). Genetic determinants of ethanol reinforcement. In P. W. Kalivas & H. H. Samson (Eds.) *The neurobiology of drug and alcohol addiction*, (pp. 302–310) New York: The New York Academy of Sciences.

Deitrich, R. A., Dunwiddie, T. V., Harris, R. A., & Erwin, V. G. (1989). Mechanism of action of ethanol: Initial central nervous system actions. *Pharmacology Review, 41*, 489–537.

Fuhrmann, G., Strosser, M. T., Besnard, F., Kempf, E., Kempf, J., & Ebel, A. (1986). Genotypic differences in age and chronic alcohol exposure effects on somatostatin levels in hippocampus and striatum in mice. *Neurochemical Research, 11*, 625–636.

Goldstein, D. B., Chin, J. H., & Lyon, R. C. (1982). Ethanol disordering of spin-labeled mouse membranes; correlation with genetically determined ethanol sensitivity of mice. *Proceedings of the National Academy of Science USA, 79*, 4231–4233.

Harris, R. A., Baxter, D. M., Mitchell, M. A., & Hitzemann, R. J. (1984). Physical properties and lipid composition of brain membranes from ethanol tolerant-dependent mice. *Molecular Pharmacology, 25*, 401–409.

Hunt, W. A. (1985). *Alcohol and biological membranes*. New York: The Guilford Press.

Klemm, W. R. (1990). Dehydration: A new alcohol theory. *Alcohol, 7*, 49–50.

Komiskey, H. L., Raemont, L. M., & Mundinger, K. L. (1988). Aging: Modulation of GABA binding sites by ethanol and diazepam. *Brain Research, 458*, 37–44.

Niesen, C. E., Baskys, A., & Carlen, P. L. (1988). Reversed ethanol effects on potassium conductances in aged hippocampal dentate granule neurons. *Brain Research, 445*, 137–141.

Ott, J. F., Hunter, B. E., & Walker, D. W. (1985). The effect of age on ethanol metabolism and on the hypothermic and hypnotic responses to ethanol in the Fischer 344 rat. *Alcoholism: Clinical and Experimental Research, 9*, 59–65.

Peinado, J. M., Collins, D. M., & Myers, R. D. (1987). Ethanol challenge alters amino acid neurotransmitter release from frontal cortex of aged rat. *Neurobiology of Aging, 8*, 241–247.

Pentney, R. J., Quackenbush, L. J., & O'Neill, M. (1989). Length changes in dendritic networks of cerebellar Purkinje cells of old rats after chronic ethanol treatment. *Alcoholism: Clinical and Experimental Research, 13*, 413–419.

Pentney, R. J., & Quackenbush, L. J. (1990). Dendritic hypertrophy in Purkinje neurons of old Fischer rats after long-term ethanol treatment. *Alcoholism: Clinical and Experimental Research, 14*, 878–886.

Pentney, R. J., & Quackenbush, L. J. (1991). Effects of long durations of ethanol treatment during aging on dendritic plasticity in Fischer 344 rats. *Alcoholism: Clinical and Experimental Research, 15*, 1024–1030.

Pentney, R. J., & Quigley, P. J. (1987). Morphometric parameters of Purkinje dendritic networks after ethanol treatment during aging. *Alcoholism: Clinical and Experimental Research, 11*, 536–540.

Pietrzak, E. R., Wilce, P. A., & Shanley, B. C. (1989). Plasticity of brain muscarinic receptors in aging rats: The adaptative response to scopolamine and ethanol treatment. *Neuroscience Letters, 104,* 331–335.

Pietrzak, E. R., Wilce, P. A., & Shanley, B. C. (1990). Interaction of chronic ethanol consumption and aging on brain muscarinic cholinergic receptors. *Journal of Pharmacology and Experimental Therapeutics, 252,* 869–872.

Ritzmann, R. F., & Springer, A. (1980). Age differences in brain sensitivity and tolerance to ethanol in mice. *Age, 3,* 15–17.

Rottenberg, H., Waring, A., & Rubin, E. (1981). Tolerance and cross-tolerance in chronic alcoholics: Reduced membrane binding of ethanol and other drugs. *Science, 213,* 583–585.

Rubin, E., & Rottenberg, H. (1982). Ethanol-induced injury and adaptations in biological membranes. *Federation Proceedings, 41,* 2465–2471.

Schroeder, F., Morrison, W. J., Gorka, C., & Wood, W. G. (1988). Transbilayer effects of ethanol on fluidity of brain membrane leaflets. *Biochimica et Biophysica Acta, 946,* 85–94.

Stout, J. G., & Kreishman, G. P. (1992). Domain-specific binding of alcohols to neuronal membranes. In R. R. Watson (Ed.), *Alcohol and neurobiology, receptors, membranes and channels,* (pp. 205–214) Boca Raton, FL: CRC Press.

Strong, R., Wood, W. G., & Samorajski, T. (1991). Neurochemistry of ageing. In M. S. J. Pathy (Ed.), *Principles and practices of geriatric medicine,* (pp. 69–97). (New York: John Wiley & Sons).

Strong, R., & Wood W. G. (1984). Membrane properties and aging: *in vivo* and *in vitro* effects of ethanol on synaptosomal τ-aminobutyric acid (GABA) release. *Journal of Pharmacology and Experimental Therapeutics, 229,* 726–730.

Sun, G. Y., Huang, H. M., Lee, D. Z., Chung-Wang, Y. J., Wood, W. G., Strong, R., & Sun, A. Y. (1987). Chronic ethanol effect on the acidic phospholipids of synaptosomes isolated from cerebral cortex of C57BL/6NNia mice—a comparison with age. *Alcohol and Alcoholism, 22,* 367–373.

Sun, G. Y., Navidi, M., Yoa, F-G, Wood, W. G., & Sun, A. Y. (1993). Effects of chronic ethanol administration on poly-phosphoinositide metabolism in the mouse brain: Variance with age. *Neurochemistry International, 23,* 45–52.

Sun, G. Y., & Sun, A. Y. (1985). Ethanol and membrane lipids. *Alcoholism: Clinical and Experimental Research, 9,* 164–180.

Taraschi, T. F., Ellingson, J. S., Wu, A., Zimmerman, R., & Rubin, E. (1986). Phosphatidylinositol from ethanol-fed rats confers membrane tolerance to ethanol. *Proceedings of the National Academy of Science USA, 83,* 9398–9402.

Taraschi, T. F., Ellingson, J. S., Wu-Sun, A., & Rubin, E. (1990). Rats withdrawn from ethanol rapidly re-acquire membrane tolerance after resumption of ethanol feeding. *Biochimica et Biophysica Acta, 1021,* 51–55.

Watson, R. R. (Ed.). (1992). *Alcohol and neurobiology, receptors, membranes, and channels.* Boca Raton, FL: CRC Press.

Wood, W. G. (1976). Age-associated differences in response to alcohol in rats and mice: A biochemical and behavioral review. *Experimental Aging Research, 2,* 543–562.

Wood, W. G., Armbrecht, H. J., & Wise, R. W. (1982). Ethanol intoxication and withdrawal among three age groups of C57BL/6NNia mice. *Pharmacology, Biochemistry and Behavior, 17,* 1037–1041.

Wood, W. G., Armbrecht, H. J., & Wise, R. W. (1984). Aging and the effects of ethanol: The role of brain membranes. In J. T. Hartford & T. Samorajski (Eds.) *Alcoholism in the elderly,* (pp. 139–151). New York: Raven Press.

Wood, W. G., Lahiri, S., Gorka, C., Armbrecht, H. J., & Strong, R. (1987). *In vitro* effects of ethanol on erythrocyte membrane fluidity of alcoholic patients: An electron spin resonance study. *Alcoholism: Clinical and Experimental Research, 11,* 332–335.

Wood, W. G., Gorka, C., Rao, A. M., & Schroeder, F. (1989a). Specific action of ethanol on lateral and vertical membrane domains. In G. Y. Sun, P. K. Rudeen, W. G. Wood, Y-H. Wei, & A. Y. Sun (Eds.) *Molecular mechanisms of alcohol.* (pp. 3–13). Clifton, New Jersey: Humana Press.

Wood, W. G., Gorka, C., & Schroeder, F. (1989b). Acute and chronic effects of ethanol on transbilayer membrane domains. *Journal of Neurochemistry, 52*, 1925–1930.

Wood, W. G., Schroeder, F., Hogy, L., Rao, A. M., & Nemecz, G. (1990). Asymmetric distribution of a fluorescent sterol in synaptic plasma membranes: Effects of chronic ethanol consumption. *Biochimica et Biophysica Acta, 1025*, 243–246.

Wood, W. G., Schroeder, F., & Rao, A. M. (1991). Significance of ethanol-induced changes in membrane lipid domains. *Alcohol and Alcoholism*, Suppl. 1, 221–225.

Wood, W. G., Rao, A. M., Igbavboa, U., & Semotuk, M. (1993). Cholesterol exchange and lateral cholesterol pools in synaptosomal membranes of pair-fed control and chronic ethanol-treated mice. *Alcoholism: Clinical and Experimental Research, 17*, 345–350.

Wood, W. G., & Armbrecht, H. J. (1982a). Age differences in ethanol-induced hypothermia and impairment in mice. *Neurobiology of Aging, 3*, 243–246.

Wood, W. G., & Armbrecht, H. J. (1982b). Behavioral effects of ethanol in animals: Age differences and age changes. *Alcoholism: Clinical and Experimental Research, 6*, 3–12.

Wood, W. G., & Schroeder, F. (1988a). Membrane effects of ethanol: Bulk lipid versus lipid domains. *Life Science, 43*, 467–475.

Wood, W. G., & Schroeder, F. (1988b). Membrane structure in aged humans and animals. In R. Strong, W. G. Wood, & W. J. Burke (Eds.) *Central nervous system disorders of aging: Clinical intervention and research* (pp. 199–209). New York: Raven Press.

Wood, W. G., & Schroeder, F. (1992). Membrane exofacial and cytofacial leaflets: A new approach to understanding how ethanol alters brain membranes. In R. R. Watson (Ed.), *Alcohol and neurobiology: Receptors, membranes, and channels* (pp. 161–184). Boca Raton, FL: CRC Press.

Yeagle, P. L. (1989). Lipid regulation of cell membrane structure and function. *FASEB Journal, 3*, 1833–1842.

York, J. L. (1982). Body water content, ethanol pharmacokinetics, and the responsiveness to ethanol in young and old rats. *Developmental Pharmacology and Therapeutics, 4*, 106–116.

11

The Effects of Aging on the Interaction of Ethanol with Chemical Neurotransmission in the Brain

PAULA BICKFORD, ANYA M.-Y. LIN,
KAREN PARFITT AND MICHAEL R. PALMER

Ethanol interacts with chemical neurotransmission in the brain to produce the physiological effects of intoxication. Thus, changes in chemical neurotransmission that result from the process of aging could alter the actions of ethanol in the aged brain. This chapter will focus on a specific action of ethanol to illustrate some of these age-related changes. First, we will discuss age-related changes in β-adrenergic receptor function. Second, we will review the actions of ethanol on β-adrenergic receptor modulation of γ-amino butyric acid$_A$ (GABA$_A$) receptor function in the cerebellar cortex. Finally, we will discuss how the age-related changes in β-receptor function affect the action of ethanol on chemical neurotransmission in the cerebellar cortex.

Catecholaminergic pathways serve as an example of systems that have been shown to be altered during aging. Several areas of the central nervous system (CNS) demonstrate decreases in catecholamine turnover and tyrosine hydroxylase activity in aging, and reductions in β-adrenergic receptor numbers have been described (Miller & Zahniser, 1988). Moreover, decreases in catecholamine-stimulated adenylate cyclase activity and cyclic nucleotide accumulation in old animals have been reported.

We have examined noradrenergic function in aging using the cerebellum as a model. The inhibitory noradrenergic input from the locus coeruleus to the cerebellum has been extensively studied in terms of its anatomy, physiology, and pharmacology (Bickford, Hoffer, & Freedman, 1986; Bickford-Wimer, Granholm, & Gerhardt, 1988). Noradrenergic fibers arising from the pontine nucleus locus coeruleus ascend through the superior cerebellar peduncle to synapse on cerebellar Purkinje neurons. Activation of this input inhibits spontaneous discharge of the cerebellar Purkinje neurons via a cyclic adenosine mono phosphate (AMP) dependent process (Bickford, Hoffer, & Freedman, 1986). However, the interaction of norepinephrine (NE) with cerebellar neuronal circuitry has been shown to be more complex than a simple effect on spontaneous discharge. NE is thought to have neuromodulatory actions, since it augments inhibitory inputs to Purkinje neurons at doses that do not affect spontaneous discharge. This can be observed when GABA, the putative neurotransmitter for the basket cell inhibition of Purkinje cells, is locally applied onto Purkinje cells. When NE or isoproterenol (a β-adrenergic receptor agonist) is administered at the same time as GABA, there is an increase in the response to GABA. This change in GABA response during NE application has been termed modulation. We will show evidence in this chapter that the modulatory actions of NE in the cerebellum are altered by the aging process.

One of the actions of ethanol in the CNS is an interaction with GABAergic receptors (Deitrich, Dunwiddie, Harris, & Erwin, 1989; Shefner, 1990). For example, ethanol has been reported to share the muscle relaxant, antianxiety, and sedative-hypnotic properties with agents, such as barbiturates, that are thought to interact with $GABA_A$ receptor/Cl⁻ channel complex (Becker & Anton, 1990; Skolnick & Paul, 1981). Furthermore, a variety of the ethanol-induced responses were potentiated by GABA agonists, such as muscimol, and antagonized by GABA antagonists, such as bicuculline (Becker & Anton, 1990; Ferko, 1990; Freund, van Horne, Harlan, & Palmer, 1993; Hinko & Rozanov, 1990; Liljequist & Engel, 1982; Martz, Deitrich, & Harris, 1983). In addition, ethanol can augment GABA responses in brain synaptoneurosomes (Allan & Harris, 1986; Allan & Harris, 1987), in cultured spinal neurons (Mehta & Ticku, 1988; Suzdak, Schwartz, Skolnick, & Paul, 1986; Suzdak et al., 1986; Ticku, Lowrimore, & Lehoullier, 1986), in feline cerebral cortex (Nestoros, 1980), in hippocampal neurons (Aguayo, 1990), and in rat dorsal root ganglion neurons (Nishio & Narahashi, 1990) as well as in *Xenopus* oocytes, which express mouse brain mRNA for the $GABA_A$ receptor-Cl⁻ channel (Wafford, Dunwiddie, & Harris, 1990). GABA antagonists have been reported to block some of these potentiating effects of ethanol (Allan & Harris, 1987; Mehta & Ticku, 1988; Suzdak, Schwartz, Skolnick, & Paul, 1986). Taken together, these data suggest that $GABA_A$ mechanisms may be involved in some actions of ethanol.

Although ethanol appears to interact with the $GABA_A$ mechanism, we and others previously found that ethanol either had no direct effect or antagonized the GABA-induced electrophysiological responses of cerebellar Purkinje neurons and hippocampal neurons (Bloom & Siggins, 1987; Carlen, Gurevich, & Durand, 1982; Freund, van Horne, Harlan, & Palmer, 1993; Harris & Sinclair, 1984; Siggins et al., 1987). However, systemically administered ethanol has been shown to potentiate GABA-induced depressions of cerebellar Purkinje neurons if these GABA responses were concomitantly modulated by applications of norepinephrine (NE) or the β-adrenergic agonist isoproterenol (ISO) at the dose that has no effect on the basal neuronal activity (Lin, Freund, & Palmer, 1991; Stowe et al., 1986). Furthermore, we recently showed that local applications of ethanol also potentiated ISO-modulated GABA responses and that catecholamine sensitization of GABA responses to the potentiating effects of ethanol is mediated by a β-adrenergic mechanism (Lin et al., 1992). We concluded that a β-adrenergic modulation plays an important role in the ethanol-induced potentiation of GABA responses of cerebellar Purkinje neurons.

This chapter will review work on how aging can alter the actions of NE at the β-adrenergic receptor. These age-related changes in β-adrenergic receptor function can then directly affect the way ethanol acts on cerebellar Purkinje neurons in aged rats.

METHODS

Electrophysiological experiments were performed on young (aged 4 to 6 months) and old (aged 18 to 20 or 24 to 25 months) male F344 rats, weighing 250 to 550 g, which were obtained from the National Institute on Aging contract colonies maintained by Harlan Laboratories. Each animal was anesthetized with urethane (0.75 to 1.25 g/kg, i.p.), intubated, and fixed in a stereotaxic instrument. Aged rats required lower doses of anesthetics; however, all rats were equivalently anesthetized at the surgical plane of anesthesia, monitored by corneal reflex and toe pinch reflex. Rectal temperature was monitored with a rectal thermistor and maintained at 37°C with a heating pad. After cisternal drainage, the skull and other superficial tissues over the cerebellar vermis were removed, the dura was carefully opened to expose the underlying brain, and the exposed brain tissue was covered with 2% agar. Three to five-barrel micropipettes were constructed as described by Palmer (1982) and were lowered into the fifth and sixth vermian lobules of the cerebellum with a micromanipulator. One 5 M NaCl-filled barrel with resistance of 5 MΩ was used to record spontaneous neuronal firing from identified cerebellar Purkinje neurons (Eccles, Ito, & Szentogothai, 1967). A second 5M NaCl-filled barrel of a multibarrel micropipette was used as a balance barrel for current neutralization during microiontophoresis. The remaining three barrels of the micropipette were used for the application of drugs into the environment of each cell by microiontophoresis or electroosmotic application (Palmer & Hoffer, 1980) or by pressure ejection (Palmer, 1982). Current for iontophoresis or electro-osmosis was controlled by operational amplifiers; the timing of drug applications was controlled by a crystal clock circuit (Smith & Hoffer, 1978).

Extracellular action potentials were recorded from single Purkinje cells, the signals were filtered, amplified, and isolated by a window discriminator. The firing rates were integrated over 1-sec time intervals, and displayed as ratemeter records on a strip chart recorder. Each neuron was required to exhibit a stable firing rate during pre- and post-drug periods, and drug responses were acceptable only if they were repeatable and reversible. The drug-induced responses were quantified using a computer and a graphics tablet to determine the percent inhibition of cell firing caused by drug applications as previously described (Palmer & Hoffer, 1980). The responses under various treatments were analyzed with multivariate analysis of variance suitable for repeated measures, and some data were analyzed by unpaired student's t-test and Fisher's exact test.

Drugs applied locally by microiontophoresis from multibarrel micropipettes included 0.5 M GABA (pH = 5, Sigma) and 0.25 M (−)-isoproterenol HCl (pH = 4, Sigma), and these drugs were dissolved in distilled water which was bubbled with nitrogen gas prior to use. Drugs dissolved in 154 mM NaCl included ethanol (750 mM, pH = 7) applied by electro-osmosis and 0.1 mM phentolamine HCl (pH = 7, Sigma) and 0.1 mM timolol maleate (pH = 7, Sigma) applied by pressure ejection.

For the studies of antagonists, an agonist dose (expressed in psi × sec) that produced a 50% or greater response was used, and responses to agonists were compared when an antagonist was and was not present. A response was considered antagonized if the original response was reduced by 80% or more in the presence of antagonist. For the aging studies, a dose of the agonist that produced an approximate 50% inhibition of Purkinje cell firing rate was tested at least three times to ensure a consistent response. Agonist doses above and below this ED_{50} dose were also tested to establish a dose-response relationship for each cell. Only data from cells that did not show a decrease in action potential amplitude during the response to the agonist and that showed recovery after exposure to the agonist were used. The drug-induced responses were quantified by computer, and the data from ratemeter displays were digitized using a Tektronix graphics tablet and were led to a computer for analysis of drug-induced changes of firing rate as described in the literature (Freedman, Hoffer, & Woodward, 1975; Palmer & Hoffer, 1980). The effects of antagonists were compared using chi-squared analysis.

When comparing dose response curves to locally applied drugs between young and aged rats, the micropipette tip diameter is a critical factor involved in determining the concentration of drug that reaches the receptor. This problem can be minimized by carefully monitoring pipette construction and by using the same pipette to record from the young rat and then the old rat. The next pipette was started in the old rat to control for the loss in pipette potency with time. In addition, more than ten pipettes were used for each animal group, which statistically lowers the contribution of any one pipette to the overall data set.

Cumulative population dose-response curves were constructed using a least-squares nonlinear regression curve-fitting program adapted by Motulsky (ISI Software, 1987). For these curves, "response" was defined as an approximate 50% inhibition of Purkinje cell firing rate. This analysis yielded the maximum percentages of responding neurons and the population ED_{50}, which is an estimate of the dose of drug that is effective in eliciting a 50% inhibition in firing rate for half of the neurons in the population of cells analyzed. Differences between the young and the 18- and 26-month age groups were compared using the Kolmogorov Smirnov statistical test, which assesses the significance of differences between populations when the data is represented in a cumulative fashion as described here.

RESULTS

Age-Induced Change in β-Adrenergic Receptors

Local application of either dobutamine, a β_1-selective agonist (Tuttle & Mills, 1975) or zinterol, a β_2-selective agonist (Gwee, Nott, Raper, & Rodger, 1972), elicited a dose-dependent inhibition of Purkinje cell firing rate. ICI 89406, a β_1-selective antagonist, blocked the effects of dobutamine in 5 out of 5 cells studied (Figure 11.1A, Table 11.1). ICI 118551, a β_2-selective antagonist, did not affect dobutamine-induced inhibitions (n = 4; Figure 11.1B, Table 11.1). Conversely, ICI 89406 did not affect zinterol-induced inhibitions (n = 4; Figure 11.2A and Table 11.1), whereas ICI 118551 blocked the β_2 effects in 8 out of 8 cells studied (Figure 11.2B, Table 11.1). Thus, dobutamine and zinterol appear to be acting selectively at β_1 and β_2 receptors, respectively, at this 1 mM barrel concentration.

Electrophysiological responses of Purkinje neurons to dobutamine and zinterol (barrel concentration 1 mM for both) were compared in young (3-month-old) and aged (18- and 26-month-old) Fischer 344 rats. Each agonist was tested in seventeen 3-month-old, eight 18-month-old, and nine 26-month-old rats; both agonists were tested on each cell, so that results for the two agonists were obtained from the same population of neurons. For each neuron, several doses of the agonists were tested to determine a dose that

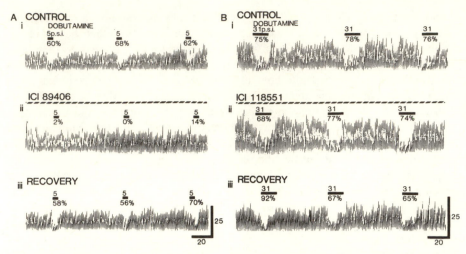

Figure 11.1. Ratemeter records showing the effects of beta$_1$- and beta $_2$-selective antagonists, ICI 89406 and ICI 118551, on dobutamine-induced inhibition of Purkinje cell spontaneous firing rate. Ratemeter records show the response of a Purkinje cell to pressure microejection pulses of dobutamine before, during, and after continuous administration of antagonist. Each vertical deflection of the ratemeter pen indicates the number of action potentials per second of the neuron being recorded. Dose of agonist in this and subsequent ratemeter records is expressed in terms of pounds per square inch (p.s.i., noted above drug applications) $\times$ seconds (as indicated by duration of solid bars above ratemeter records). Numbers below the bars indicate the percent inhibitory response to agonist applications. (A) ICI 89406 was able to block dobutamine-induced inhibitions at doses that did not affect spontaneous activity. Recovery to control levels of response was observed when the antagonist was discontinued. (B) ICI 118551 was not able to block dobutamine-induced inhibition. Calibrations: vertical—25 action potentials per second; horizontal—20 seconds.

produced a 40 to 60% (an approximate 50%) decrease in Purkinje cell spontaneous activity; this ED$_{50}$ dose was tested at least three times to ensure a consistent response.

Figure 11.3 is a ratemeter record from a typical experiment, showing the response of Purkinje neurons to dobutamine from a 3-month old (A), and a 26-month-old (B) F344 rat to local, pressure-ejected applications of dobutamine. In order to eliminate variance due to differences in release of drug from different micropipettes, the same pipette was used to record from a 3-month-old and a 26-month-old rat (Figure 11.3A and B). Figure 11.3A shows that a dose of 2 psi $\times$ 2 sec (or 4 psi $\times$ sec) produced an approximate 50% inhibition in spontaneous discharge rate of the cell from a young rat. In contrast, Figure 11.3B illustrates the failure of a neuron from a 26-month-old rat to

Table 11.1. Effects of Selective β Adrenergic Antagonists on Dobutamine and Zinterol

Agonist	Antagonist	N	Blockade	No Blockade
Dobutamine	ICI 89406	5	5	0
	ICI 118551	4	0	4
Zinterol	ICI 89406	4	0	4
	ICI 118551	8	8	0

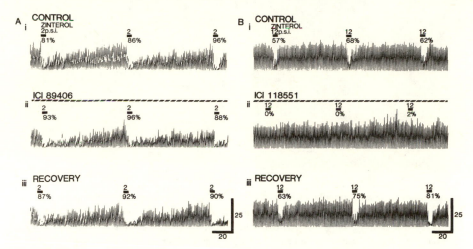

Figure 11.2. Effects of ICI 89406 and ICI 118551 on zinterol-induced inhibition of Purkinje cell spontaneous firing rate. (A) ICI 89406 was not able to block the effects of zinterol. (B) ICI 118551 was able to block the zinterol-induced inhibitions at doses that did not affect spontaneous activity. Recovery to control levels of response was observed when the antagonist was discontinued. Calibrations: vertical—25 action potentials per second; horizontal—20 seconds.

respond to even very high doses (1550 psi × sec) of the β_1 agonist from the same micropipette.

Figure 11.4 shows cumulative population dose-response curves from all the groups tested (3-month, 18-month, and 26-month) for the number of Purkinje cells responding to dobutamine. Comparison of these curves revealed significant age-related decreases

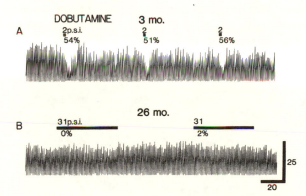

Figure 11.3. Ratemeter records showing the responses of cerebellar Purkinje neurons of 3-month (A) and 26-month (B) Fischer 344 rats to local application of dobutamine. Several doses of the agonist were tested to determine a dose that produced an approximate 50% inhibition of Purkinje cell firing rate. A paired-pipette paradigm was used, in which the pipette in (A) was the same as that used in (B). The Purkinje neuron of the 26-month rat failed to respond to even very high doses of dobutamine (1550 p.s.i. × sec.), whereas a relatively low dose of the beta$_1$ agonist (8 p.s.i. × sec. was capable of eliciting an approximate 50% decrease in spontaneous firing rate in the pipette-matched 3-month-old rat. Calibrations: vertical—25 action potentials per second; horizontal—20 seconds.

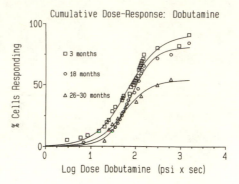

Figure 11.4. Cumulative population dose-response curves of Purkinje neuron responses to local application of dobutamine in 3-, 18-, and 26-month-old Fischer 344 rats. Dose-response curves from the 26-month-old groups differed from the 3-month-old group with significance levels of $p < 0.01$ using the Kolmogorov-Smirnov statistic. The number of cells represented is N = 70 (3 months), N = 33 (18 months) and N = 37 (26 months). The ordinate represents the percentage of cells tested responding to a given dose of the agonist with an approximate 50% inhibition of firing rate. The abscissa corresponds to the log dose of agonist in p.s.i. × seconds. The data are presented in a cumulative fashion.

in responsiveness to this β_1 agonist. Fifty percent of the neurons did not respond even to the highest doses of dobutamine in the 26-month-old age group, but there was no significant shift in the population ED_{50}s for those cells that did respond [51.6 psi × sec, 95% confidence interval (CI) = 38.5 to 69.3; 83.2 psi × sec, 95% CI = 67.0 to 103.4; 57.99 psi × sec, 47.5 to 70.7 for 3-month-old, 18-month-old, and 26-month-old, respectively]. The cumulative population dose-response curves from the 26-month age group differed significantly from the 3-month group ($p < 0.01$, Kolmogorov-Smirnov statistic).

In contrast, comparison of the cumulative dose-response curves for zinterol (Figure 11.5) reveals no significant age-related change in response to the β_2 agonist; there was

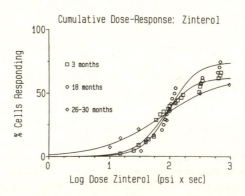

Figure 11.5. Cumulative population dose-response curves of Purkinje neuron responses to locally applied zinterol in 3-, 18-, and 26-month-old Fischer 344 rats. Dose-response curves from the 18- and 26-month-old group did not differ significantly from the 3-month-old group using the Kolmogorov-Smirnov statistic. The number of cells represented is N = 68 (3 months), N = 32 (18 months) and N = 34 (26 months).

no evidence of change in the population ED_{50} with aging (113.7 psi $\times$ sec, 95% CI = 90.5 to 142.9; 129.2 psi $\times$ sec, 95% CI = 99.9 to 167.0; 123.7 psi $\times$ sec, 95% CI = 69.4 to 220.4 for 3-, 18- and 26-month-old, respectively), nor was there a change in the total number of cells responding.

Interaction of Ethanol with β-Receptor Modulation of GABA$_A$ Receptors

In young F344 rats, we observed an ethanol-induced potentiation of the ISO-facilitated GABA$_A$ responses similar to what has been previously observed in young Sprague-Dawley rats (Lin, Freund, & Palmer, 1991; Lin et al., 1992). GABA was applied iontophoretically onto a cerebellar Purkinje neuron (Figure 11.6A) and the dose was adjusted to obtain a 32% ± 1% inhibition of spontaneous firing of 31 cerebellar Purkinje neurons studied. Microiontophoretic application of ISO facilitated (positively modulated) GABA responses (Figure 11.6B), and the dose of ISO was adjusted to augment GABA responses to a submaximal potentiation of GABA responses so that an additional effect of ethanol might be observed. The subsequent coadministration of ethanol with ISO caused a further augmentation of GABA responses (Figure 11.6C) in 31 out of 55 cerebellar Purkinje neurons tested in young F344 rats. The GABA responses returned

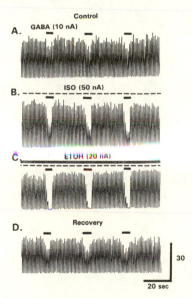

Figure 11.6. A local application of EtOH potentiated the ISO-facilitated GABA-induced depressions in a cerebellar Purkinje neuron of a young (5-months-old) F344 rat. Drug applications are indicated by horizontal bars over the ratemeter records. Sequential ratemeter records of a single cerebellar Purkinje neuron illustrate (A) the control depressant responses to microiontophoretically applied GABA (10 nA, 5 sec) alone; (B) a facilitation (positive modulation) of GABA responses by a local application of ISO (50 nA, continuous application, dotted line); and (C) a potentiation of the ISO-modulated GABA inhibitions after a local application of ethanol (20 nA, continous application, dashed line). Calibration: vertical—30 action potentials per sec; horizontal—20 sec.

to control levels when the applications of both ISO and ethanol were terminated (Figure 11.6D).

Aging and Ethanol Interactions

The same strategy was used to study the interaction of ethanol with the ISO-modulated GABA responses in aged (24 to 25 months old) F344 rats. Unlike the young animals, only 13 out of the 59 cerebellar Purkinje neurons studied in the aged F344 rats demonstrated an ISO-induced facilitation of GABA responses. Furthermore, among these neurons from aged rats showing an ISO-induced modulation of GABA responses, the responsiveness to ISO appeared subsensitive. ISO facilitated GABA responses from an average 33% ± 3% inhibition to an average 43% ± 3% inhibition; however, the dose of ISO used to elicit the facilitation of GABA responses was 20 nA ± 2 nA in young F344 rats and 45 nA ± 4 nA in aged F344 rats (Mean ± SEM, $p < 0.001$ by unpaired student's test).

In contrast to the ISO-induced potentiation of GABA responses in young F344 rats,

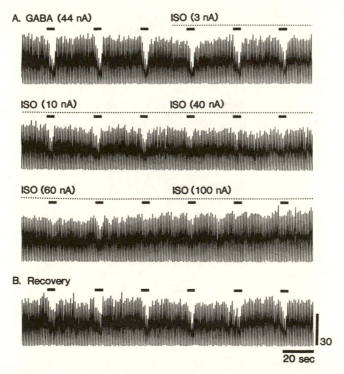

Figure 11.7. GABA-induced depressions of the spontaneous firing of cerebellar Purkinje neurons of aged F344 rats were attenuated (negatively modulated) by continuous applications of ISO. Sequential ratemeter records of neuronal firing of a cerebellar Purkinje neuron in an aged F344 rat show that (A) depressant responses by GABA applications were partially attenuated by low doses of ISO (continuous iontophoretic application, 3 and 10 nA, dotted line). Increasing the dose of ISO from 40, 60, to 100 nA completely eliminated GABA responses; (B) the GABA responses gradually returned to control levels after termination of ISO application. Calibration: vertical—30 action potentials per sec; horizontal—20 sec.

ISO either had no effect or even antagonized the GABA responses of 46 out of the 59 neurons recorded from aged F344 rats (Figure 11.7). The application of ISO attenuated GABA responses (Figure 11.8A, B) in 33 out of the 59 neurons from aged F344 rats; this submaximal response was chosen so that any differential effect of ethanol could be observed. Subsequent ethanol application further decreased these attenuated GABA responses (Figure 11.8C). The GABA responses returned to control levels after terminating the applications of ethanol and ISO (Figure 11.8D).

The responses to ISO and GABA in young and aged rats were divided into four categories that are illustrated in Figure 11.9. The first category contains responses from neurons where ethanol potentiated the ISO-faciliated GABA responses as previously

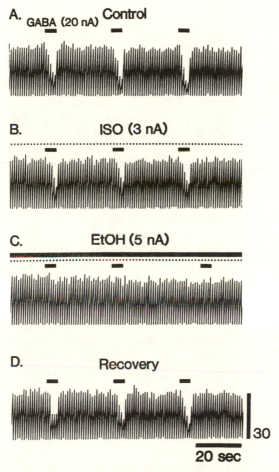

Figure 11.8. The local application of EtOH decreased ISO-attenuated GABA responses of a cerebellar Purkinje neuron of an aged (24-month) F344 rat. Sequential ratemeter records illustrate that (A) the control GABA applications (20 nA, 5 sec) depressed the spontaneous firing of the neuron; (B) continuous application of ISO (3 nA, dotted line) partially antagonized GABA responses; (C) a local application of ethanol (5 nA, continuous application) blocked completely the ISO-attenuated GABA responses; (D) the GABA response returned to control levels after termination of both ISO and EtOH applications. Calibration: vertical—30 action potentials per sec; horizontal—20 sec.

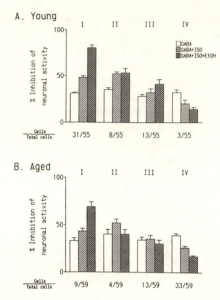

Figure 11.9. One hundred fourteen cerebellar Purkinje neurons collected from young and old F344 rats were categorized according to the differential effects of ISO and EtOH on GABA responses. The control depressant responses by GABA applications (blank bars) were differentially affected by ISO (hatched bars), and EtOH further affected the ISO-modulated GABA responses (crossed bars). Fifty-five cerebellar Purkinje neurons from young F344 rats (A) and 59 neurons from aged F344 rats (B) were classified into four different groups: I, II, III, and IV as described under "Results." Briefly, the control GABA responses in the first group were facilitated by ISO, and EtOH further potentiated the modulated GABA responses; those in groups II and III were not significantly affected by either ISO or EtOH; and the GABA responses in the fourth group were inhibited by ISO and EtOH. Values are mean ± S.E.M.

described in young Sprague-Dawley rats. Responses from neurons in Category II were characterized by a facilitation of GABA responses by ISO but no further augumentation with ethanol. Category III responses were characterized by no significant interaction of ISO with GABA responses and by no changes in responses to GABA with subsequent applications of ethanol. The fourth type of response was opposite to that observed in Category I; that is, ISO attenuated the GABA responses and ethanol further diminished the ISO-attenuated GABA responses.

The frequency distribution of these four types of response recorded from 114 Purkinje neurons from young and aged F344 rats is illustrated in Figure 11.10. There was a significant shift in the types of responses observed in cerebellar Purkinje neurons from aged F344 rats. With respect to the effect of age on the ISO-induced modulation of GABA responses, the GABA responses of 71% of the neurons recorded from young F344 rats were modulated by ISO; in aged F344 rats, however, only 22% of the neurons demonstrated augmentation of GABA responses by ISO. On the other hand, a large percentage (78%) of neurons in aged F344 rats showed no effect of ISO or a reversal of the effects seen in young F344 rats. The same split is observed with the ethanol-induced potentiation of the modulated GABA responses. The predominant response elicited by ethanol in young F344 rats was a further potentiation of the ISO-facilitated GABA responses; whereas in aged F344 rats, the opposite effect was observed, either

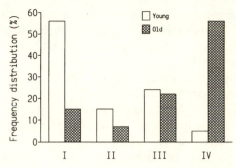

Figure 11.10. Frequency distribution of 114 Purkinje neurons collected from young (blank bars) and aged (crossed bars) F344 rats. Groups I, II, III, and IV underlying each pair of bars represent four different responses that could be recorded from cerebellar Purkinje neurons to combinations of GABA, ISO, and ethanol (see text for explanation). Most cerebellar Purkinje neurons from young F344 rats are represented in group I; these neurons demonstrated an ISO-induced facilitation of GABA-induced depressions of spontaneous firing that were further potentiated by ethanol (as shown in Figure 11.6). Most of the cerebellar Purkinje neurons from aged F344 rats, on the other hand, were classified as group IV; these neurons demonstrated an ISO-induced attenuation of GABA responses that were further decreased by ethanol (see Figure 11.9).

no effect of ethanol on the ISO-modulated GABA response or a further diminution of the ISO-attenuated GABA responses. Thus, the critical factor for determining the responses to ethanol was the effect of ISO on the GABA responses.

DISCUSSION

In this chapter we have presented evidence that concurrent with the aging process there is a decline in the function of β-adrenergic receptors in the cerebellum of F344 rats. One of the actions of alcohol in the central nervous system is mediated through the β-adrenergic receptor. Ethanol can potentiate the modulatory effects of ISO on GABA mediated inhibitions. In aged rats, this action of ethanol is altered such that the opposite effect is observed, i.e., ethanol diminishes the effect of GABA in the presence of ISO. The underlying cause of the change in ethanol actions is the altered action of the β-adrenergic receptor. Ethanol will potentiate the action of ISO on GABA-mediated responses in both young and aged rats; it is the action of ISO that changes in the aged rats.

The age related decline in the β_1 adrenergic receptor function most likely underlies the change in ethanol responses that have been reported here. It is the β_1 receptor subtype that is thought to mediate modulation of GABAergic neurotransmission in the cerebellum (Yeh & Woodward, 1983). The ability of NE to modulate afferent inputs to Purkinje cells in the cerebellum may play a critical role in information processing within the cerebellar cortex. The cerebellum is thought to be involved in balance, coordination, and motor learning (Watson & McElligott, 1984; McElligott, Ebner, & Bloedel, 1986; Bickford et al., 1992). Furthermore, alterations in β-adrenergic receptor function are hypothesized to underlie some of the age-related declines in motor learning observed in aged rats (Bickford, 1993).

At least two explanations are possible for the alteration in the ISO modulation of GABA responses that is observed in the aged rats. First, the negative modulation of GABA responses may result from alterations in the GABA$_A$ receptor/Cl⁻ channel complex during aging. The GABA$_A$ receptor is a hetero-oligomeric complex composed of several distinct polypeptide subunits, including α, β, γ, and δ (Olsen & Tobin, 1990); α, β, and γ have been reported to contain consensus sequences for protein phosphorylation and are phosphorylated by protein kinases such as PKC and PKA (Browning et al., 1990; Leidenheimer, Browning, & Harris, 1991; Leidenheimer et al., 1991). However, the functional importance of phosphorylation of GABA$_A$ receptors in unclear in that it has been reported either to increase or decrease GABA$_A$ receptor function (Cheun & Yeh, 1991; Leidenheimer, Browning, & Harris, 1991; Leidenheimer et al., 1991; Porter et al., 1990). In the present study, the modulatory actions of ISO on GABA$_A$ receptor function are mediated via c-AMP activation of PKA, which in turn phosphorylates either GABA$_A$ receptors or some other protein, resulting in the augmentation of the GABA$_A$ receptor function. If the differential subunit composition of the GABA$_A$ receptor complex underlies the discrepancies observed with respect to the functional consequence of phosphorylation, then an age-related change in subunit composition of the GABA$_A$ receptor complex could explain the change from ISO augmentation of GABA in young rats to ISO attenuation of GABA in aged rats.

The second possible explanation is that the ISO-attenuated GABA responses result from age-related decreases in β-adrenergic receptor coupled second messenger pathway, (Parfitt, Hoffer, & Browning, 1991; Schmidt, 1981; Walker & Walker, 1973). Several studies have shown that activation of PKC decreases the activity of the GABA$_A$ receptor that was expressed in *Xenopus* oocytes (Sigel & Baur, 1988). Thus, an age-associated disequilibrium between phosphorylation of the GABA$_A$ receptor complex by PKA and PKC could underlie the age-related change in the modulatory effects of ISO.

In conclusion, as a result of normal aging in rodents there is a decline in the physiological effects of β-noradrenergic receptors. This change is specific to the β_1 noradrenergic receptor subtype. It is the β_1 subtype that is associated with the neuromodulatory actions of NE upon GABA responses in the cerebellum. One of the actions of alcohol in the CNS is mediated via the neuromodulatory effect of NE on GABA$_A$ receptors. The result is that the actions of ethanol in the aged brain are different than the actions of alcohol in the young brain. The cerebellum is known to be involved with motor coordination and motor learning (Watson & McElligott, 1984; McElligott, Ebner, & Bloedel, 1986; Bickford et al., 1992), and the age-related changes in motor learning that have been observed in rats are correlated with changes in function of β-noradrenergic receptors (Bickford, 1993). The actions of ethanol on motor learning have not been examined, however, and ethanol could potentially disrupt this key learning process in aged animals. In summary, aging results in alterations in neurotransmission that affect the actions of ethanol in the aged brain.

References

Aguayo, L. G. (1990). Ethanol potentiated the GABA$_a$-activated Cl⁻ current in mouse hippocampal and cortical neurons. *European Journal of Pharmacology, 187*, 127–130.

Allan, A. M., & Harris, R. A. (1986). Gamma-aminobutyric acid and alcohol actions: Neurochemical studies of long sleep and short sleep mice. *Life Sciences, 39*, 2005–2015.

Allan, A. M., & Harris, R. A. (1987). Involvement of neuronal chloride channels in ethanol intoxication, tolerance, and dependence. In M. Galanter (Ed.), *Recent developments in alcoholism, volume 5* (pp. 313–325). New York: Plenum Press.

Becker, H. C., & Anton, R. F. (1990). Valproate potentiates and picrotoxin antagonizes the anxiolytic action of ethanol in a nonshock conflict task. *Neuropharmacology, 29*, 837–843.

Bickford, P. (1993). Motor learning deficits in aged rats are correlated with loss of cerebellar noradrenergic function. *Brain Research, 620*, 133–138.

Bickford, P., Heron, C., Young, D. A., Gerhardt, G. A., & de la Garza, R. (1992). Impaired acquisition of novel locomotor tasks in aged and norepinephrine-depleted F344 rats. *Neurobiology of Aging, 13*, 475–481.

Bickford, P. C., Hoffer, B. J., & Freedman, R. (1986). Diminished interaction of norepinephrine with climbing fiber inputs to cerebellar Purkinje neurons in aged Fischer 344 rats. *Brain Research, 385*, 405–410.

Bickford-Wimer, P. C., Granholm, A. C., & Gerhardt, G. A. (1988). Cerebellar noradrenergic systems in aging: Studies *in situ* and in *in oculo* grafts. *Neurobiology of Aging, 9*, 591–599.

Bloom, F. E., & Siggins, G. R. (1987). Electrophysiological action of ethanol at the cellular level. *Alcohol, 4*, 331–337.

Browning, M. D., Bureau, M., Dudek, E. M., & Olsen, R. (1990). Protein kinase C and cAMP-dependent protein kinase phosphorylate the B subunit of the purified g-aminobutyric acid A receptor. *Proceedings of the National Academy of Sciences, 87*, 1315–1318.

Carlen, P. L., Gurevich, N., & Durand, D. (1982). Ethanol in low doses augments calcium-mediated mechanisms measured intracellularly in hippocampal neurons. *Science, 215*, 306–309.

Cheun, J. E., & Yeh, H. H. (1991). Cyclic-AMP-dependent protein kinase: An intermediary in the modulation of GABA$_a$ receptor function on cerebellar Purkinje cells. *Society for Neuroscience Abstracts, 17*, 602(abstract).

Deitrich, R. A., Dunwiddie, T. V., Harris, R. A., & Erwin, V. (1989). Mechanism of action of ethanol: Initial central nervous system action. *Pharmacology Review, 41*, 489–537.

Eccles, J. C., Ito, M., & Szentogothai, J. (1967). *The cerebellum as a neuronal machine.* New York: Springer.

Ferko, A. P. (1990). The interaction between ethanol and cysteine on the central depressant effects of ethanol in mice. *Pharmacology and Biochemistry of Behavior, 36*, 619–624.

Freedman, R., Hoffer, B. J., & Woodward, D. J. (1975). A quantitative microiontophoretic analysis of the responses of central neurones to noradrenaline: Interactions with cobalt, manganese, verapamil and dichloroisoprenaline. *British Journal of Pharmacology, 54*, 529–539.

Freund, R. K., van Horne, C. G., Harlan, J. T., & Palmer, M. R. (1993). Electrophysiological interaction of ethanol with GABAergic mechanisms in the rat cerebellum *in vivo*. *Alcoholism, Clinical and Experimental Research, 17*, 321–328.

Gwee, M. C. E., Nott, N. W., Raper, C., & Rodger, I. W. (1972). Pharmacological actions of a new beta-adrenoceptor agonist, MJ-9184-1, in anaesthetized cats. *British Journal of Pharmacology, 46*, 375–385.

Harris, D. P., & Sinclair, J. G. (1984). Ethanol-GABA interactions at the rat Purkinje cell. *Gen Pharmacology, 15*, 449–454.

Hinko, C. N., & Rozanov, C. (1990). The role of bicuculline, aminooxyacetic acid and gabaculine in the regulation of ethanol-induced motor impairment. *European Journal of Pharmacology, 182*, 261–271.

ISI Software. (1987). *Graphpad: Plot, analyze data and digitize graphs.* San Diego: Author.

Leidenheimer, N. J., Machu, T. K., Endo, S., Olsen, R. W., Harris, R. A., & Browning, M. D. (1991). Cyclic AMP-dependent protein kinase decreases gamma-aminobutyric acid$_a$ receptor-mediated Cl uptake by brain microsacs. *Journal of Neurochemistry, 57,* 722–725.

Leidenheimer, N. J., Browning, M., & Harris, R. A. (1991). GABA$_a$ receptor phosphorylation: Multiple sites, actions and artifacts. *Trends in Pharmacological Sciences, 12,* 84–87.

Liljequist, S., & Engel, J. (1982). Effects of GABAergic agonists and antagonists on various ethanol-induced behavioral changes. *Psychopharmacology, 78,* 71–75.

Lin, A. M.-Y., Friedemann, M., Bickford, P. C., Gerhardt, G. A., Freund, R. K., & Palmer, M. K. (1992). Pre- and postsynaptic effects of ethanol on the interaction of norepinephrine with GABA responses in the cerebellum of young and old F344 rats: Electrophysiological and *in vivo* electrochemical studies. *Society for Neuroscience Abstracts, 18,* 1236(abstract).

Lin, A. M.-Y., Freund, R. K., & Palmer, M. R. (1991). Ethanol potentiation of GABA-induced electrophysiological responses in cerebellum: Requirement for catecholamine modulation. *Neuroscience Letters, 122,* 154–158.

Martz, A., Deitrich, R. A., & Harris, R. A. (1983). Behavioral evidence for the involvement of G-aminobutyric acid in the actions of ethanol. *European Journal of Pharmacology, 89,* 53–62.

McElligott, J. G., Ebner, T. J., & Bloedel, J. R. (1986). Reduction of cerebellar norepinephrine alters climbing fiber enhancement of mossy fiber input to the Purkinje cell. *Brain Research, 397,* 245–252.

Mehta, A. K., & Ticku, M. K. (1988). Ethanol potentiation of GABAergic transmission in cultured spinal cord neurons involves gamma-aminobutyric acid$_a$-gated chloride channels. *Journal of Pharmacology and Experimental Therapeutics, 246,* 558–564.

Miller, J. A., & Zahniser, N. R. (1988). Quantitative autoradiographic analysis of 125I-pindolol binding in Fischer 344 rat brain: Changes in beta-adrenergic receptor density with aging. *Neurobiology of Aging, 9,* 267–272.

Nestoros, J. N. (1980). Ethanol specifically potentiates GABA-mediated neurotransmission in feline cerebral cortex. *Science, 209,* 708–710.

Nishio, M., & Narahashi, T. (1990). Ethanol enhancement of GABA-activated chloride current in rat dorsal root ganglion neurons. *Brain Research, 518,* 283–286.

Olsen, R. W., & Tobin, A. J. (1990). Molecular biology of GABA$_a$ receptors. *The FASEB Journal, 4,* 1469–1480.

Palmer, M. R. (1982). Micro pressure-ejection: A complimentary technique to microiontophoresis for neuropharmacological studies in the mammalian central nervous system. *Journal Electrophysiological Techniques, 9,* 123–139.

Palmer, M. R., & Hoffer, B. J. (1980). Catecholamine modulation of enkephalin-induced electrophysiological responses in cerebral cortex. *Journal of Pharmacology and Experimental Therapeutics, 213,* 205–215.

Parfitt, K. D., Hoffer, B. J., & Browning, M. D. (1991). Norepinephrine and isoproterenol increase the phosphorylation of synapsin I and synapsin II in dentate slices of young but not aged Fisher 344 rats. *Proceedings of the National Academy of Sciences, 88,* 2361–2365.

Porter, N. M., Twyman, R. E., Uhler, M. D., & Macdonald, R. L. (1990). Cyclic AMP-dependent protein kinase decreases GABA$_a$ receptor current in mouse spinal cord neurons. *Neuron, 5,* 789–796.

Schmidt, M. J. (1981). The cyclic nucleotide system in the brain during aging. In S. J. Enna, T. Samorajski, & B. Beer (Eds.), *Brain neurotransmitters and receptors in aging and age-related disorders,* (pp. 171–193). New York: Raven Press.

Shefner, S. A. (1990). Electrophysiological effects of ethanol on brain neurones. In R. R. Watson

(Ed.), *Biochemistry and physiology of substance abuse* (2nd ed.), (pp. 25–53). Boca Raton, FL: CRC Press.

Sigel, E., & Baur, R. (1988). Activation of protein kinase C differentially modulates neuronal Na^+, Ca^+, and gamma-aminobutyrate type A channel. *Proceedings of the National Academy of Sciences, 85*, 6192–6196.

Siggins, G. R., Bloom, F. E., French, E. D., Madamra, S. G., Mancillas, J., Pittman, Q. J., & Rogers, J. (1987). Electrophysiology of ethanol on central neurons. *Annals of the New York Academy of Sciences, 492*, 350–366.

Skolnick, P., & Paul, S. M. (1981). Benzodiazepine receptors. *Annual Review of Medicinal Chemistry, 16*, 21–29.

Smith, B. M., & Hoffer, B. J. (1978). A gated, high voltage iontophoresis system with accurate current monitoring. *Electroencephalography and Clinical Neurophysiology, 44*, 398–402.

Stowe, Z. N., Lee, R. S., Smith, S. S., Chapin, J. K., Waterhouse, B. D., & Woodward, D. J. (1986). Effect of systemic ethanol on responses of rat cerebellar Purkinje neurons to iontophoretically applied norepinephrine and GABA. *Society for Neuroscience Abstracts, 12*, 994(abstract).

Suzdak, P. D., Glowa, J. R., Crawley, J. N., Schwartz, R. D., Skolnick, P., & Paul, S. M. (1986). A selective imadazobenzodiazepine antagonist of ethanol in the rat. *Science, 234*, 1243–1247.

Suzdak, P. D., Schwartz, R. D., Skolnick, P., & Paul, S. M. (1986). Ethanol stimulates gamma-aminobutyric acid receptor mediated chloride transport in rat brain synaptoneurosomes. *Proceedings of the National Academy of Sciences, 83*, 4071–4075.

Ticku, M. K., Lowrimore, P., & Lehoullier, P. (1986). Ethanol enhances GABA-induced $^{36}Cl^-$ influx in primary spinal cord cultured neurons. *Brain Research Bulletin, 17*, 123–126.

Tuttle, R., & Mills, J. (1975). Development of a new catecholamine to selectively increase cardiac contractility. *Circulation Research, 36*, 185–196.

Wafford, K. A., Dunwiddie, T. V., & Harris, R. A. (1990). Genetic differences in the ethanol sensitivity of GABA$_a$ receptors expressed in *Xenopus oocytes. Science, 249*, 291–293.

Walker, J. B., & Walker, J. P. (1973). Properties of adenylate cyclase from senescent rat brain. *Brain Research, 54*, 391–396.

Watson, M., & McElligott, J. G. (1984). Cerebellar norepinephrine depletion and impaired acquisition of specific locomotor tasks in rats. *Brain Research, 296*, 129–138.

Yeh, H. H., & Woodward, D. J. (1983). Beta-1 adrenergic receptors mediate noradrenergic facilitation of Purkinje cell responses to gamma-amminobutyric acid in cerebellum of rat. *Neuropharmacology, 22*, 629–639.

III

TREATMENT OF ALCOHOL PROBLEMS

12

Older Alcoholics:
Entry Into Treatment

EDITH S. LISANSKY GOMBERG

In historical perspective, clinical studies of alcoholics[1] came before epidemiological study of alcohol use and problems. It is, in fact, often argued that epidemiological findings about large population samples are more valid than clinical studies which focus on the selected subgroup that enters treatment (Cohen & Cohen, 1984). The ratio of untreated to treated alcohol abusers is estimated to range from 3:1 to 13:1, (Sobell, Sobell, & Tonneato, 1992); clearly most alcoholics are never seen by researchers or therapists. It is sometimes said that only the most severely disturbed enter treatment so that generalizations from such a sample would be limited to one end of the distribution.

But just how different are the problem drinkers who do not enter treatment from those who do? Are the problem drinkers encountered in treatment facilities different from those who are not in treatment, and in what ways different? If the alcoholic persons encountered in treatment are very similar in most measurable ways to those who do not enter treatment, are our generalizations about alcoholics made from clinical study reasonably valid?

When individuals reach that stage of drinking that is termed alcohol abuse or dependence, they must fit several criteria. To sum up the criteria spelled out in the most recent Diagnostic and Statistical Manual of the American Psychiatric Association (DSM IV, 1994) people who are diagnosable as alcoholics (a) drink a good deal and frequently, (b) show loss-of-control behavior, e.g., fruitlessly swear off drinking or try to moderate the amount, (c) manifest alcohol-related consequences and continue drinking despite the consequences, and (d) show withdrawal and tolerance behaviors. There may be some people who manifest such behavior for a particular period and then pass from the alcoholic into the nonalcoholic population. Others will continue the behavior until there is an intervention. Still others will die of alcohol-related causes.

A question with which some researchers struggle is a basic one: Is treatment better than no treatment? Can we be sure that particular treatments are always better than no treatment when we have so little information about no-treatment outcomes? For that matter, our information about those who are treated and the outcome of that treatment is not impressive.

Once it is clear that there is a diagnosable, verifiable alcohol disorder, there are a number of different outcomes possible:

1. The problem drinker enters treatment (inpatient, outpatient, various modalities, self-help organization, etc.) and achieves "recovery." Recovery is usually defined as sobriety.
2. The problem drinker enters treatment that fails to modify his drinking behaviors.
3. The problem drinker does not enter treatment and continues drinking and experiencing alcohol-related problems.
4. The problem drinker does not enter treatment but achieves recovery with no apparent formal intervention. This is termed *spontaneous remission* or *spontaneous recovery*.

Sobell and her colleagues call it *natural recovery* (Sobell et al., 1993). There may be a informal, noninstitutionalized intervention, e.g., a warning from a physician or employer or spouse, alcohol-related medical and physical problems, self-disgust, etc. The criteria for defining spontaneous remission will vary from one investigator to another. Knupfer (1972) defined spontaneous recovery for a group of studied ex-problem drinkers, excluding religious conversion, serious illness, prolonged psychiatric treatment, and/or involvement in Alcoholics Anonymous. Smart (1975–1976) in his review of spontaneous recovery studies, concluded that investigations should "focus on . . . informal 'treatment' by friends, relative, and Alcoholics Anonymous."

SPONTANEOUS REMISSION STUDIES

Early on, Drew pointed out that the incidence of male alcoholism dropped after age 40, and he described alcoholism as, "a self-limiting disease" (Drew, 1968). Drew indicated that although mortality and morbidity account for some of the diminution, "a significant proportion of this disappearance is probably due to spontaneous recovery" (Drew, 1968, p. 965).

Emrick (1975) reviewed the outcomes of "psychologically oriented treatments" and the effectiveness of no-treatment versus treatment. Comparing an untreated group with "a minimally treated" group, he reported very modest changes in outcome and concluded that there was no evidence to suggest that "change processes" with treatment and without treatment were different.

There are some investigators who do not accept the phenomenon of spontaneous remission. Eysenck and Beech (1971) took the position that spontaneous remission "is theoretically expected to be entirely absent," and clinical experience showed that lack of treatment "almost always" meant lack of improvement.

Knupfer (1972) reported on a community sample of recovered problem drinkers with strict criteria in the definition of spontaneous recovery (excluding religious conversion, etc.). She found 25% of the problem drinkers reported spontaneous remission which was, in her sample, "at least three-fourths of all recoveries."

Tuchfeld and his colleagues studied ex-problem drinkers who had had no formal treatment in order to explore the processes involved (Tuchfeld, Simuel, & Schmitt, 1976; Tuchfeld, 1981). Their description of the processes involved the following major components: serious health problems, educational materials, distress at identification with a negative role model, a humiliating event, and recognition of the drinking problem.

Smart (1975–1976) summarized the results of nine studies of spontaneous remission conducted from 1942 to 1975. The report of positive results ranged from 10% recovery among untreated alcoholics (Newman, 1965) to 42% (Goodwin, Crane, & Guze, 1971). Smart concluded that it is uncertain whether spontaneous remission "equals or exceeds" recovery with treatment.

Saunders and Kershaw (1979) reported results of a community survey in England which showed that "not only does spontaneous remission occur in alcoholism, but . . . [it] occurs most readily in less severe cases." Not everyone agrees that spontaneous remission is likely in less severe alcohol dependence. Vaillant (1983) asks the question: How important is access to treatment in recovery from alcoholism? The response is that "men who achieved successful abstinence did not differ from severe alcoholics in general. The treatment encounters experienced by the currently abstinent men were not more frequent, nor was the severity of their alcoholism any less (Vaillant, p. 183)."

The problem of defining alcoholism in epidemiological studies is coupled with the further problem that there is "no natural boundary" between remission and nonremission (Roizen, Cahalan, & Shanks, 1978). Roizen et al. demonstrated that by varying the criteria for outcome and the selection of the to-be-studied problem drinking group, improvement rates can be shown to vary from 11% to 71%. The traditional clinical image of alcoholism as stable and lasting needs some rethinking; there may be one subgroup of alcoholics who manifest the symptoms over long periods in their lifetime, and other subgroups who enter and then leave the alcoholic population.

Cognitive processes associated with spontaneous remission were investigated by Ludwig (1985), who interviewed 29 former alcoholics. Factors associated with abstinence included medical problems, physical aversion to alcohol, changes in lifestyle, and spiritual mystical experiences. Once abstinence had been achieved, maintaining sobriety was "overwhelmingly" involved with negative associations to drinking which might include unpleasant, sickening, humiliating, or distasteful experiences of a personal nature.

Sobell and her collaborators have produced the most recent work on natural recovery (Sobell, Sobell, & Toneatto, 1992; Sobell, Cunningham, Sobell, & Toneatto, 1993). Comparison of drinking history and life events was made of 92 recovered alcoholics who had never sought formal help, 28 treated-and-recovered alcoholics, and 62 alcoholics who were not in treatment. Recovered alcoholics who had not sought help were divided into those who were currently abstinent and those who were currently nonabstinent, and there were demographic differences among spontaneously recovered alcoholics: More women were currently nonabstinent and more older individuals were currently abstinent. From the interview data, the investigators concluded that a "cognitive evaluation"—an appraisal of the pros and cons of drinking—may initiate the process, and that "spousal support" is a strong factor in maintenance of the sobriety.

All the studies reported above deal with problem drinkers in a wide age range. While some research subject groups may have included older alcoholics, there is little said or written about spontaneous remission among older problem drinkers. Atkinson, Ganzini, and Bernstein (1992) comment "There is no information about rates of spontaneous remission in older alcoholics." A review of longitudinal studies of alcohol use across the life span reports considerable variation in spontaneous remission across the life course by age and gender (Fillmore, 1988). Age trajectories of male drinkers indicate that recovery is most frequent in youth and in old age.[2]

It should be added that the 7th Special Report to Congress (Alcohol and Health, 1990) noted that 1.43 million persons were in treatment in 5,586 alcoholism treatment units in the 12-month period ending October, 1987—85% in outpatient care and 15% in inpatient or residential settings. Whatever the ratio of untreated to treated alcohol abusers, there is a very sizable population of problem drinkers in treatment. The question remains: Why do some get into treatment and others do not?

WHO ENTERS TREATMENT?

Research attention has focused less on the question of who enters or initiates treatment and more on the related question of, having entered, who *remains* in a treatment program for the whole course (e.g., Leigh, Ogborne, & Cleland, 1984). Baekeland and Lundwall (1977), in a classic paper, have described a composite picture of an alcoholic patient "most likely to drop out of treatment." The characteristics of the likely dropout include being a "highly symptomatic, socially isolated lower-class person of poor social stability who is highly ambivalent about treatment and has psychopathic features." A study of 1,503 patients admitted to Hazelden, a treatment facility (Kammeier & Laudergan, 1977), showed an average stay of 33 days for completers and 16 days for dropouts; almost 80% of admissions completed the treatment program, and more women than men (25% and 19%) dropped out.

Weisner (1993) has offered a model of alcohol treatment entry. Comparing problem drinkers in treatment with problem drinkers "in the general population" (presumably untreated), ages 18 to 56 and older, discriminant function analyses showed significant differences between treated and untreated for both men and women. For women, treatment history, employment, and ethnicity contributed a major portion to the model; for men, treatment history, employment, and social consequences were major contributors. Weisner juxtaposed *severity* and *the number of social consequences*. Severity is the accumulation of symptoms indicating alcohol dependence, and social consequences are the difficulties encountered with family or community. Which is more predictive of entering treatment? The author concluded that recent work has found social consequences to play a more important role in entering treatment.

Pressure from social networks as a critical variable in entering treatment has been elucidated in several research reports (Finlay, 1966; Strug & Hyman, 1981). Finlay's (1966) study involved 69 clinical patients who were in treatment and 35 new patients; the data are drawn from tape-recorded interviews. Strug and Hyman (1981) utilized a technique of social-network analyses with 54 alcoholic men in inpatient treatment and 48 alcoholic men in a detoxification center who had had no formal treatment and no intention of seeking treatment. The authors concluded that alcoholics who enter treatment "do so not after ties and attachments to networks are lost, but rather as a result of pressure from network members and especially confidents who discourage their drinking" (Strug & Hyman, 1981, p. 882).

Motivation for treatment is a concept that has been a major issue for clinicians. In a classic article, Sterne and Pittman (1965) described the concept as a source of "institutional and professional blockage in the treatment of alcoholics.'' A recent review of the literature on motivation for treatment (Miller, 1985) examined and rejected a trait model of motivation: Patient characteristics play a modest role in predicting treatment participation and adherence. Instead, he posited a model in which the therapist's perception of patient motivation and the therapist's perception of prognosis are linked to outcome, to treatment compliance, to participation, and to adherence. This model, however, speaks to retention of the patient and, to completion of a course of treatment, but not to the question of how the patient came to enter treatment in the first place.

A study of the motivation of alcoholics to enter treatment (Pfeiffer, Feuerlein, & Brenke-Schulte, 1991) investigated factors among alcoholics who do enter treatment: sociodemographic and alcoholism-related factors, and attitudes toward current life situation and toward alcohol problems. Drawn from a psychiatric outpatient clinic, 239 patients diagnosed as alcohol-dependent were evaluated and followed. Those who entered treatment were compared with those who did not. They found that those who entered treatment (1) expressed feelings of less control over their current life situation, (2) found their alcohol problems more harmful and uncontrollable, (3) were more conscious of suffering because of their alcohol problems, (4) more actively sought help, and (5) saw the outcome of therapy more positively.

Krampen (1989) obtained responses from 140 male and 51 female alcoholics entering treatment to a list of 14 reasons for accepting treatment. The list contained several severity items but was largely composed of social consequences. Krampen's study supports the earlier work of Lemere, O'Hollaren, and Maxwell (1958) which concluded that ''few if any alcoholics decide to stop drinking until some pressure is put on them.''

Chan, Pristach, and Welte (1991) studied three groups: alcoholics in treatment, patients at health clinics, and a general population sample. When the alcoholics were compared with heavy drinkers in the other two groups, differences were minimal for age, self-reported daily alcohol intake, and recent illicit drug use. Significant differences between alcoholics in treatment and the heavy drinkers in the other groups appeared in MAST scores, alcohol-related health problems, and depression symptoms. The inference was that alcohol-related illness and depression had served as at least part of the motivation to enter treatment.

RELEVANT STUDIES OF OLDER ALCOHOLICS

Schuckit and Miller (1976) studied admission to a veterans' hospital of patients 65 and older, and reported 18% as alcoholic. A survey of another veterans' hospital found, among men 60 and older, 15% were currently and actively alcoholic (Gomberg, 1975) although an even larger percentage reported a past history of alcohol problems, now remitted.

Referral sources may vary with age. Hoffman (1976) compared patients 65 and older referred to a state hospital with younger patients. Older patients were more likely to be referred by physicians, by family members, and by law enforcement agencies. In a different setting, Corrigan (1974) studied people who called an information/referral facility in New York City with concern about their own or someone else's drinking ''among those aged 60 or over, more than twice as many problem drinkers were called about [than self-reporting callers]. In this we may be seeing the concern expressed by family and friends" (Corrigan, 1974, page 15). Finlayson, Hurt, Davis, & Morse (1988) noted that the most common factor in motivating elderly alcohol-dependent people to seek treatment was the concern of family and friends.

Referral sources will vary with the kind of institution or facility reporting. State hospitals and veterans' hospitals are likely to see lower income people, and referral may often be by law enforcement agencies. The social network, i.e., family and friends, are mentioned more often in middle- and upper-income facilities.

Kofoed et al. (1984) examined patients at an outpatient program for elderly substance abusers in a veterans' medical center. Most referrals were from the legal system (57%); 19% of referrals were from the health care system and 17% from family.

It is of some interest that Graham and Tinney (1986), evaluating a Toronto outpatient program for alcoholics, comment that their patients "typically enter the program for help with other problems and not for addictions treatment." Their patients may be described as homeless people, referred to the program by health agencies.

Of 250 persons referred to a mental health outreach program for older people, 50 were judged to be manifesting alcohol-related problems (Hubbard, Santos, & Santos, 1979). Eliminating those who were being victimized by heavy drinking by significant others, almost half were chronic long-term alcoholics, often living alone. Twelve referrals, 28%, were of relatively recent onset among people who had a history of moderate drinking, although the question was raised about earlier, sporadic episodes of heavy drinking. A quarter of the group, 25%, were apparently responding to the synergistic effect of alcohol and medication.

A study of 216 patients admitted to the Mayo Clinic was reported by Finlayson, Hurt, Davis, & Morse (1988). These patients, 65 and older, were both early-onset and recent-onset problem drinkers. Those with recent onset were more likely to report a precipitating life event than those whose problem drinking was of long duration. Early- and recent-onset patients were not distinguished by comorbid psychiatric diagnoses, and 14% of the 216 patients had an associated drug abuse problem, in all instances problems involving legally prescribed drugs.

A study of the characteristics, diagnosis, and treatment of elderly alcoholism (Curtis, et al., 1989) was designed to investigate whether hospital physicians screened and referred elderly alcoholics. Elderly problem drinkers were less likely to be diagnosed if they were white, female, or well-educated. Elderly problem drinkers were less likely than younger patients to have treatment recommended, and if treatment was recommended, it was less likely to be initiated.

Short-term remission among elderly problem drinkers was studied utilizing three groups: remitted problem drinkers, unremitted problem drinkers, and nonproblem controls (Moos, Brennan, & Moos, 1991). At initial assessment, those who remitted later showed several differences from the group that continued to drink problematically: (1) they consumed less alcohol, (2) they reported fewer drinking problems, (3) they had friends who approved less of drinking, (4) they were more likely to seek mental health help, and (5) they were likely to be recent-onset problem drinkers. The authors concluded that recent-onset problem drinkers are more reactive to physical health stressors and social influence than early-onset drinkers.

The question of elder-specific treatment programs has been raised. Janik and Dunham (1983) compared patients drawn from 550 different treatment programs. From this national data base, patients who were 60 and older are distinguishable on a number of points from patients who were 59 and younger. They differed on use of drugs other than alcohol (younger patients more), on driving arrests (younger more), on social stability (older patients more), and on attendance at Alcoholics Anonymous (older patients more). Although these differences were noted, Janik and Dunham concluded that the differences between age groups did not warrant special, elder-specific programs. This was challenged by Kofoed and his collaborators (1987), who reported that patients in an elder-specific program were more likely to complete the course of treatment than older patients in mixed age groups.

Many aspects of elderly alcoholism and drug dependence are discussed in a volume by Gottheil, Druley, Skoloda, and Waxman (1985). These include stress and life events, differential drug effects on the aging brain, coping tactics, and treatment strategies. The question of different outcomes and who enters treatment is not raised.

It is generally agreed among those working with older alcoholics that there are problems of detection and screening. Older persons are less likely to be visible in the workplace. They may be widowed and living alone. It is also true that older persons tend not to seek treatment (Atkinson, 1990); the study of factors that facilitate treatment entry and those that serve as barrier to treatment entry is critical.

HYPOTHESES ABOUT TREATMENT ENTRY

From the information gleaned from studies of motivation to enter treatment and from studies of older alcoholics, a number of hypotheses emerge about which elderly alcoholics are likely to seek treatment.

Severity of Alcohol Abuse Dependence

Self-Identification

The prediction is that alcoholics who manifest "higher perceived illness severity" are more likely to enter treatment (Bardsley & Beckman, 1988). The reasoning here is that problem drinkers are more likely to enter treatment if they perceive their problems as severe. Related to perceived illness severity is self-identification as an alcoholic (Skinner, Glaser, & Annis, 1982). Those who identify themselves as alcoholic report a wider range of problems related to alcohol, greater consumption of alcohol, and more likelihood of attendance at Alcoholics Anonymous, than those who do not identify themselves as alcoholics.

Negative Consequences

In a study of Boston residents who had sought treatment for drinking problems compared with those who did not (Hingson et al., 1980; Hingson et al., 1982), the significant distinction was the belief that alcohol was adversely affecting health, family relationships, friendships and work. Those who held such belief saw their drinking problems as more severe and sought treatment because of the consequences. Chan, Pristach, and Welte (1991) also noted treatment/nontreatment differences in terms of more reported alcohol-related problems in the former group. More depressive symptomatology has also been noted among people who have sought treatment (Woodruff, Guze, & Clayton, 1973; Chan, Pristach, & Welte, 1991).

Social Response and Consequences

Those seeking treatment are individuals more likely to hold beliefs of negative consequences of alcohol. In contrast with hypotheses about the person holding these beliefs, the following hypotheses focus on concern with others' response, with the response of significant others and society toward the client's drinking.

Network Pressure

Those more likely to seek treatment are those who have been under pressure from their social networks. It has been noted that "concern of family and friends" was the most common factor motivating patients for treatment (Finlayson, Hurt, Davis, & Morse, 1988). A study of those who telephone about their own or someone else's problem drinking (Corrigan, 1974) showed that among those 60 and older, more than twice as many problem drinkers were called about than was true of other age groups; Corrigan interpreted this as "the concern expressed by family and friends" about alcoholism among the retired older people or about problems of long duration.

Response from Others (Nonfamily)

Here we would include pressure from people on the job, from legal authorities, and from the community, e.g., neighbors, social agency, or medical personnel, etc.

Data Sources for Hypotheses

It should be noted that not all the studies on which these hypotheses are based draw from the same research subject populations. Most of them draw from clinical samples, from people referred for alcohol-related problems (Bardsley & Beckman, 1988; Skinner, Glaser & Annis, 1982; Woodruff, Guze, & Clayton, 1973; Finlayson, Hurt, Davis, & Morse, 1988); but Hingson and his collaborators reported from a community survey (Hingson et al., 1980; Hingson et al., 1982) and Corrigan's (1974) data came from calls to an information and referral service.

A CURRENT STUDY OF OLDER ALCOHOLICS

One hundred and seventy-one male alcoholics, 55 and older, were interviewed. There were 104 alcoholics in treatment and 67 who were not in treatment. The men in treatment were unremitted alcoholics whose problem drinking occurred within the last 12 months and, in most instances, was part of a considerably longer pattern. The alcoholics not in treatment were men who had been drinking alcoholically for at least one year, who were not in treatment, and who had not sought any treatment during the past year. Both groups were drawn from the general ward of a university hospital, a veterans' hospital ward, substance abuse treatment facilities both urban and suburban, community advertising, senior citizen housing, senior community centers, and meetings of Alcoholics Anonymous.

Preliminary screening to determine eligibility for participation was done with a brief mental status examination (Folstein, Folstein, & McHugh, 1975), a brief medical and psychiatric history, the CAGE (Ewing, 1984) and MAST (Seltzer, 1971) tests. Those who participated in the study were then administered the Diagnostic Interview Schedule (Robins et al., 1981) and the MRC2,[3] a structured interview developed for the study to collect information about life events, social supports, drinking history and practices, health status, and perceptions of drinking severity and consequences.

A demographic comparison of the two groups showed little difference. Mean age for the treatment group was 63.3, for the not-in-treatment group, 64.8. Educational achievement was virtually identical and marital status showed no significant differences. There was some difference in current work status: More of the men in treatment were still in the labor market (38% and 21%) and more of the men not in treatment were retired (64% and 44%).

Examination of drinking history and patterns showed few differences. Age at onset averaged 32 for the treatment group and 27 for the men not in treatment; duration was actually more for the group not in treatment, but differences are not significant. The lifetime daily drinking average (computed as the lifetime average quantity during the years the respondent drank regularly) was not significantly different (6.7 for the treatment group and 7.1 for the group not in treatment). There were some small differences between the two groups: The men in treatment showed more preference for high alcohol content beverages, they reported greater likelihood of drinking at home or on the job, and they were more likely to drink alone.

Self-Identification

Table 12.1 lists items culled from patient interviews, items dealing with self-description and self-identification as an alcoholic drinker. The results are quite clear: Those in

Table 12.1. Self-Description

	In treatment $N = 104$	Not in treatment $N = 67$	P Value
Best describes you at present?			
Alcoholic/problem drinker.	39%	15%	
Currently an abstainer	32%	9%	.0001
Daily/heavy drinker	22%	44%	
Infrequent/moderate drinker	8%	32%	
Do you feel you are a normal drinker? No	78%	48%	.0001
Can you stop drinking without a struggle after one or two drinks? No	54%	24%	.0001
Are you able to stop drinking when you want to? No	53%	15%	.0001

treatment identified themselves and described their drinking differently from those heavy/problem drinkers who did not enter treatment. Asked if they consider themselves "normal drinkers," more than three-quarters of the men in treatment replied negatively.

The criteria for alcohol dependence, the DSM IIIR nine criteria for the diagnosis of alcohol dependence, are again a matter of self-report (Table 12.2). In terms of the nine criteria, the men in treatment much more readily defined themselves as highly dependent: Twice as many men in treatment reported themselves as high dependent, and twice as many of the men not in treatment reported themselves as low dependent.

Negative Consequences

Table 12.3 lists negative consequences of heavy drinking, reported by the men in treatment and by the men not in treatment. The consequences fell into three groups: (1) items dealing with medical or health consequences of heavy drinking, (2) a few items about family and friends, and (3) items dealing with the psychological consequences of heavy drinking.

Other consequences of heavy drinking queried were feeling sick or dizzy, unexplained bruises, falls, and continued drinking with the knowledge that it worsened health. Replies showed minute differences between the two groups of men. There was one consequence reported significantly more often by those who were *not* in treatment—hospitalization during the past year: 24% of those in treatment and 61% of those not in treatment answered affirmatively, a difference significant at the $p = .0001$ level. Because of this, data were analyzed to see if more not-in-treatment men had been drawn

Table 12.2. DSM IIIR: Criteria for Alcohol Dependence

Criteria	In treatment $N = 104$	Not in treatment $N = 67$	P Value
Withdrawal symptoms	82%	42%	.0001
Reduced/given up activities in order to drink	45%	22%	.002
A.M. drinking to prevent hangovers/shakes	55%	34%	.008
So much time drinking, little time for anything else	53%	32%	.009
Drank much more than you expected when you began	80%	58%	n.s.
Tried to quit/cut down on drinking more than once	62%	38%	n.s.
Drinking kept you from working or child care	28%	17%	n.s.
Continued to drink despite problems	59%	41%	n.s.
Tolerance, increased amount to get an effect	43%	58%	n.s.
LOW DEPENDENCE			
3 TO 6 signs positive	33%	68%	
HIGH DEPENDENCE			
7 to 9 signs positive	66%	30%	.002

Table 12.3. Reported Negative Consequences

	In treatment N = 104	Not in treatment N = 67	P value
Alcohol-related serious health problems	60%	35%	.002
Emergency room use	47%	25%	.004
Loss of appetite	63%	32%	.0001
Accidents at home	37%	23%	n.s.
Friends stopped visiting	21%	11%	n.s.
Children worried	83%	54%	.0001
Increasingly depressed	52%	29%	.005
Increasingly lonely	47%	28%	.015
Trouble making any decisions	41%	20%	.006

from inpatient services but, surprisingly, there was little difference between those in treatment and those not in treatment.

Network Pressure

Here the possible social pressures from networks of family and friends are examined. Since the not-in-treatment men were presumably still drinking, the question of events that seem to precipitate a cessation of drinking were asked of the men in treatment (see Table 12.4). The report of the men in treatment usually indicated more than one item as operative in treatment seeking, but it is of interest that the urging of family and friends had the highest percentage of affirmative response (68%). Close behind is the existence of a disturbing event; these events were classified, and the most frequently cited disturbing events dealt either with a medical problem or with problems with spouse/family/friends.

Nonfamily Social Response

These precipitants to treatment-seeking were the pressures and the response from community institutional figures rather than family or friends. Pressure to get treatment may have come from an employer, from the police, or from a physician or a facility like a hospital emergency room. From Table 12.5, it appears that there was really very little

Table 12.4. Men in Treatment: Events

When you stopped drinking this time, were any of the following going on? Yes.	
Urging of family and friends	68%
Disturbing event	65%
Feeling very low and depressed	56%
Many medical problems	47%
Shakiness blackouts, passing out	47%
Relatives fed up with you	36%
Marital problems	36%

Table 12.5. Social Consequences of Drinking

	In treatment $N = 104$	Not in treatment $N = 67$	P Value
Objections at work	34%	24%	n.s.
Lost a job	19%	20%	n.s.
Fights while drinking	25%	32%	n.s.
Drunk driving accident	28%	34%	n.s.
Trouble with police	49%	42%	n.s.
Talked to physician about the drinking problem	71%	29%	.0001
Entered detoxification program	83%	17%	.0001
Emergency room hospital use	47%	25%	.004

difference in such pressures reported by the men in treatment and those not in treatment. The response of employers and police to the mens' drinking did not differentiate those who sought treatment and those who did not. What did distinguish them was the response of others who were part of the health care network system. This included physicians, emergency room personnel, and detoxification program personnel. It is difficult to say whether these represented pressure for treatment or whether the alcoholic men who were more ready to utilize any health resources were more likely to enter treatment for their alcoholism.

An earlier report of some of the findings above (Gomberg, Nelson, Iacob, & Young, 1993) included a multiple regression analysis to examine the association of different theoretically etiological variables with the in-treatment/not-in-treatment status of the research subjects. These are found in Tables 12.6 and 12.7. Self-description or identification of oneself as an alcoholic or problem drinker was the best predictor of entry into treatment. An excellent constellation of predictors was also derived from a model that included dependence severity (see Table 12.2 items from DSM-III-R), preferred beverage (men in-treatment preference for high alcohol content beverages), and presence in the labor market (high proportion of men in treatment who were working or looking for work).

Table 12.6. Inter-Relationships of Candidate Predictors

	Labor Market	Location	Alone	Social Consequences	Dependence Severity	Negative Effects	Problem Years	Self-Description
In labor market	—	—	—	—	—	—	—	—
Location	(.07)	—	—	—	—	—	—	—
Alone	(−.01)	(.34)**	—	—	—	—	—	—
Social consequences	(.26)	.17*	(.29)	—	—	—	—	—
Dependence severity	(.19)	.26**	(.24)	.59**	—	—	—	—
Negative effects	(.16)	.25**	(.26)	.59**	.69**	—	—	—
Problem years	(.36)**	.08	(.19)	−.02	−.06	−.04	—	—
Self-description	(.24)	.09	(.25)*	.33**	.53**	.51**	−.15	—
Preferred beverage	(0)	(.21)	(.05)	(.20)	(.16)	(.18)	(.23)*	(.20)

( ) Denotes Cramer's V; all others are Spearman correlations.

*$p < .05$ **$p < .01$

Table 12.7. Predictors of Treatment Group

Variable	Beta	S.E.	P-Value
A. Best model with self-description and eight other candidate predictors [Correlation between predicted and observed group (Somers D) = .579]			
Self-description	.872	.147	.0001
B. Best model without self-description [Correlation between predicted and observed group (Somers D) = .468]			
Dependence severity	.3691	.0973	.0001
Preferred beverage	.7898	.3617	.0290
In labor market	.7949	.4237	.0607

Note: Model X^2 (3) = 24.582, p = .0001

When we examine the four sets of hypotheses seeking to predict who will enter treatment and who will not, there is strong support for the hypotheses of self-identification and of negative consequences. The severity of the alcoholism is clearly greater among those who enter treatment, and they show more dependence-on-alcohol signs than do the men who do not enter treatment.

Support for hypotheses dealing with social response to problematic drinking is not as clear. When subjects were asked directly about events or circumstances that apparently precipitated their entry into treatment, two-thirds of them said that the urging of family and friends was a major factor. Feeling depressed, "increasingly depressed," ranks high as a precipitant. But social response and pressure at work or from legal authority does not seem to be significant in the decision to enter treatment, and this may be related to the fact that this is an *older* sample of problem drinkers.

Health consequences loom large and the pressure from family and friends seems significant. The social pressure that may come from physicians and other health workers is significant, but before it can be applied the alcoholic must show help-seeking behavior. Treatment may be encouraged, but first the man must appear in the emergency room, in a detoxification program, or in a physician's examining room. One may raise the question of attitude and behavior patterns called health-care-seeking. When the men were interviewed, they were asked about "hassles" or "irritants" and the ways they habitually cope with these, and this was followed by an open-ended question about dealing with "an unhappy situation." There were small differences between the men in treatment and those not in treatment, although the latter more often took a positive approach or tried to distract themselves. Those responses classified as "seeking help outside of the self" were offered by 45% of the men in treatment and 23% of those not in treatment. It was also noted that the significantly higher Michigan Alcoholism Screen Test scores of the men in treatment seemed to lean heavily on three items, each given a score of 5. These were:

8. Have you ever attended a meeting of Alcoholics Anonymous?
19. Have you ever gone to anyone for help with your drinking?
20. Have you ever been in a hospital because of drinking?

The MAST responses that indicate help-seeking behavior and the men's in-treatment response to the question about coping with unhappy situations by "seeking help outside of the self," definitely suggested more health-care-seeking behavior among those who entered treatment.

SUMMARY

How may we describe the elderly male alcoholic who is likely to enter a treatment program?

1. He is self-identified as a problem drinker or alcoholic.
2. He shows high severity on the criteria of alcohol dependence.
3. He is likely to report urging of family and friends to seek help.
4. He is likely to prefer alcoholic beverages with high alcohol content.
5. He is likely to be in the labor market, although he may be unemployed and looking for work.
6. He manifests health-care-seeking behaviors.

With current high interest in prevention, future work on the factors that contribute to treatment entry could make a real contribution to secondary prevention, i.e., to intervention before the negative effects of heavy drinking become irreversible. From the point of view of the clinician and practitioner, more information that increases the effectiveness of casefinding will be useful and necessary.

Notes

1. The terms alcoholic, alcohol abuser, alcohol-dependent and problem drinker are used here to describe those drinkers whose excessive alcohol intake represents a problem to themselves and others.

2. It is relevant to note that the Wilsnacks (1991), reporting longitudinal epidemiological study of female drinking, have found that younger women, 21 to 34, were most likely "to move out of problem drinking," at Time 2, and middle aged women, 35 to 49, "showed most chronicity."

3. Those interested in the interview schedule (MRC 2, The Coping Strategies of Older People) may write to the authors for a copy.

References

American Psychiatric Association. (1987). *Diagnostic and Statistical Manual IIIR*. Washington, D.C.

American Psychiatric Association. (1994). *Diagnostic and Statistical Manual IV*. Washington, D.C.

Atkinson, R. M. (1990). Aging and alcohol use disorders: Diagnostic issues in the elderly. *International Psychogeriatrics, 2*, 55–72.

Atkinson, R. M., Ganzini, L., & Bernstein, M. J. (1992). Alcohol and substance-use disorders in the elderly. In *Handbook of Mental Health and Aging*, 2nd ed. (pp. 515–555). New York: Academic Press.

Alcohol and Health (1990), 7th Special Report to the U.S. Congress. DHHS Publ. No. (ADM) 90-1656. Washington, DC: Government Printing Office.

Baekeland, F., & Lundwall, L. K. (1977). Engaging the alcoholic in treatment and keeping him there. In B. Kissin and H. Begleiter (Eds.), *The Biology of Alcoholism, Vol. 5. Treatment and Rehabilitation of the Chronic Alcoholic* (pp. 161–195). New York: Plenum.

Bardsley, P. E., & Beckman, L. J. (1988). The health belief model and entry into alcoholism treatment. *The International Journal of the Addictions, 23*, 19–28.

Chan, A. W. K., Pristach, E. A., & Welte, J. W. (1991). Detection of alcohol problems and heavy drinking in three populations. (Abstract). *Alcoholism: Clinical and Experimental Research, 15*, 375. (Abstract No. 383).

Cohen, P., & Cohen, J. (1984). The clinician's illusion. *Archives of General Psychiatry, 4*, 1178–1182.

Corrigan, E. M. (1974). *Problem drinkers seeking treatment* (Monograph No. 8). Rutgers Center of Alcohol Studies. New Brunswick, NJ: RCAS Publications Division.

Curtis, J. R., Geller, G., Stokes, E. J., Levine, D. M., & Moore, R. D. (1989). Characteristics, diagnosis and treatment of alcoholism in elderly patients. *Journal of the American Geriatrics Society, 37*, 310–316.

Drew, L. R. H. (1968). Alcoholism as a self-limiting disease. *Quarterly Journal of Studies on Alcohol, 29*, 956–967.

Emrick, C. S. (1975). A review of the psychologically oriented treatment of alcoholism. II. The relative effectiveness of different treatment approaches and the effectiveness of treatment versus no treatment. *Quarterly Journal of Studies on Alcohol, 36*, 88–108.

Ewing, J. A. (1984). Detecting alcoholics, the CAGE questionnaire. *Journal of the American Medical Association, 252*, 1905–1907.

Eysenck, H. J., & Beech, R. (1971). Counterconditioning and related methods. In A. E. Bergen, & S. L. Garfield (Eds.), *Handbook of psychotherapy and behavior change: An experimental analysis.* New York: Wiley.

Fillmore, K. M. (1988). *Alcohol use across the life span: A critical review of 70 years of international longitudinal research.* Toronto: Addiction Research Foundation.

Finlay, D. G. (1966). Effect of role network pressure on an alcoholic's approach to treatment. *Social Work*, 71–77.

Finlayson, R. E., Hurt, R. D., Davis, L. J., & Morse, R. M. (1988). Alcoholism in elderly persons: A study of the psychiatric and psychosocial features of 216 patients. *Mayo Clinic Proceedings, 63*, 761–768.

Folstein, M. F., Folstein, S. E., & McHugh, P. R. (1975). Mini-mental state: A practical method for grading the cognitive status of patients for the clinician. *Journal of Psychiatric Research, 12*, 189–198.

Gomberg, E. S. L. (1975). Prevalence of alcoholism among ward patients in a veterans administration hospital. *Journal of Studies on Alcohol, 36*, 1458–1467.

Gomberg, E. S. L., Nelson, B. W., Jacob, A., & Young, J. (1993). Elderly male alcoholics: Who enters treatment. *Alcoholism: Clinical and Experimental Research, 17*, 490. Abstract 293.

Goodwin, D. W., Crane, J. B., & Guze, S. B. (1971). Felons who drink: An 8-year follow-up. *Quarterly Journal of Studies on Alcohol, 32*, 136–147.

Gottheil, E., Druley, K. A., Skoloda, T. E., & Waxman, H. M. (Eds.) (1985). *The combined problems of alcoholism, drug addiction and aging.* Springfield, IL: C. C. Thomas.

Graham, K., & Timney, C. (1986). *Evaluation of the COPA project.* Unpublished manuscript.

Hingson, R., Scotch, N., Day, N., & Culbert, A. (1980). Recognizing and seeking help for drinking problems; a study in the Boston metropolitan area. *Journal of Studies on Alcohol, 41*, 1102–1117.

Hingson, R., Mangione, T., Meyers, A., & Scotch, N. (1982). Seeking help for drinking problems, A study in the Boston metropolitan area. *Journal of Studies on Alcohol, 43*, 273–288.

Hoffman, H. (1976). *Referral sources, prehospital events, and after-care of young and old alcoholics.* Wilmar State Hospital, Wilmar, MN. Unpublished manuscript.

Hubbard, R. W., Santos, J. F., & Santos, M. A. (1979). Alcohol and older adults: Overt and covert influences. *Social Casework, 60*, 166–170.

Janik, S. W., & Dunham, R. G. (1983). A nationwide examination of the need for specific alcoholism treatment programs for the elderly. *Journal of Studies on Alcohol, 44*, 307–317.

Kammeier, S. M. L., & Laundergan, J. C. (1977). *The outcome of treatment: Patients admitted to Hazelden in 1975.* Center City, MN: Hazelden Foundation.

Knupfer, G. (1972). Ex-problem drinkers. In M. Roff, L. N. Robins, & M. Pollack (Eds.), *Life history research in psychopathology, Volume 2* (pp. 256–284). Minneapolis: University of Minnesota Press.

Kofoed, L. L., Tolson, R. L., Atkinson, R. M., Toth, R. L., & Turner, J. A. (1987). Treatment compliance of older alcoholics: An elderly-specific approach is superior to "mainstreaming." *Journal of Studies on Alcohol, 48*, 47–51.

Kofoed, L. L., Tolson, R. L., Atkinson, R. M., Turner, J. A., & Toth, R. F. (1984). Elderly groups in an alcoholism clinic. In R. M. Atkinson (Ed.), *Alcohol and drug abuse in old age* (pp. 35–48). Washington, DC: American Psychiatric Press.

Krampen, G. (1989). Motivation in the treatment of alcoholism. *Addictive Behaviors, 14*, 197–200.

Leigh, G., Ogborne, A. C., & Cleland, P. (1984). Factors associated with patient dropout from an outpatient alcoholism treatment service. *Journal of Studies on Alcohol, 45*, 359–362.

Lemere, F., O'Hollaren, P., & Maxwell, M. A. (1958). Motivation in the treatment of alcoholism. *Quarterly Journal of Studies on Alcohol, 19*, 428–431.

Ludwig, A. M. (1985). Cognitive processes associated with "spontaneous" recovery from alcoholism. *Journal of Studies on Alcohol, 46*, 53–58.

Miller, W. R. (1985). Motivation for treatment: A review with special emphasis on alcoholism. *Psychological Bulletin, 98*, 84–107.

Moos, R. H., Brennan, P. L., & Moos, B. S. (1991). Short-term processes of remission and nonremission among late-life problem drinkers. *Alcoholism: Clinical and Experimental Research, 15*, 948–955.

Newman, A. R. (1965). *Alcoholism in Fronteac County.* Unpublished doctoral dissertation, Queens University, Kingston, Ontario.

Pfeiffer, W., Feuerlein, W., & Brenk-Schulte, E. (1991). The motivation of alcohol dependents to undergo treatment. *Drug and Alcohol Dependence, 29*, 87–95.

Robins, L. N., Helzer, J. E., Croughan, J., Williams, J. B. W., & Spitzer, R. I. (1981). *N.I.M.H. Diagnostic Interview Schedule, Version III* (May, 1981). Rockville, MD: National Institute of Mental Health.

Roizen, R., Cahalan, D., & Shanks, P. (1978). "Spontaneous remission" among untreated problem drinkers. In D. Kandel (Ed.), *Longitudinal research in drug use: Empirical findings and methodological issues* (pp. 197–221). Washington, DC: Hemisphere Press.

Saunders, W. M., & Kershaw, P. W. (1979). Spontaneous remission from alcoholism: A community study. *British Journal of Addiction, 74*, 251–265.

Schuckit, M. A., & Miller, P. L. (1976). Alcoholism in elderly men: A survey of a general medical ward. *Annals of the New York Academy of Sciences, 273*, 558–571.

Selzer, M. L. (1971). The Michigan Alcoholism Screening Test: The quest for a new diagnostic instrument. *American Journal of Psychiatry, 127*, 1653–1658.

Skinner, H. A., Glaser, F. B., & Annis, H. M. (1982). Crossing the threshold: Factors in self-identification as an alcoholic. *British Journal of Addiction, 77*, 51–64.

Smart, R. G. (1975–1976). Spontaneous recovery in alcoholics: A review and analysis of the available research. *Drug and Alcohol Dependence, 1*, 277–285.

Sobell, L. C., Cunningham, J. A., Sobell, M. B., & Toneatto, T. (1993). A life-span perspective on natural recovery (self-change) from alcohol problems. In J. S. Baer, G. A. Marlatt, & R. J. McMahon (Eds.), *Addictive behaviors across the life span: Prevention, treatment and policy issues* (pp. 34–66). Newbury Park, CA: Sage.

Sobell, L. C., Sobell, M. B., & Toneatto, T. (1992). Recovery from alcohol problems without treatment. In N. Heather, W. R. Miller, & J. Greeley (Eds.), *Self-control and addictive behaviors* (pp. 198–242). New York: Maxwell Macmillan.

Sterne, M. W., & Pittman, D. J. (1965). The concept of motivation: A source of institutional and professional blockage in the treatment of alcoholics. *Quarterly Journal of Studies on Alcohol, 26*, 41–57.

Strug, D. L., & Hyman, M. M. (1981). Social networks of alcoholics. *Journal of Studies on Alcohol, 42*, 855–884.

Tuchfeld, B. S. (1981). Spontaneous remission in alcoholics. *Journal of Studies on Alcohol, 42*, 626–641.

Tuchfeld, B. S., Simuel, J. B., & Schmitt, M. L. (1976). *Changes in patterns of alcohol use without the aid of formal treatment. An exploratory study of former problem drinkers.* Springfield, VA: National Technical Information Service.

Vaillant, G. E. (1983). *The natural history of alcoholism, causes, patterns, and paths to recovery.* Cambridge, MA: Harvard University Press.

Weisner, C. (1993). Toward an alcohol treatment entry model: A comparison of problem drinkers in the general population and in treatment. *Alcoholism: Clinical and Experimental Research, 17*, 746–752.

Wilsnack, S. C., & Wilsnack, R. W. (1991). Epidemiology of women's drinking. *Journal of Substance Abuse, 3*, 133–157.

Woodruff, R. A., Jr., Guze, S. B., & Clayton, P. J. (1973). Alcoholics who see a psychiatrist compared with those who do not. *Quarterly Journal of Studies on Alcohol, 34*, 1162–1171.

13

Treatment Programs
for Aging Alcoholics

ROLAND M. ATKINSON

As the general population ages, the number of older alcoholics is increasing, but little systematic information exists on the natural course of alcoholism and problem drinking in aging persons, the best treatments for them, or valid methods to evaluate treatment outcome in older alcoholics (Atkinson, 1990). New information on these themes is emerging rapidly, however, and this chapter will attempt to review this nascent literature critically. First I will address several factors other than treatment that can influence outcome and its measurement. The better studies of treatment programs for older alcoholics will then be reviewed in detail. Results, however, will be presented descriptively, not quantitatively. The studies vary so greatly in clientele served, treatment provided, follow-up duration, and measures used to determine outcome or compliance, that it would be highly misleading to compare outcome or compliance statistics among them directly. After reviewing treatment studies, I will discuss some of the issues requiring special attention in the treatment of older problem drinkers, based on clinical experience, and will end with conclusions about what we know and what we need to find out about treatment through future clinical research.

DEFINITIONS

Terms like alcoholism, treatment compliance, and outcome are defined, as I will use them, in Table 13.1. Age cutoffs demarcating "older" patient groups vary widely in the reports to be reviewed, from age 45 to age 65, reflecting the differing perspectives of alcoholism experts and gerontologists about what "old" means (Atkinson et al., 1990). These differences from study to study will be noted in the discussion to follow, for they are not trivial. One report, for example, noted different treatment outcomes for a group age 45 to 60 when compared to a group older than 60 (Kashner et al., 1992, below), and others detected differences in compliance depending upon whether patients age 55 to 59 years were included along with older patients.

Table 13.1. Definitions of Terms Used in This Chapter

- **Heavy drinking** This term is used primarily by epidemiologists and is variously defined, usually as daily drinking, ranging from one drink-equivalent/day (a highball or shot glass of hard liquor, 4 oz. glass of table wine, or 12 oz. beer) in some studies, to drinking the equivalent of 50 grams/day of pure ethanol, about 4 to 5 drink equivalents, in other studies. Because of age-associated changes in biological sensitivity, functional decline, and pharmacokinetics, the distinction between heavy drinking and biomedically hazardous drinking tends to narrow with age (Atkinson, 1984; Atkinson, 1990).
- **Problem Drinking** A term also used primarily by epidemiologists, it refers to focal problems—social, legal, occupational, or health—engendered or aggravated by alcohol use. The more problems, the more likely an alcohol use disorder or alcoholism exists.
- **Alcohol Use Disorders** Diagnostic group developed by the American Psychiatric Association, in their diagnostic manual of mental disorders (American Psychiatric Association 1994 and previously), that sets forth explicit criteria for the diagnosis of alcohol dependence and alcohol abuse; criteria cover faulty control of drinking, biomedical consequences (including tolerance and withdrawal), and social consequences of drinking (Atkinson, 1990).
- **Alcoholism** The National Council on Alcoholism and the American Society of Addiction Medicine recently defined this term as follows: " . . . a primary, chronic disease with genetic, psychosocial, and environmental factors influencing its development and manifestations. The disease is often progressive and fatal. It is characterized by impaired control over drinking, preoccupation with the drug alcohol, use of alcohol despite adverse consequences, and distortions in thinking, most notably denial. Each of these symptoms may be cotinuous or periodic." (Morse & Flavin, 1992). It is probably a broader definition of alcoholism than the DSM-IV definition of alcohol dependence. For patients typically seen in alcoholism treatment settings, the terms "problem drinking," "alcohol dependence," and "alcoholism" are likely to define the same individuals. For narrative style, in this chapter I will usually use the terms "alcoholism" and "alcoholic" to represent all cases in treatment.
- **Compliance** Treatment compliance refers to the patient's fulfillment of prescribed activities and goals *during* treatment. In alcoholism treatment, prescribed activities commonly include participation in planned sessions, e.g., attending scheduled counseling sessions, AA meetings and educational classes, remaining in the program until a specified endpoint, and taking prescribed medication such as disulfiram and/or psychiatric medications. Compliance also includes fulfillment of program expectations concerning drinking behavior during treatment, e.g., either abstaining from alcohol or meeting specific goals for reduced intake, and avoiding previous drinking settings. Treatment personnel and records can collect most data needed for compliance studies in the routine course of patient care.
- **Outcome** Treatment outcome refers to the patient's continuing fulfillment of prescribed activities and goals *following completion* of treatment. Drinking behavior is the most commonly measured outcome variable, e.g., continuing abstinence or adherence to a reduced drinking goal, number and degree of drinking relapses, or quantity and frequency of drinking compared to pretreatment. Social adaptation and/or functional status may also be measured, especially focusing on alcohol-related social, legal, occupational, and/or health impairments. Holding the gains made during treatment for a significant period after treatment is obviously a more stringent test of treatment efficacy; thus outcome studies are more valuable in determining the usefulness of an experimental treatment program. They are, however, much more costly to conduct, since research personnel and data systems, not treatment staff, must collect the data. For that reason outcome studies often report 6-month or 1-year followup, falling short of the 2- or 3-year interval considered by many workers to be a minimum threshold for "successful arrest" of alcoholism (Glatt, 1956) or "secure abstinence" (Vaillant, 1983). Pretreatment predictors of outcome may not be the same as predictors of compliance (Gilbert, 1988).
- **Response** This term has two meanings in treatment research. It refers to the answers given by patients, collaterals, and staff to questions about compliance or outcome. One may refer to patients as "respondents" and systematic inaccuracies in their answers as "response bias." Response also is a term used by some workers to refer to both program attendance/completion, which I call compliance, and patient satisfaction, as measured by questionnaires probing patient attitudes about the treatment program (Moos & Finney, 1988). No study of older alcoholics has reported patient satisfaction data.

187

NONTREATMENT FACTORS INFLUENCING TREATMENT OUTCOME AND EVALUATION

Clinical Issues

The Course of Alcoholism and Heavy Drinking in Later Life

There is sparce but consistent evidence that, with age, long-term light to moderate drinkers tend to continue their earlier consumption patterns, whereas heavy drinkers, problem drinkers, and alcoholics tend to reduce or terminate their drinking in later life, often without formal treatment (spontaneous abstinence or reduced drinking) (Hermos et al., 1988; Liberto et al., 1992; Nordström & Berglund, 1987). In the only reported longitudinal study of alcoholics in their sixties and seventies, conducted among male military veterans over three years, two of nine patients who were securely abstinent at the start relapsed, two of nine patients who were drinking at the start subsequently became abstinent without treatment, and 5% of elderly medical clinic nonalcoholic "controls" developed drinking problems for the first time (Schuckit et al., 1980). Late-onset problem drinking may have an especially evanescent course: High rates of both recent problem onset and rapid spontaneous problem resolution were reported by late middle-aged (55 to 64 years) community dwellers in one study (Moos et al., 1991).

These findings, while fragmentary, suggest that problem drinking status for many at-risk aging persons is quite unstable. On the one hand, this may favor positive treatment outcome, at least over the short term. However, this instability in drinking status also suggests that treatment could be falsely credited for reduction in alcohol consumption or abstinence that would have occurred spontaneously, especially in late-onset cases. Given the apparently fluctuating nature of alcohol consumption in many older problem drinkers, neither compliance during treatment nor short-term outcome after treatment may be good indicators of longer term prognosis.

Medical and Psychiatric Comorbidity

More so in aging persons than others, comorbid medical illness can complicate the course and treatment of alcoholism (Hurt et al., 1988; Moos et al., 1993). The importance of these comorbidities is enhanced by the fact that often elderly alcoholics do not enter treatment until associated medical problems necessitate hospitalization (Rosin & Glatt, 1971; Schuckit & Miller, 1976). Major diseases caused or aggravated by alcohol, such as cirrhosis and dementia, are associated with high short-term mortality rates in older patients who continue to drink heavily, although alcoholism treatment reduces mortality of older patients with alcoholic liver disease (Atkinson, 1990; Hurt et al., 1988; Woodhouse & James, 1985). Death from comorbid medical disorders during alcoholism treatment, even among compliant patients, is predictably more common in older than younger patients, and occurred in 5% of men patients age $\geq$ 55 years during a one-year Veterans Affairs (VA) outpatient program (Atkinson et al., 1993). Deteriorating health status also may force patients to discontinue treatment prematurely, and painful disorders such as arthritis can be a drinking relapse risk factor.

Psychiatric comorbidity (so-called "dual disorder" or "dual diagnosis" cases) can complicate the course and treatment of alcoholism at any age. Very few studies have reported careful evaluation of psychiatric comorbidity in older alcoholic patients using modern diagnostic criteria. Pooled VA inpatient data collected in 1987 showed that 29% of 6,592 substance abusing veterans age 65 years or older had a concomitant psychiatric diagnosis (Moos et al., 1993). Depressive (7.8%) and organic (7.5%) disorders were the most common. Many of these patients were evaluated in medical detoxification or extended care settings in which psychiatric evaluations may not have met an adequate standard. Among 216 patients age ≥ 65 years evaluated after admission to an alcohol treatment unit in a nonprofit community teaching hospital, lifetime DSM-III comorbid nonsubstance-related mental disorders were found in nearly half of patients (Finlayson et al., 1988). Effects of recent drinking would be expected to influence mental status under these circumstances. Organic mental disorders were twice as frequent as affective disorders, the second most common diagnostic group (25% versus 12%).

In an age-specific social group treatment program located in a VA alcoholism outpatient clinic, where assessments were made at least 30 days after last drinking and an effort had been made to screen out patients with major mental disorders, only 32%, 16 of 50 patients age ≥ 60 years, had lifetime DSM-III comorbid mental disorders (Atkinson & Tolson, 1992). Mild to moderate mood disorders (dysthymic, cyclothymic, and adjustment disorders) were far more common than organic disorders in these outpatients (22% versus 6%). Mild or focal cognitive deficits, insufficient to fulfill diagnostic criteria for an organic mental disorder or syndrome, were discerned in an additional 19% of a hospitalized cohort (Finlayson, et al., 1988) and 16% of an outpatient cohort (Atkinson & Tolson, 1992). Two-thirds of the affective disorder cases in the hospitalized sample were major depressive episodes versus none in the outpatient sample.

In a recent study of pooled data from a 4-week survey of all veterans seeking outpatient mental health services at VA facilities nationwide, comorbid diagnoses were reported for subgroups of 3,986 men age 60 to 69 years, and 543 men age ≥ 70 years, who had a diagnosis of "alcoholism" (Blow et al., 1992). About half of these patients (45% of the 60 to 69 group and 51% of the ≥ 70 group) had comorbid nonsubstance mental disorders. Affective disorders were most frequent (21% in both older age groups), followed by organic mental disorders (9% of the 60 to 69 group and 18% of the ≥ 70 group) and anxiety disorders (10% in both groups). As might be expected, since the setting was mental health rather than alcoholism clinics, rates for schizophrenia (9% and 8% in the two older age groups, respectively) and major depression (9% and 12%, respectively) were prominent compared to the older age alcoholism clinic cohort described earlier. These findings, like the pooled VA inpatient data cited earlier (Moos et al., 1993) are based on unusually large samples of aging alcoholics. But this data must be evaluated cautiously because there was no training, supervision, or testing to assure uniform thoroughness of clinical evaluations or adherence to diagnostic criteria. Nevertheless, the findings do add weight to the view that psychiatric comorbidity is highly prevalent in elderly alcoholics. Whether psychiatric comorbidity is more common in elderly alcoholics than in other geriatric cohorts—for example, patients admitted to geriatric evaluation and management units, or to nursing homes—is conjectural.

Depression and anxiety tend to be associated more with early-onset alcoholism than with late-onset (Atkinson et al., 1990; Atkinson & Tolson, 1992; Schonfeld & Dupree, 1991), and early-onset patients may be more likely to drop out of treatment (see below), possibly as a function of psychiatric comorbidity or greater pessimism about improvement. Presence of a comorbid mental disorder may increase the likelihood of patients receiving post-inpatient discharge follow-up care (Moos et al., 1994). However, one can expect that elderly patients with comorbid mental problems will have a less favorable treatment outcome than others (Moos et al., 1994), unless these disorders are specifically considered.

Structural and Setting Variables

Demographic characteristics (gender, racial or ethnic group, socioeconomic status, and attained age within the long span of older adulthood) might affect compliance and outcome, and in fact this review will demonstrate some structural effects. Social and environmental factors can lead to compliance problems such as reduced attendance at scheduled meetings and dropout from treatment. Program location and size, patient eligibility and finances, transportation, and family collaboration may all have high impact on treatment continuation, compliance, and outcome. For some persons, attending any program located in an alcoholism treatment setting may be too embarrassing to sustain, and the community may not offer an acceptable alternative, say one located in a senior center or geriatric clinic. While many alcohol clinics operate nearly exclusively at night, older clients prefer to attend appointments during daylight hours, for reasons of perceived personal safety and ability to see more clearly.

Measurement Issues

While characterization and measurement of elderly alcoholism is not the focus of this chapter, it is an issue that is highly relevant to the problem of evaluating treatment effects. If traditional methods of eliciting alcohol consumption information are faulty when used for the elderly, as has been suggested (Graham, 1986), it follows that these same methods may yield faulty information on changes in consumption with treatment. And parameters of successful social rehabilitation used for younger persons (for example, return to the work force or cessation of alcohol-related arrests) have less relevance for many older problem drinkers (Graham, 1986).

Measuring Alcohol Consumption in the Elderly

The validity of alcohol consumption measurement in alcoholics of all ages remains controversial (Babor et al., 1987; Fuller et al., 1988). Factors such as lack of awareness of consumption level, faulty memory, embarrassment, lack of knowledgeable collaterals, and family collusion may mitigate accurate reporting of consumption for elderly problem drinkers in particular (Graham, 1986; Wattis, 1981). On the other hand, alcohol consumption, measured in ways that minimize response biases, still may be a relatively simple and valid indicator of changes in overall biomedical and psychosocial adjustment following alcoholism treatment (Babor et al., 1988).

Several recent reports suggest that, using proper methodologic safeguards, it is possible to obtain a reasonably accurate portrayal of alcohol consumption by elderly persons, including alcohol abusers. Such procedural safeguards can be stated as principles of measurement and include the following major points: (a) a prospective rather than retrospective approach yields more valid and reliable consumption data; (b) in either case, frequent samples of brief time frames yield better information on consumption than infrequent samples of longer time frames; (c) prospective diary keeping, also called self-monitoring, probably yields better data than quantity-frequency questionnaires; (d) multiple methods used together, e.g., data from patient and from a collateral (relative, friend, or caseworker), or questionnaire data augmented by interview or diary, yield better data than single methods; (e) respondents need extensive training in the methods to be used; and (f) assurances of confidentiality and minimization of negative consequences for reporting drinking should be made (Isacsson et al., 1987; Tucker et al., 1991; Werch, 1989). Interviews, especially using the time-line-follow-back method, have been recommended by some as superior to questionnaire approaches (Sobell et al., 1979), although some elderly persons may report higher consumption on a questionnaire than in an interview (Isacsson et al., 1987).

Measuring Functional Status

A few projects (e.g., Dupree et al., 1984; Thomas-Knight, 1978) have employed sophisticated batteries of outcome measures addressing psychosocial and functional status, some borrowed from studies of younger alcoholics and nonalcohol-related gerontology research and others contrived for the particular study. But to date there has been no report of an elder-specific alcohol treatment outcome measure that has been tested for validity and reliability. Any such measure needs to augment the traditional focus on employment and social deviance with measures covering age-related manifestations of excess alcohol use (for example, falls and confusion, overall physical health status, instrumental activities of daily living, social network as construed for older persons, and use of discretionary or leisure time). Cognitive testing is essential and, for those patients with significant memory impairment, measures of collaterals' reports of functional status are crucial.

EFFECT OF AGE ON THE OUTCOME OF ALCOHOLISM TREATMENT IN MIXED-AGE SETTINGS

The proportion of patients over age 60 enrolled in alcoholism treatment programs varies from about 1% to 10% (Atkinson & Kofoed, 1982; Kola et al., 1980). There is evidence from pooled VA data that older alcoholics may be selectively shunted away from substance abuse inpatient treatment programs and cared for in alternative settings such as medical detoxification and extended care units, perhaps in part because of their medical comorbidities (Moos et al., 1993). These older alcoholic veterans are also are less likely than younger patients to receive outpatient substance abuse aftercare services following hospital discharge. Given their "minority status" in alcohol treatment programs and their special needs as usually perceived by caregivers in other aging services, how do older patients fare in typical mixed-age alcoholism treatment settings? This question has been addressed in several reports of compliance and outcome that stratified subjects by age group. Such efforts began with studies of inpatient alcoholism treatment units in the 1950s in Western Europe and continued through the 1960s and 1970s in the United States and elsewhere. Several of the studies that are commonly cited in discussions of age and outcome of alcoholism treatment in fact included few or no patients over age 50 or 60. They are not considered here. A very few studies in outpatient settings have been reported more recently, paralleling the gradual shift in emphasis of alcoholism treatment toward ambulatory approaches.

Treatment of Alcohol Withdrawal

In the most thoroughly studied large cohort of hospitalized older alcoholics, 216 patients age $\geq$ 65 years, 9 (4%) developed withdrawal delirium (Finlayson et al., 1988), a rate similar to that seen in younger patients (Atkinson, 1988). In the only systematic published report on the treatment of alcohol withdrawal disorders, 24 patients, ages 21 to 33 years, were compared with 26 patients, ages 58 to 77 years, on a scale measuring severity of alcohol withdrawal (Liskow et al., 1989). Although they reported consuming less alcohol in the 30-day and 24-hour periods preceding admission, the older group had more severe withdrawal and also required higher doses of sedative medication (chlordiazepoxide) to control symptoms. Longer duration of alcoholism and history of more complicated prior withdrawal episodes in the older cohort, rather than age, could have accounted for these differences in withdrawal severity.

The authors speculated that because of both phenomena (severity of withdrawal and higher sedative need), entry into alcohol treatment could be delayed in older patients, insofar as effective participation in educational and psychotherapeutic activities requires intact cognitive processes. Since withdrawal and its treatment represent relatively straightforward biomedical processes, provided the unit staff members are attuned to general issues of acute illness in the elderly and geriatric consultation is available, there is little basis for arguing that age-specific detoxification programs are necessary. Nevertheless, it can be argued that medically complex or frail elderly alcoholics might receive safer and generally more effective care during withdrawal if treated on a specialized geriatric evaluation and management (GEM) unit, and this practice occurs in some GEMs (J. W. Campbell, personal communication, November, 1992).

Inpatient/Residential Treatment

Medical comorbidity, often aggravated by drinking, frequently requires acute medical treatment in hospital, where not uncommonly the identification of alcoholism first occurs. The focus of this chapter, however, concerns specific treatment for alcoholism, and inpatient treatment for this disorder presumes that acute medical problems have been resolved and chronic medical problems stabilized before the patient is referred along or transferred to an alcoholism treatment unit (ATU). Many ATUs do accept patients at risk for severe alcohol withdrawal and treat this in the early days of the admission.

Most reports of age and ATU outcome have found that older patients fare as well as, or slightly better than, younger patients, but these studies, the best of which are represented in Table 13.2, all have serious limitations. They vary in definition of the older age group, and most, irrespective of how the older group is defined, report small numbers of older patients. They also presumably vary in the definition of alcoholism, typically omitting reference to this as well as to other inclusion or exclusion criteria, comorbidities in general, and cognitive status in particular. They vary further in methods of obtaining follow-up information, criteria for recovery or improvement (although most limit their focus to alcohol consumption and often ignore functional status), and duration of follow-up. Finally, no attempt was made in most of these studies to quantify or control for post-ATU outpatient treatment or participation in Alcoholics Anonymous.

The variation in findings in these reports is perhaps best epitomized by a study that used the same methods to evaluate 18-month outcome from two programs for alcoholics in Belfast, Northern Ireland. In one program (psychiatric hospital, with shorter stay and emphasis on management of alcohol withdrawal) age was associated with favorable outcome, while in the other (ATU emphasizing group therapy, alcohol education, and AA linkage, in addition to managing withdrawal) age was unrelated to outcome (Blaney et al., 1975).

Outpatient Treatment

An early study in Edinburgh compared 1-year drinking status for 50 men and women who received several weeks' inpatient ATU treatment followed by outpatient treatment versus another 50 patients who received only outpatient treatment (Ritson, 1968). The sample included 37 patients age $\geq$ 50 years, with just 7 $\geq$ 60 years. Treatment assignments were nonrandom. Patients were encouraged to remain in treatment throughout the year, although there was an unspecified number of dropouts, making this a compliance, not an outcome, study. Older age favored compliance, as measured by reduced drinking and better home adjustment, in both treatment conditions.

In the largest survey of age effects on alcoholism treatment, pooled data from about 550 programs throughout the United States, reporting to NIAAA during 1977 through 1979, was analysed according to age group, comparing 3,163 subjects age $\geq$ 60 years versus 3,190 younger adults (Janik & Dunham, 1983). Multiple treatments were included, but these were specified and quantified as (a) hours spent in detoxification, (b) total days of inpatient treatment, (c) total hours spent in and times received outpatient treatment, and (d) number of monthly service reports submitted, an estimate of duration of treatment. "Initial outcome" was measured 180 days after initiation of treatment. Not only was there no requirement for completion of treatment or for a specific interval before follow-up, but the proportion of patients still in treatment at 180 days was not reported, although presumably it was fairly high. Strictly speaking, this too was not a study of outcome but of compliance.

It was also not reported whether any of the programs represented in the pooled data included elder-specific treatment tracks. If so, their numbers probably would have been small and their effects diluted in the massed data. Dependent measures employed at baseline and at 180 days included patient and counselor assessments of the alcohol problem, a quantity-frequency drinking measure, an impairment index, and (at 180 days) the counselor's global assessment of changes in the client's alcohol problem. As for any large-scale survey of pooled data, one is justified in having reservations about the rigor and reliability of measures quantifying treatment effects. This survey found no age-related differences in treatments given, or in results on the dependent measures of drinking behavior and other features, at 180 days. On most measures, including baseline alcohol-related symptoms and status at 180 days, subjects in the group age 40

Table 13.2. Studies of Age and Treatment Outcome from Mixed-Age, Hospital-Based Inpatient Alcohol Treatment Units*

Study, Location, Dates of Index ATU Treatment	Older Subgroup Age Cutoff	Number of Pts. in Subgroup	Category of Study	Followup Method (Interval)	Findings and Comments
Glatt (1956) London Several month admission men, 1952–1954	> 50	29	Outcome	Various (6 months to 3 1/2 years)	Outcome of older men slightly superior to others, but similar when "psychopaths" (most of whom were younger) were excluded.
Ellis & Krupinski (1964) Victoria, Australia ATU 2–23 days, men, 1960	≥ 50 ≥ 60	117 30	Outcome	Readmission for alcohol treatment (2 years)	Age unrelated to outcome.
Myerson & Mayer (1966) Boston, ATU + halfway house Skid-road men, 1952	> 50	23	Outcome	Various (8–10 years)	Age unrelated to outcome.
Bateman and Petersen (1971) U.S. Southern State program 28 days, men, 1962–1964	≥ 45	202	Outcome	Mail survey (6 months)	Older subgroup reported significantly more frequent abstinence, but method makes the finding questionable and followup was short.
Blaney et al. (1975) Belfast, N. Ireland ATU v. psychiatric hospital men and women, 1968	≥ 50 ≥ 60	83 24	Outcome	Structured interviews by researcher (18 months)	Outcome was more favorable with age from psychiatric facility; age did not affect outcome from ATU. Results were confounded by differing lengths of stay (tended to be much longer in ATU).

Study	Age	N	Type	Measure	Findings
Schuckit (1977) Washington State; pooled data for 9 programs and 32 clinics men and women, 1975	≥ 60	41	Compliance	Standardized reports by treatment staff (completion)	Older group was significantly more likely to complete treatment. But study favored success in older group, who were more often treated in hospital rather than clinic (100% v. 79%) and for briefer duration to achieve completion (0.6 month v. 1.2 months).
Wiens et al. (1982–83) Portland, Oregon, private ATU 10–11 days + 4–6 op visits men and women, 1978–1979	≥ 65	78	Outcome	Various (12 months)	Older group was "treated as successfully, even a bit more so, as younger patients." However, report included no data on younger patients, instead citing other reports by the authors.
Fitzgerald & Mulford (1992) Iowa drinking drivers, pooled data, various ip & op programs 88% men, 1985–1987	≥ 55 ≥ 65	156 51	Outcome	Phone, mail survey (2 years)	Older subgroups fared as well as or better than persons under age 55 in reported abstinence, heavy drinking episodes, and rearrests. Most treatment was nonresidential; older groups spent less time in residential care, equivalent time in outpatient and AA sessions.
Moos et al. (1994) National VA pooled data, all inpatient care for substance abuse; 95% men; 1986–1987	≥ 55	22,678	Outcome	Readmissions to VA system (12 months)	Among older patients, prior admissions, unmarried status, and psychiatric comorbidity predicted readmission, either for substance abuse, or, psychiatric care. Treatment was in psychiatric, medical detox., extended care or substance abuse units. No comparison to younger patients' outcome was reported, 90% of cases alcoholic.

*All programs were public except the one studied by Wiens et al. ip = inpatient/residential treatment; op = outpatient treatment to 59 years scored somewhat worse than either the group $\geq$ age 60 or the group age 21 to 39. On several dependent measures at 180 days, men in all age groups tended to score worse than women.

The authors concluded that their findings did not support the need for elder-specific alcoholism treatment. Like all prior studies of age effects in mixed-age programs, however, they had no elder-specific program data for comparison, nor did their data permit analysis of interaction effects, that is, age-by-specific-treatment modality. Nor did they consider the typical circumstances in mixed-age programs, where older persons represent a small minority of the total for whom the program is presumably tailored (see below). The milieu in a typical "mainstream" program may not be conducive to effective engagement and treatment of this older minority, which militates against the possibility of a more favorable outcome (Kofoed et al., 1987; Schonfeld & Dupree, 1991). The authors' methods made it impossible, in the final analysis, to answer the question whether older patients might have had superior outcome, compared to younger patients, if treated in an age-specific program and/or by methods especially suited for the older alcoholic.

Recent interest in the general issue of matching patients to treatment has extended to older outpatients. In a recent prospective study, in the setting of an alcoholism outpatient clinic based at a nonprofit psychiatric hospital in the northeast United States, 42 patients age $\geq$ 50 years were compared with 134 patients 30 to 49 years old, and 53 patients 18 to 29 years old, in their drinking status 3 months after beginning one of three randomly assigned outpatient treatment conditions (Rice et al., 1993). One-third of patients were women. DSM-III alcohol use disorder diagnoses were made on the basis of a nationally used, well-standardized structured interview, the Diagnostic Interview Schedule. All treatment conditions were age-mixed, but the use of different modalities permits assessment of an age group-by-modality interaction effect. Since treatments were scheduled over about 4 months, this report is more a compliance than an outcome study.

Although there were some common features across all three treatment conditions, one condition focused on individual issues of improved problem solving and assertiveness in order for patients to reduce their risk of relapse. The second condition focused on relationships and included sessions with the patient's domestic partner. The third condition focused on vocational/occupational issues in addition to some focus on relationships and individual issues. Alcohol consumption for this 3-month report was measured by telephone interview using the time-line-follow-back method and corroborated by a knowledgeable collateral, again using telephone interviews (face-to-face interviews are planned at 6-month intervals in future outcome follow-ups of this cohort).

Overall, there were no main age or treatment condition effects on compliance. However, there were significant age group-by-modality effects. For older patients, the number of days abstinent was greatest, and the number of heavy drinking days fewest, among those treated in the individual-focused condition, while middle-aged patients did better in the relationship-focused condition. For the young adults, there were no differences in compliance across treatment conditions. The authors rightly concluded that age is a variable that needs to be considered when testing patient-treatment matching hypotheses. This is the first, and to date only, reported demonstration of an interaction between age and the specific content and focus of therapeutic rehabilitation approaches to alcoholism.

What Can We Learn from Mixed-Age Studies?

These studies tell us something about what age contributes, operating as a subject or 'structural' variable, to alcoholism treatment compliance and outcome. Despite the great variation in setting, subjects, design and quality of the various studies over the past 35 years, there is one invariable finding: No study has shown that age confers a special liability for poor treatment outcome. Given what we know about age-associated medical and psychiatric comorbidities and relative lack of social supports, and given some of the prevailing prejudices about the presumed inadaptability of older people to psychosocial and psychoeducational treatments, this is a rather remarkable finding.

One might object that mixed-age programs may have screened out many elderly alcoholics because of comorbidities, so that older subjects in these studies are not representative of all older alcoholics (Moos et al., 1993b). Granting this objection, it can still be asserted that such screening, if it occurred, may have in fact operated to equalize comorbidities across age groups, in a sense controlling for them and making the influence of age *per se* more likely to be apparent in the outcome results.

There is no evidence from mixed-age studies to support one particular inpatient approach over another, except for the difficult-to-interpret finding in the Belfast study that older patients treated in a general psychiatric ward setting had better drinking outcomes than those treated in an ATU (Blaney et al., 1975). Just one study was designed to demonstrate interaction effects between age and specific outpatient treatment approaches. Its findings have face validity: In the older age group, that was presumably less reliant on job or domestic partner because of losses if for no other reason, a treatment condition emphasizing individual mastery of drinking—using techniques such as improved problem solving, self-assertion, and identification of drinking antecedents to reduce risk of relapse—was more successful than approaches based on enhancing occupational skills or relationships.

What we cannot learn from these mixed-age reports is whether older patients would fare better if clustered in age-specific treatment settings than they do when treated together with younger persons, an issue that I will discuss next.

AGE-SPECIFIC TREATMENT FOR OLDER ALCOHOLICS

Why should age-specific treatment be considered for older alcoholics? Answers to this question, considered further in the next section, include the following. (a) There may be different age-associated etiologies, perpetuating factors, and risk factors for relapse in late-life problem drinking that can be better addressed on an elder-specific basis. (b) Cognitive, social and value differences may require staff with special interpersonal qualities and training, and special approaches, e.g., slower pacing, repetition, and emotionally supportive rather than confrontive style by counselors. (c) Social bonding with age peers is likely to facilitate identification with a group and promote shared reminiscence, and thus may enhance program compliance and improve outcome. (d) The health and social status of older patients may preclude certain treatment approaches (e.g., routine use of disulfiram), and favor methods rarely used for a younger group (e.g., community outreach and home visitation strategies, social services, and advocacy).

Types of Elder-Specific Programs

Most elder-specific programs have arisen to meet perceived clinical and social needs in a particular community. Many of these programs began with no preconceived outcome evaluation design. Reports are often limited to a simple descriptive narrative, with or without supporting statistical data, while a few include systematic evaluation, and fewer yet offer controlled comparisons of one treatment "condition" with another, or of one patient subgroup with another treated in the same program.

Several prototypic elder-specific models for formal alcoholism treatment have been reported. The most widely described outpatient models are those using (a) supportive social programs (Zimberg, 1978) that often emphasize group and family therapy, either in a "freestanding" program (Dunlop et al., 1982; Williams, 1983) or in an alcoholism outpatient clinic (Atkinson et al., 1993; Kofoed et al., 1984), and (b) cognitive-behavioral therapy, offered in a group format as part of a day treatment program in an aging services setting (Dupree et al., 1984; Schonfeld & Dupree, 1991). Such programs may receive referrals from, or work in conjunction with, mixed-age, hospital-based ATUs (Atkinson et al., 1993; Dunlop, 1990). Elder-specific residential ATUs have also been established (Gordon, 1988; Kashner et al., 1992; Thomas-Knight, 1978) and will be described further below.

Alcoholism is often a hidden problem for which elders themselves do not seek treatment (Atkinson, 1990). For this reason, nontraditional community outreach programs have been developed in several localities to promote case finding (Fredriksen, 1992; Hubbard et al., 1979; Jinks & Raschko, 1990), individual and group social and educational activities and referral to alcoholism treatment (Fredriksen, 1992), and in-home therapeutic visitation for housebound and reticent elderly problem drinkers (Graham et al., 1990). Another strategy designed to engage aging problem drinkers in natural settings, that is, in settings where they are more likely to congregate, is the special primary medical care clinic ("Alcohol-Related Disorders Clinic"), run conjointly by medical and alcoholism clinicians for the treatment of older alcoholics with significant medical comorbidities (Willenbring, 1992; see also Chapter 16 in this book). This model may prove especially important in settings like the VA that tend to shunt older alcoholics away from substance abuse programs toward primary medical care (Moos et al., 1993b).

Anecdotal reports of other initiatives, gleaned from oral presentations, newsclips, and brief articles in paraprofessional sources, suggest that a number of other strategies are being tried to assist elderly problem drinkers. These include such diverse initiatives as broad-based community education, tenant assistance training for boarding house managers, adding substance abuse specialists to interdisciplinary geriatric teams, age-specific chapters of AA, alcohol-free adult foster care, and one-to-one, in-home elderly peer counseling. For articles describing several of these recent initiatives, see issue number 361 of the magazine *Aging* (Administration on Aging, 1990).

Comparisons Among Patient Subgroups Treated in the Same Age-Specific Treatment Condition

A few single-condition studies were designed to make comparisons possible between subgroups of the older patients treated in a single age-specific program, e.g., those with late-onset versus early-onset problem drinking, or such studies have taken place in settings that permit some comparison in compliance or outcome to younger age cohorts treated in the same location.

Comparisons of Compliance of Older versus Younger Patients

In a recent report of compliance of 205 military veterans, age $\geq$ 55 years, with a 1-year, age-specific VA outpatient alcoholism social group treatment program, the proportion of patients completing treatment was twice that of younger men treated in groups during the same time frame within the same clinic (Atkinson et al., 1993). In part, this sizable difference in retention very likely reflected different program policies about management of drinking slips (tolerated more in the elder-specific program provided the trend was toward smaller, less frequent slips) and apparent drop outs (in the elder-specific program unannounced home visits frequently were made to patients who missed group meetings resulting in the patients' return to treatment).

Comparisons of Compliance of Older Patients Based on Treatment and Referral Variables

Patients under court supervision after drinking driving offenses were more likely to complete treatment and had higher attendance rates at weekly group meetings than other patients in the VA outpatient study just described (Atkinson et al., 1993). They also reported less family alcoholism and lower levels of anxiety and depression at intake than others. Thus lower psychiatric comorbidity, rather than court supervision *per se*, could have accounted for the differences in compliance. Regardless of referral source, married patients whose spouses agreed to engage in therapeutic program activities for at least a month were more likely to complete treatment than those whose spouses refused such treatment. Marital therapy was not randomly assigned, and even though no differences were found between the two subgroups of married patients on several alcohol-related, demographic, and psychiatric symptom variables, the differences in their treatment compliance may reflect differences in natural family cohesion and support (marked by willingness of the spouse to participate) more than marital therapy effects. Rates of documented drinking relapses during treatment, based on information collected from multiple sources by treatment personnel, were not influenced by either court supervision or marital therapy.

Comparisons of Compliance of Older Patients Based on Late versus Early Onset of Alcohol Problems

Whether alcohol problems that arise for the first time in middle or late life are more amenable to treatment than longstanding problems has been controversial. Several reports in the 1970s that either supported or failed to support this notion were based on either anecdotal case reports or limited systematic data (Atkinson et al., 1990; Brody, 1982). Information is now available from two elder-specific outpatient treatment programs that shed some new light on this controversy.

Using a *post hoc*, matched-pairs design, 46 women and men $\geq$ age 60 years, whose problem drinking began either before age 50 (early onset, $n = 23$) or after age 50 (late onset, $n = 23$), were compared on rates of completion of a 6-month day-treatment program located in a public, academically oriented aging services setting (Schonfeld & Dupree, 1991). The program incorporated an 80-session cognitive-behavioral group educational sequence designed to improve self-efficacy in managing life problems and antecedents to drinking. The treatment approach seems similar to, but more extensive than, that described above as individual-focused treatment in a study comparing outpatient treatment modalities (Rice et al., 1993). Late-onset alcoholics were significantly more likely to complete treatment. However, in a larger pool of 148 similarly treated patients, age ≥ 55 years, from which the first sample of 46 was drawn, there were no differences in completion rate based on onset age.

In the elder-specific VA project discussed above, compliance with a 1-year program of weekly social support group meetings was determined in 132 alcoholic men age ≥ 60 years, who were also assessed on several non-alcohol and alcohol-related variables, including age at onset of the first alcohol problem (Atkinson et al., 1990). The cohort was subdivided into early onset (≤ age 40 years, $n = 50$), midlife onset (41 to 59, $n = 62$), and late onset (≥ 60, $n = 20$) subgroups. In univariate analyses onset age group was significantly related to program completion and to attendance rates at weekly meetings, the older the better. In a later report, age at onset was used as a continuous variable in a stepwise regression analysis of the contribution of 12 independent variables to outpatient group treatment compliance in 128 men ≥ age 55 (Atkinson et al., 1993). In this analysis, onset age did not contribute to variance in program completion, but did contribute significantly to variance in attendance rate. Rates of documented drinking relapses during treatment did not differ with onset age.

The information from these two programs is consistent in suggesting that there probably are effects of late onset on treatment compliance, if one considers patients age ≥ 60 years at entry to treatment. In each program, curiously, inclusion of somewhat younger patients, age 55 to 59, reduced the relationship between late onset and improved compliance.

What Can We Learn from Studies of Single Age-Specific Treatment Conditions?

If proper attention is given in advance to specific hypotheses and to careful measurement of variables under study, much can be learned from studies that include no control or comparison treatment conditions. Among factors that have been or could be studied usefully in this manner to assess their effects on treatment compliance and outcome are (a) clinical variables, for example, medical and psychiatric comorbidities, and alcohol-related variables, for example, medical and psychiatric comorbidities, and alcohol-related variables such as late onset; (b) referral and treatment variables; and (c) ethnic, racial, and gender variables (virtually no information is available on these dimensions). Later onset of problem drinking appears to be associated with better treatment compliance among patients age 60 and older, but perhaps not among patients age 55 to 59. As is true for younger alcoholics, older ones appear to benefit from strong third-party (judicial or domestic) support for treatment. As yet no reports of treatment outcome (rather than compliance) have focused on any of these variables in single-condition studies.

Another useful product of single-condition studies can be the development of treatment guides and manuals to transfer information to other programs and facilitate efforts to replicate treatment results. To date only one program has generated such products, the Gerontology Alcohol Project in Tampa, Florida (Schonfeld & Dupree, 1990).

What we cannot learn from single-condition studies are the answers to such fundamental questions as whether outcome of treated patients is superior to no treatment, whether age-specific treatment is superior to mixed-age treatment, and which age-specific modalities work best for the elderly.

Comparative Studies: Relative Efficacy of Different Treatment Conditions

Control in treatment outcome research implies that a given modality or condition is being compared to either a no-treatment condition (typically delayed or placebo treatment) or to some other modality of treatment. In the best studies, subjects are selected from a common pool of potential participants who meet inclusion/exclusion criteria and agree in advance to take part in any of the treatment conditions under study, and subsequently are randomly assigned to one of these treatment conditions. As in psychotherapy research, treatments should proceed according to explicit procedural manuals, clinicians should be trained on these, and actual delivery of treatments should be unobtrusively monitored, using video- or audiotapes for later review to assure adherence to intended methods. The same compliance or outcome measures and time frames should be used for all conditions, with information ideally collected by research personnel who are not affiliated with the treatment programs.

In view of the fluctuating, unstable natural course of alcohol use in older problem drinkers, particularly late-onset drinkers (see above), one might expect a fairly high rate of short-term abstinence in a no-treatment condition (spontaneous abstinence). It is therefore frustrating, if ethically understandable, that no studies have been reported that compare an elder-specific alcoholism treatment condition with a no-treatment control condition. Less justifiable is the fact that to date there have also been no studies designed to test one elder-specific treatment condition against another (for example, supportive social group treatment versus cognitive-behavioral treatment in outpatient settings).

There are reports of three studies in which an elder-specific condition was compared with a mixed-age condition. But random treatment assignment from a common subject pool was made in just one of these studies, and it is the only one of the three that approaches being a true outcome evaluation study. None used explicit treatment guides, training, or monitoring of delivery. These three studies will now be reviewed.

Comparison Studies of Age-Specific versus Mixed-Age Programs

In an outpatient study of problem drinking men and women, $\geq$ age 54 years, in a VA alcoholism clinic, all patients received weekly group therapy for one year and were expected to remain abstinent (Kofoed et al., 1987). Compliance was compared for a cohort treated in age-specific therapy groups ($n = 25$) versus a cohort treated in mixed-age groups (with other patients as young as age 20 years) ($n = 24$). Assignments to the two conditions were nonrandom, but no more than two older patients were assigned to any one mixed-age therapy group. Cohorts were similar on a number of non-alcohol and alcohol-related variables, except that the age-specific cohort had later onset age for the first alcohol problem (44 years versus 34 for the mixed-age cohort).

Mixed-age groups tended to use confrontive techniques to promote "here-and-now," affectively charged exchanges aimed at reducing denial of substance-abuse and life problems, and more honest relationships and self-appraisals. Age-specific groups were more slow paced and emotionally supportive, tolerated non-self-disclosure, joking, and story telling, and encouraged shared reminiscence (Atkinson & Tolson, 1984; Kofoed et al., 1984). Patients in the age-specific treatment cohort significantly more often completed treatment and had higher rates of attendance at group meetings. There was no difference between groups in rates of documented drinking relapses, based on information collected from multiple sources by treatment personnel. The investigators judged that the difference in onset age did not account for the differences in compliance (Atkinson et al., 1985; Kofoed et al., 1987).

The earliest reported controlled study of age-specific versus mixed-age treatment took place at another VA hospital, where a special residential ATU (the Older Alcoholic Rehabilitation [OAR] program) was designed for older patients to offer education and therapy programs that addressed the interaction between aging and alcoholism (Thomas-Knight, 1978). "Age consciousness raising" was promoted, and special attention was given in education and discussion groups to themes like death and dying, sexuality, loss of loved ones, health, religious concerns, and community resources for the aged. Alcoholic male military veterans age $\geq$ 55 years were assigned nonrandomly either to the OAR program or another, mixed-age ATU in the same hospital. Length of treatment was not clearly stated, but inferred to be approximately 30 days in each ATU.

Instruments were chosen to measure "positive changes" in terms of mood, self-actualization, life satisfaction, and purpose in life. These attitudes and feelings were assessed at the end of treatment in 14 completers of the OAR program and 17 completers of the mixed-age ATU program. Whether tests were administered by personnel affiliated with the ATUs was not stated. Responses of the OAR treatment cohort demonstrated significantly more change on all measures when compared to patients treated in the mixed-age ATU. Since patient responses were reflective of OAR program philosophy and goals, they may have represented a response bias based on social desirability and investigator expectations. This strong possibility and the timing of measurement at the point of program completion mark this as a compliance study. While the author concluded that older alcoholics "progress" more when treatment addresses the interaction between aging and alcoholism, the relationship between changes on the measured parameters and drinking behavior or social adaptation remained unstudied and conjectural.

The most recent and best controlled comparison of age-specific treatment to mixed-age treatment comes from the same VA hospital as the 1978 study just reviewed, and indeed seems to be an extension of that study, although it was not cited in the new report (Kashner et al., 1992). Male military veterans age $\geq$ 45 years (age 45 to 59: $n = 64$; age 60 to 69: $n = 62$; age $\geq$ 70: $n = 11$; total: $n = 137$) who had been consecutively discharged from a detoxification unit and who agreed to participate were randomly assigned to either an age-specific ATU (called the OAR program, as in the 1978 study; $n = 72$) or a mixed-age ATU in the same facility ($n = 65$). Patients who agreed to participate in the study were found to be demographically similar to refusers, but, curiously, data was not reported that compared the two participating patient cohorts on demographic, alcohol-related, or other variables. All treatments were, however, carefully quantified, including number of hours of various forms of therapy given during ATU treatment. Length of stay for OAR patients averaged 33 days versus 35 days for patients on the mixed-age ATU. Dropout rates were 10% from OAR and 5% from the mixed-age program, a nonsignificant difference. During ATU treatment, OAR patients received more peer group sessions, training as peer advisers to other patients, and relaxation therapy, and less physical recreation than patients in the mixed-age ATU. All patients were offered outpatient aftercare for one year: OAR patients averaged 8 visits, mixed-age ATU patients 5 visits over that period.

Outcome was assessed according to several prestudy hypotheses and was measured in several ways, 6 months and 1 year after ATU discharge. Since 1-year outpatient aftercare was a part of the program, one could argue that this was a compliance study, but visits were fairly infrequent and similar in number and content for patients in the two conditions. I conclude, therefore, that the investigators accurately portrayed this as an outcome study. Data on alcohol consumption were gathered in face-to-face interviews using a structured quantity-frequency questionnaire administered by master's-level personnel not affiliated with either ATU. Days of ATU care, numbers of various treatment sessions and outpatient visits, and VA care costs were determined from hospital records and computer files. Data on costs of non-VA care were collected from patient interviews.

Overall, OAR patients were 2.9 times more likely at 6 months and 2.1 times more likely at 1 year to report abstinence than their counterparts who received more traditional treatment on the mixed-age ATU. These differences increased with patient age: Patients who were age 50, 55, 60, and 70 years old were, respectively, 0.5, 1, 1.6 and 5.1 times more likely to abstain from drinking following OAR treatment than after the traditional ATU program. Put another way, at 12 months the odds of reporting abstinence increased 2.5 times for every 10 years of patient age in the OAR cohort. By comparison, age weakly influenced abstinence rates among patients assigned to the traditional ATU: The odds increased only 1.6 times for every 10 years of patient age. Compared to mixed-age ATU care, the OAR was also more "productive," that is, produced more abstinence per treatment unit cost.

While this study is to date the one best designed to test the efficacy of age-specific treatment for older alcoholics, it does suffer from two critical weaknesses: use of a single measure of alcohol consumption based on a quantity-frequency questionnaire, administered only to patients, and lack of reported data to assure that the two patient groups were similar at entry to treatment.

What Can We Learn from Comparative Studies of Age-Specific Treatment?

Despite the modest number of controlled comparison studies to date, they are consistent in suggesting that age-specific treatment is superior to mixed-age or "mainstreamed" treatment for older alcoholics. These findings beg for further and more refined replication, with greater emphasis on studies of outcome, rather than compliance, and on studies in non-VA settings, since all three of the controlled studies have been conducted in VA programs that typically treat medically indigent male military veterans. Studies comparing age-specific treatments to a delayed treatment (no-treatment) condition are unlikely to materialize for ethical reasons: The length of treatment delay is too great for the outpatient conditions, and the typical degree of acuity of illness is too severe to justify delayed entry into residential (ATU) programs. Studies comparing outpatient age-specific modalities are also needed to answer questions about the relative value of such modalities as cognitive-behavioral training, family and marital therapy, and emotionally supportive socialization groups in the rehabilitation of older alcoholics.

SPECIFIC TREATMENT FOR OLDER ALCOHOLICS:
THEMES TO BE ADDRESSED

While the main purpose of this chapter has been to review systematic studies of alcoholism treatment compliance and outcome for older problem drinkers, I want to complement this material with some discussion of certain "desiderata" for treatment programs—issues that have emerged out of the collective anecdotal clinical experience of my group and others but that in most cases still await more systematic, quantitative study. Three broad goals of treatment for all older adult problem drinkers can be stated: (a) reduction or cessation of alcohol consumption, (b) resolution or stabilization of comorbid medical and psychiatric disorders, and (c) optimization of the social and home environment. Success in achieving these goals depends on the availability of proper services and staff.

Risk Factors for Drinking Relapse and Treatment Dropout

Whether older patients are treated in age-specific or mixed-age settings, their treatment may need to address risk factors that are, if not uniquely associated with old age, at least more commonly noted in older alcoholic patients. In my experience with over 400 older male alcoholic military veterans, risk factors that have repeatedly been apparent, although typically occurring in varying combinations and degrees of prominence, include (a) excess discretionary time, or lack of skills to use time constructively, often epitomized in the patient's complaint of boredom, (b) excess discretionary money (alcohol consumption (Barnes, 1979) and late-onset problem drinking (Atkinson, 1984) in older persons tend to increase with income and socioeconomic status), (c) chronic medical disorders like arthritis or obstructive pulmonary disease that produce chronic pain, insomnia, depressed mood, and/or anxiety, (d) life stress—both major events and chronic strains—in relation to faulty coping mechanisms and social supports, especially influencing late-onset problem drinking or relapse in abstinent earlier onset alcoholics (Atkinson, 1994; Finney & Moos, 1984; Moos et al., 1991), (e) predisposing factors, for example, family history of alcoholism and prior personal substance use, (f) psychiatric comorbidity, especially antisocial personality, chronic mood disorders and adjustment disorders with depressed mood, and cognitive deficits, (g) reduced "social controls," that is, social role-related expectations of conformity by family, coworkers, and friends (Peck, 1979), and (h) drinking partners and colluders, including domestic partners, adult children and other relatives, and retired friends.

Many of these same issues may also be risk factors for older women alcoholics, but social and public drinking is far less common in women, for whom a major risk factor is instead social isolation and reclusiveness (Dunlop, et al., 1982; Fredriksen, 1992; Graham et al., 1990). Another major factor, especially for minority elderly women, is economic deprivation and poverty (see Gomberg's discussion in Chapter 12 this book).

Managing Comorbidities

The high prevalence of comorbid disorders makes it imperative that older patients routinely receive thorough medical evaluation, a screening test for cognitive impairment, and screening for the presence of other mental disorders. Hospital or outpatient care for more extensive evaluation and ongoing treatment of medical and psychiatric disorders must be arranged when indicated. For patients with nonsevere mental disorders, or where distressing and disruptive symptoms can be held in check with psychiatric medications, an age-specific outpatient "dual disorders" program in an alcoholism clinic setting may be ideal, but models for such care have not been tested. Patients with severe comorbid mental disorders, for example, frank dementia or schizophrenia, probably are better managed in a geriatric mental health setting, perhaps one that combines mental health day treatment with foster or residential care, than in an alcoholism program.

Staffing, Case Management, and Psychosocial Program Requirements

A daunting array of tasks is often required in order to help older patients reduce their alcohol use, avoid relapse from abstinence, prevent dropping out of treatment, arrange necessary medical and psychiatric care, optimize social and living arrangements, and assure access to and payment for all of these and other services. While no one caregiver may be able to provide all needed services, patients in more complex circumstances often need a case manager, someone who is comfortable working in interdisciplinary geriatric team settings and is able to function as an advocate, expediter, and broker in helping older patients and their families acquire necessary services from various sources throughout the community. In outpatient or aftercare settings in particular, help is often required to solve problems of transportation, housing, deficient social supports and finances, and legal problems (Erckenbrack & Klug, 1989). The capacity and skill to work effectively with patients' family members, including family psychotherapy, is also essential in the rehabilitation of many aging alcoholics (Atkinson et al., 1993; Dunlop, 1990; Dunlop et al., 1982).

Compared to younger patients, elderly alcoholics tend to be more submissive, feel the need for more interpersonal involvement with the professional staff, and benefit more from simple encouragement and support (Linn, 1978). The ideal caregiver for an aging alcoholic, whether in a case manager or alcoholism counselor role, is a professional with some prior training and experience in the three fields of social gerontology or geriatrics, mental health, and alcoholism treatment. Such a caregiver should be comfortable in interactions requiring a slow pace, repetition of information, and the imparting of considerable emotional support. A number of other points about staffing and program requirements germane to managing these tasks have already been mentioned in earlier sections and will not be repeated here. Ten to 15 years ago, neither mixed-age alcoholism programs (Kola et al., 1980) nor aging services agencies (Kola et al., 1984) tended to view the recognition or treatment of alcoholism in older adults as significant issues, and therefore they saw little need for specialized policies, staffing, or training. One can hope that the recent surge of information on aging and alcoholism is altering these perceptions, and there is some encouraging data to suggest this is the case (Schonfeld et al., 1993).

CONCLUSIONS

What We Know

It is clear that aging confers no special liability for poor outcome following alcoholism treatment. Moreover, older patients tend to benefit more if treated in age-specific, rather than mixed-age, settings and should be offered treatment in such settings when available. Treatment of the aging alcoholic will likely be informed by staff trained to recognize the special features of alcoholism in this age group and the associated special general health and social needs.

What We Need to Find Out

I would rank the following themes or questions among those deserving the highest priority for future research about treatment: (a) determination of the characteristics of older persons who need treatment for problem drinking versus those needing only simple advice or natural peer supportive intervention, (b) development of relatively simple elder-specific alcoholism treatment outcome measures covering alcohol consumption and functional status, (c) determination of the actual effects of putative age-associated risk factors for relapse, especially cognitive impairment, depression, and chronic medical illness, (d) determination of the comparative efficacy—based on at least 2-year outcomes—of individual-focused, cognitive-behavioral outpatient alcoholism treatment for patients age ≥ 60 years randomly assigned to receive this treatment in either an age-specific or mixed-age condition, (e) determination of the comparative efficacy—based on at least 2-year outcomes—of age-specific outpatient treatment conditions, for patients age ≥ 60 years, that feature individual-focused, cognitive-behavioral therapy versus supportive social group therapy, with or without family therapy in each condition, in a randomized 2×2 design, (f) testing of comparative models for treating older "dual diagnosis" patients, (g) further testing of the efficacy of age-specific residential ATU programs, (h) determination of the differential treatment needs of aging women, and of ethnic and racial minorities, and (i) testing of comparative models for treating aging persons with active alcohol problems who enter long-term health care facilities with a rehabilitation emphasis, that is, where there is high likelihood of eventual discharge to the community.

The strong support of leaders in the fields of social gerontology, clinical geriatrics, mental health and alcoholism, and older citizen advocacy groups will be needed to fulfill this ambitious research agenda.

References

Administration on Aging. (1990). *Aging*, 361. Washington, DC: Office of Human Development Services, U.S. Department of Health and Human Services.

American Psychiatric Association. (1987). *Diagnostic and statistical manual of mental disorders*, (3rd ed., revised). Washington, DC.

Atkinson, R. M. (1984). Substance use and abuse in late life. In R. M. Atkinson (Ed.), *Alcohol and drug abuse in old age* (pp. 1–21). Washington, DC: American Psychiatric Press.

Atkinson, R. M. (1988). Alcoholism in the elderly population. (Editorial). *Mayo Clinic Proceedings, 63*, 825–829.

Atkinson, R. M. (1990). Aging and alcohol use disorders: diagnostic issues in the elderly. *International Psychogeriatrics, 2*, 55–72.

Atkinson, R. M. (1994). Late onset problem drinking in older adults. *International Journal of Geriatric Psychiatry, 9*, 321–326.

Atkinson, R. M. & Kofoed, L. L. (1982). Alcohol and drug abuse in old age: A clinical perspective. *Substance and Alcohol Actions/Misuse, 3*, 353–368.

Atkinson, R. M. & Tolson, R. L. (1984). Substance abuse by the elderly. *Medical Aspects of Human Sexuality, 18*, 100, 104, 107.

Atkinson, R. M., & Tolson, R. L. (1992). Late onset alcohol use disorders in older men. Research poster presented at the annual meeting of the American Association for Geriatric Psychiatry, San Francisco, February.

Atkinson, R. M., Tolson, R. L., & Turner, J. A. (1990). Late versus early onset problem drinking in older men. *Alcoholism: Clinical and Experimental Research, 14*, 574–579.

Atkinson, R. M., Tolson, R. L., & Turner, J. A. (1993). Factors affecting outpatient treatment compliance of older male problem drinkers. *Journal of Studies on Alcohol, 54*, 102–106.

Atkinson, R. M., Turner, J. A., Kofoed, L. L., & Tolson, R. L. (1985). Early versus late onset alcoholism in older persons: Preliminary findings. *Alcoholism: Clinical and Experimental Research, 9*, 513–515.

Babor, T. F., Dolinsky, Z., Rounsaville, B., & Jaffe, J. (1988). Unitary versus multidimensional models of alcoholism treatment outcome: An empirical study. *Journal of Studies on Alcohol, 49*, 167–177.

Babor, T. F., Stephens, R. S., & Marlatt, G. A. (1987). Verbal report methods in clinical research on alcoholism: Response bias and its minimization. *Journal of Studies on Alcohol, 48*, 410–424.

Barnes, G. M. (1979). Alcohol use among older persons: Findings from a western New York State general population survey. *Journal of the American Geriatrics Society, 27*, 244–250.

Bateman, N. I., & Petersen, D. M. (1971). Variables related to outcome of treatment for hospitalized alcoholics. *The International Journal of the Addictions, 6*, 215–224.

Blaney, R., Radford, I. S., & MacKenzie, G. (1975). A Belfast study of the prediction of outcome in the treatment of alcoholism. *British Journal of Addiction, 70*, 41–50.

Blow, F. C., Cook, C, A, L,, Booth, B. M., Falcon, S. P., & Friedman, M. J. (1992). Age-related psychiatric comorbidities and level of functioning in alcoholic veterans seeking outpatient treatment. *Hospital and Community Psychiatry, 43*, 990–995.

Brody, J. A. (1982). Aging and alcohol abuse. *Journal of the American Geriatrics Society, 30*, 123–126.

Dunlop, J. (1990). Peer groups support seniors fighting alcohol and drugs. *Aging, 361*, 28–32.

Dunlop, J., Skorney, B., & Hamilton, J. (1982). Group treatment for elderly alcoholics and their families. *Social Work in Groups, 5*, 87–92.

Dupree, L. W., Broskowski, H., & Schonfeld, L. (1984). The Gerontology Alcohol Project: A behavioral treatment program for elderly alcohol abusers. *The Gerontologist, 24*, 510–516.

Ellis, A. S., & Krupinski, J. (1964). The evaluation of a treatment programme for alcoholics: A follow-up study. *The Medical Journal of Australia, 1*, 8–13.

Erckenbrack, N. L., & Klug, C. (1989). What's missing from elderly aftercare? *The Counselor, 7(2)*, 16–18.

Finlayson, R. E., Hurt, R. D., Davis, L. J., & Morse, R. M. (1988). Alcoholism in elderly persons: A study of the psychiatric and psychosocial features of 216 inpatients. *Mayo Clinic Proceedings, 63*, 761–768.

Finney, J. W., & Moos, R. H. (1984). Life stressors and problem drinking among older persons.

In M. Galanter (Ed.), *Recent developments in alcoholism*, Vol. 2 (pp. 267–288). New York: Plenum Press.

Fitzgerald, J. L., Mulford, H. A. (1992). Elderly vs. younger problem drinker 'treatment' and recovery experiences. *British Journal of Addiction, 87*, 1281–129?.

Fredriksen, K. I. (1992). North of Market: Older women's alcohol outreach program. *The Gerontologist, 32*, 270–272.

Fuller, R. K., Lee, K. K., & Gordis, E. (1988). Validity of self-report in alcoholism research: Results of a Veterans Administration cooperative study. *Alcoholism: Clinical and Experimental Research, 12*, 201–205.

Gilbert, F. S. (1988). The effect of type of aftercare follow-up on treatment outcome among alcoholics. *Journal of Studies on Alcohol, 49*, 149–159.

Glatt, M. M. (1956). Treatment results in an English mental hospital alcoholic unit. *Acta Psychiatrica Scandinavica, 37*, 143–168.

Gordon, M. (1988). Sage Crossing. A treatment program designed for elders. *Generations. Journal of the American Society on Aging*, Summer Issue: 82–83.

Graham, K. (1986). Identifying and measuring alcohol abuse among the elderly. Serious problems with existing instrumentation. *Journal of Studies on Alcohol, 47*, 322–326.

Graham, K., Saunders, S. J., Flower, M. C., Timney, C. B., White-Campbell, M., & Zeidman, A. (1990). Outcome findings from a study of an innovative outreach addiction treatment program for the elderly. Paper presented at the annual scientific meeting of the Canadian Medical Society on Alcohol and Other Drugs, Montreal, October.

Hermos, J. A., LoCastro, J. S., Glynn, R. J., Bouchard, G. R., & DeLabry, L. O. (1988). Predictors of reduction and cessation of drinking in community-dwelling men: Results from the Normative Aging Study. *Journal of Studies on Alcohol, 49*, 363–368.

Hubbard, R. W., Santos, J. F., & Santos, M. A. (1979). Alcohol and older adults: Overt and covert influences. *Social Casework, the Journal of Contemporary Social Work, 60*, 166–170.

Hurt, R. D., Finlayson, R. E., Morse, R. M., & Davis, L. J. (1988). Alcoholism in elderly persons: Medical aspects and prognosis of 216 inpatients. *Mayo Clinic Proceedings, 63*, 753–760.

Isacsson, S-O., Hanson, B. S., Janzon, L., Lindell, S-E., & Steen, B. (1987). Methods to assess alcohol consumption in 68-year-old men: Results from the population study "Men born in 1914", Malmö, Sweden. *British Journal of Addiction, 82*, 1235–1244.

Janik, S. W., & Dunham, R. G. (1983). A nationwide examination of the need for specific alcoholism treatment programs for the elderly. *Journal of Studies on Alcohol, 44*, 307–317.

Jinks, M., & Raschko, R. (1990). A profile of alcohol and prescription drug abuse in a high-risk community-based elderly population. *DICP—Annals of Pharmacotherapy, 24*, 971–975.

Kashner, T. M., Rodell, D. E., Ogden, S. R., Guggenheim, F. G., & Karson, C. N. (1992). Outcomes and costs of two VA inpatient treatment programs for older alcoholic patients. *Hospital and Community Psychiatry, 43*, 985–989.

Kofoed, L. L., Tolson, R. L., Atkinson, R. M., Toth, R. L., & Turner, J. A. (1987). Treatment compliance of older alcoholics: An elder-specific approach is superior to "mainstreaming." *Journal of Studies on Alcohol, 48*, 47–51; correction *48*: 183.

Kofoed, L. L., Tolson, R. L., Atkinson, R. M., Turner, J. A., & Toth, R. L. (1984). Elderly groups in an alcoholism clinic. In R. M. Atkinson (Ed.), *Alcohol and drug abuse in old age*, (pp. 35–48). Washington, DC: American Psychiatric Press.

Kola, L. A., Kosberg, J. I., & Joyce, K. (1984). The alcoholic elderly client: Assessment of policies and practices of service providers. *The Gerontologist, 24*, 517–521.

Kola, L. A., Kosberg, J. I., & Wegner-Burch, K. (1980). Perceptions of the treatment responsibilities for the alcoholic elderly client. *Social Work in Health Care, 6*, 69–76.

Liberto, J. G., Oslin, D. W., & Ruskin, P. E. (1992). Alcoholism in older persons: A review of the literature. *Hospital and Community Psychiatry, 43*, 975–984.

Linn, M. W. (1978). Attrition of older alcoholics from treatment. *Addictive Diseases, 3*, 437–447.

Liskow, B. I., Rinck, C., Campbell, J., & DeSouza, C. (1989). Alcohol withdrawal in the elderly. *Journal of Studies on Alcohol, 50*, 414–421.

Moos, R. H., & Finney, J. W. (1988). Alcoholism program evaluations: The treatment domain. In D. J. Lettieri (Ed.), *Research strategies in alcoholism treatment assessment*, (pp. 31–51). New York: Haworth Press.

Moos, R. H., Brennan, P. L., & Moos, B. S. (1991). Short-term processes of remission and nonremission among late-life problem drinkers. *Alcoholism: Clinical and Experimental Research, 15*, 948–955.

Moos, R. H., Brennan, P. L., & Mertens, J. R. (1994). Diagnostic subgroups and predictors of one-year readmission among late-middle-age and older substance-abuse patients. *Journal of Studies on Alcohol, 55*, 173–183.

Moos, R. H., Mertens, J. R., & Brennan, P. L. (1993). Patterns of diagnosis and treatment among late-middle-aged and older substance abuse patients. *Journal of Studies on Alcohol, 54*, 479–487.

Morse, R. M., & Flavin, D. K. (1992). The definition of alcoholism. *Journal of the American Medical Association, 268*, 1012–1014.

Myerson, D. J., & Mayer, J. (1966). Origins, treatment and destiny of Skid-Row alcoholic men. *New England Journal of Medicine, 275*, 419–425.

Nordström, G., & Berglund, M. (1987). Ageing and recovery from alcoholism. *British Journal of Psychiatry, 151*, 382–388.

Peck, D. G. (1979). Alcohol abuse and the elderly: Social control and conformity. *Journal of Drug Issues, 9*, 63–71.

Rice, C., Longabaugh, R., Beattie, M., & Noel, N. (1993). Age group differences in response to treatment for problematic alcohol involvement. *Addiction, 88*, 1369–1375.

Ritson, B. (1968). The prognosis of alcohol addicts treated by a specialized unit. *British Journal of Psychiatry, 114*, 1019–1029.

Rosin, A. J., & Glatt, M. M. (1971). Alcohol excess in the elderly. *Quarterly Journal of Studies on Alcohol, 32*, 53–59.

Schonfeld, L., & Dupree, L. W. (1990). Older problem drinkers—long-term and late-life onset abusers: What triggers their drinking? *Aging, 361*, 5–11.

Schonfeld, L., & Dupree, L. W. (1991). Antecedents of drinking for early- and late-onset elderly alcohol abusers. *Journal of Studies on Alcohol, 52*, 587–592.

Schonfeld, L., Rohrer, G. E., Zima, M., & Spiegel, T. (1993). Alcohol abuse and medication misuse in older adults as estimated by service providers. *Journal of Gerontological Social Work, 21*, 113–125.

Schuckit, M. A. (1977). Geriatric alcoholism and drug abuse. *The Geronotologist, 17*, 168–174.

Schuckit, M. A., & Miller, P. L. (1976). Alcoholism in elderly men: A survey of a general medical ward. *Annals of the New York Academy of Sciences, 273*, 558–571.

Schuckit, M. A., Atkinson, J. H., Miller, P. L., & Berman, J. A. (1980). A three year follow-up of elderly alcoholics. *Journal of Clinical Psychiatry, 41*, 412–416.

Sobell, L. C., Maisto, S. A., Sobell, M. B., & Cooper, A. M. (1979). Reliability of alcoholics' self-reports of drinking and related behaviors one year prior to treatment in an outpatient treatment program. *Behavior: Research and Therapy, 17*, 147–160.

Thomas-Knight, R. (1978). Treating alcoholism among the aged: The effectiveness of a special treatment program for older problem drinkers. *Dissertation Abstracts International* B 39:3009, order no. 7823210.

Tucker, J. A., Vuchinich, R. E., Harris, C. V., Gavornik, M. G., & Rudd, E. J. (1991). Agreement between subject and collateral verbal reports of alcohol consumption in older adults. *Journal of Studies on Alcohol, 52*, 148–155.

Vaillant, G. E. (1983). *The natural history of alcoholism.* Cambridge, Massachusetts: Harvard University Press.

Wattis, J. P. (1981). Alcohol problems in the elderly. *Journal of the American Geriatrics Society, 29*, 131–134.

Werch, C. E. (1989). Quantity-frequency and diary measures of alcohol consumption for elderly drinkers. *The International Journal of the Addictions, 24*, 859–865.

Wiens, A. N., Menustik, C. E., Miller, S. I., & Schmitz, R. E. (1982–83). Medical-behavioral treatment of the older alcoholic patient. *American Journal of Drug and Alcohol Abuse, 9*, 461–475.

Willenbring, M. (June, 1992). Treatment intervention for late life drinkers seen in primary care. Paper presented in a symposium on Physiologic and Clinical Research on Aging and Alcohol Use at the annual meeting of the Research Society on Alcoholism, San Diego, CA.

Williams, M. (1983). Senior program stresses peer, family involvement. *NIAAA Information and Feature Service, 106*, 1.

Woodhouse, K. W., & James, O. F. W. (1985). Alcoholic liver disease in the elderly: Presentation and outcome. *Age and Ageing, 14*, 113–118.

Zimberg, S. (1978). Psychosocial treatment of elderly alcoholics. In S. Zimberg, J. Wallace, & S. B. Blume (Eds.), *Practical approaches to alcoholism psychotherapy* (pp. 237–251). New York: Plenum Press.

14

Cognitive Therapy
With Elderly Alcoholics

MEYER D. GLANTZ

Several cognitive therapy approaches have been developed specifically for use with elderly patients (c.f., Glantz, 1989, for a review), and some cognitive therapy programs have been developed specifically for the treatment of alcoholics (Sanchez-Craig, 1975, 1990; Glantz & McCourt, 1983; Glantz, 1987; Oei, Lim, & Young, 1991; Monti et al., 1990). However, there have been no cognitive therapy approaches specifically designed for elderly alcohol abusers, and such a targeted approach is likely to be more effective.

The purpose of this chapter is to provide a working basis for those with some relevant expertise to extend their intervention skills and experience to include elderly problem drinkers. Therefore, while the principles of a cognitive therapy approach to the treatment of elderly alcohol abuse are discussed here, this discussion is not intended as an exhaustive protocol. It is recommended that a psychotherapist considering using the approach described here should have had the appropriate supervised training and experience with cognitive therapy and some expertise in treating both the elderly and alcoholics.

PATTERNS OF ELDERLY PROBLEM DRINKING

The basic principles underlying abusive drinking are the same for the elderly as they are for other age groups, but the common circumstances are significantly different and therefore so are the overt patterns and the appropriate interventions. The pattern and problematic nature of the elderly person's drinking is often more subtle and hard to determine than is the case with younger adult alcoholics (c.f., Atkinson & Schuckit, 1983). While a given elderly individual may well drink less than he or she did when younger, this does not necessarily mean that the person does not have an alcohol use problem; metabolic, maturational, and related psychosocial changes may influence the changes in pattern and consequences of alcohol use. ''Maturing out'' of alcohol abuse occurs but is probably less common than previously believed. Maintenance drinking, a lower but fairly frequent intake of alcohol, is a more common pattern among the elderly than binge (high quantity or high frequency) drinking. While denial in general is very common among alcoholics, an additional problem may occur with elderly problem drinkers. Younger adult alcoholics may be alerted to the problematic nature of their drinking by such consequences as blackouts, decreases in concentration, cognitive and/ or memory function, loss of coordination and difficulties with balance, mobility and other aspects of physical function, lower general performance, competence and problem solving skills, job loss and increase in employment and family problems, social disengagement, perceived changes in the responses and respect received from others, automobile accidents and traffic violations, etc. An elderly problem drinker might experience any of these problems and attribute them not to the consequences of alcohol abuse but to the consequences of aging. Therefore, an elderly person and/or his family and friends might recognize some of the signs of alcoholism, but interpret them as the signs of "old age" or "senility." This is a particularly severe identification problem with late-onset alcoholism.

Many researchers and clinicians have found it useful to distinguish between early- and late-onset geriatric alcoholics. As first proposed by Glatt and Rosin (1964), early-onset drinkers, those elderly alcoholics who developed their alcoholism earlier in their lives and continued it into old age, were more likely to have more characterological psychopathologies and personality dysfunctions than late-onset elderly alcohol abusers who began alcoholic drinking late in life. Rosin and Glatt (1971) felt that these late-onset elderly alcoholics typically used alcohol as a coping mechanism to adapt to the stresses and problems of old age. Many researchers and clinicians have agreed with this observation (e.g., Atkinson, Tolson, & Turner, 1990), and several studies have looked at the prevalence of the two onset patterns. It appears that of those elderly persons with alcohol problems, between one-third and one-half developed the problems later in life.

Carruth et al. (1975) described three groups of older problem drinkers, "late-onset" drinkers, "late-onset (intermittent) exacerbation" drinkers, and "early-onset" drinkers. Gomberg (1980) drew a similar distinction between "reactive problems drinkers" whose problem drinking began late in life, "intermittent problem drinkers" whose periodic intervals of drinking include old age, and "survivors" whose long history of drinking extends into old age. It has been the experience of this author that the three-category onset classification is more descriptive and useful. Late-onset alcoholism appears to be more often reactive and therefore to have a better prognosis; psychotherapy for this group concentrates on conceptualization changes, coping and related skills training, and behavior changes to ameliorate social and environmental circumstances. It should be noted that the majority of late-onset alcohol abusers do demonstrate some concomitant anxiety and/or depression, and this must be a focus of treatment; however, with late-onset drinkers, the affective pathology is often also of more recent origin and therefore more tractable.

Early-onset alcoholism appears to be associated with greater comorbid psychopathology and dysfunction and a much more extensive lack of resources and support. There are two reasons for this. First, substance abusers who begin drug or alcohol abuse earlier in their lives may be more deviant and dysfunctional to begin with; they typically develop more extensive patterns of substance abuse, and they do so for reasons related to having poorer coping and function, less support and success, and more severe concomitant and characterological psychopathologies. Second, longer term alcoholism provides more time for more severe and encompassing losses and consequences to develop and compound each other. This makes it much more difficult to successfully treat early-onset alcoholism as psychotherapy requires not only intervention directed at those foci identified for the late-onset drinker but must also deal with the comorbid psychopathology, the other areas of impairment, and the long compounded history of problems (c.f., Blow et al., 1992). This is made even more difficult as there often are few strengths and limited environmental and interpersonal resources to build on.

While the majority of all alcoholics are actually intermittent drinkers in that most have had periods of sobriety and controlled limited drinking, intermittent elderly alcoholics tend to have had longer and more stable periods of nonalcoholism and to have had multiple experiences of believing that they had overcome their drinking problem but then subsequently relapsing. Some elderly intermittent alcohol abusers are reactive drinkers who respond to and cope with stresses in their later years by heavy drinking, just as they did when they were younger. Other elderly intermittent alcohol abusers seem to be similar to a type of alcoholic within the categorization that Schuckit (1979, 1982) described as a ''secondary alcoholic.'' This term refers to a patient who has a primary preexisting psychopathology that causes the secondary condition of alcohol abuse. While some ''secondary alcoholics'' are early-onset drinkers, some develop a pattern of intermittent drinking. This may be because their psychopathology is less severe, cyclical, related to variations in stress or support, etc. The importance of distinguishing and identifying these intermittent elderly drinkers lies in the need to identify and treat the primary psychopathology which, because of its nature, may be missed or assumed to be secondary to the drinking and therefore not a major focus of treatment. Because these patients are prone to use alcohol as a coping mechanism, they are extremely vulnerable to rapid relapse to previous levels of alcohol abuse once reliance on alcohol for coping is reinitiated.

A further distinction often made in relation to the elderly is that of ''young'' versus ''frail'' elderly. In general, the term ''young elderly'' describes older adults whose physical and mental functioning is relatively intact and complete and usually refers to adults 60 to 74 years of age. The term ''frail'' elderly refers to those elderly adults characterized by diminished function, illness, and/or impairment and is usually applied to adults 75 years of age and older. The cognitive therapy approach described here was developed primarily through experience with fairly healthy and functional adults in their sixties and seventies.

Classification encourages the assumption of homogeneity, and there is a tendency in our society to think of the elderly in terms of a few limited stereotypes. In fact, the elderly are the most heterogeneous of age groups, ranging the full spectrum of most characteristics, and elderly alcoholics are similarly diverse. As is true with all patient groups, the more severe the primary condition, the more extensive the comorbid and collateral problems, the longer term the problems, and the fewer the resources and supports, the worse the prognosis and the more likely the need for more extensive and longer lasting intervention. Treatment planning for elderly alcoholics must be individualized to take into account the needs and circumstances of the individual patient.

SCREENING, PATIENT SELECTION, AND INITIAL SESSION(S)

Therapy starts during the process of patient screening. At the beginning of the first session, potential patients are asked to fill out a confidential information form, which includes a request for standard identifying information; descriptions of educational, employment, and familial status and background; a "description of the reason for seeking treatment"; health and prescription drug use information; short descriptions of their primary family relationships; and "any other things" they think the therapist should be aware of. Specific drug and alcohol quantity-frequency questions are asked, as are yes/no questions about sexual abuse, suicidal behavior, physically harming others, etc. The average adult fills out the form in 15 minutes.

This experience is particularly useful in establishing some expectations for the elderly. The form has a medical history "feel" and deals with specific and at least to some extent "personal" facts. This is a familiar context and begins to contradict the stereotype of psychotherapy as "laying on a couch and free associating." It also establishes the expectation of talking about problems, disclosing information, and directly addressing alcohol (and drug) use.

After greeting, the patient is asked by the therapist if they might address him or her by their first name. Patients almost invariably agree. The point is to establish that the patient will be treated with respect and that their preferences will be considered; it also facilitates the context of personal discussion. Patients are invited to address the therapist in whatever manner they feel comfortable; the majority choose the formal address of last name and title.

Patients are then asked in a very broad and open-ended style to tell a little about themselves and the reason they have come for therapy. Questions are asked only when clarification is necessary or when the prospective patient needs prodding to continue. If the patient cannot seem to respond to open-ended questions, increasingly specific questions are asked until the patient is able to respond informatively. One area that is always probed for if not spontaneously addressed is the history of and current pattern of drinking. When it is possible, a small test for insight is tried. After the patient has provided substantial information, a question is asked whose answer requires some insight.

At this point a decision must be made as to whether the patient is an appropriate candidate for cognitive therapy. Most young elderly adults with drinking problems and no severe intellective impairments are appropriate candidates. Generally speaking, screening criteria for cognitive therapy are not different from those employed with other forms of psychotherapy. The requirements include that the patients have a treatable condition, that they have generally fully functional cognitive abilities, that they have no physical or environmental limitation that would interfere with their engaging in the treatment, that they demonstrate no other obstacle or problem that would prevent them from participating, and that they agree to abide by the rules of the treatment setting and to commit themselves to the therapy program. A strong desire to control their drinking problem, insight, a high degree of motivation, extensive interpersonal support, and adequate or better resources and environmental circumstances are highly desirable, but they are not exclusory criteria. Interestingly and contrary to some therapists' initial expectations, patients who have a high degree of verbal facility, a philosophical orientation, and/or high levels of general intelligence do not have a better prognosis in cognitive therapy than other patients.

Appropriate candidates are told that they are appropriate patients for this therapy protocol and inappropriate ones are referred to other programs. For appropriate patients, the therapy is briefly described. This helps establish reasonable expectations and conveys to the patients that they will be treated in therapy not as passive recipients of a treatment but as active collaborators with responsibility for their own progress and input into the process. Patients are told some version of the following:

Cognitive therapy is based on the fact that people have a great deal of direct control over their thoughts, often much more than they realize. This power can be used to solve problems, including those involving feelings and behaviors. Cognitive therapy has this name because it emphasizes (1) improving this cognitive ability, (2) recognizing that there are different ways to look at things, (3) removing cognitive obstacles which often come from the ways in which people think about things, and (4) using thoughts or cognitions to control feelings and behaviors.

Cognitive therapy is a relatively short-term active therapy in which patient and therapist work together to resolve problems. Part of this involves learning and improving certain skills, including problem analyzing and solving skills. One of the major goals of this therapy is for you to develop skills to the point that you can "become your own therapist," leave therapy, continue to make progress on your own, and prevent or handle future problems. This means you have a lot of control in this therapy and you will not need to worry about becoming dependent on the therapy or on me. Since the therapy is relatively short term, after patients finish, it is not unusual for them to come back for a session or two if they need to, and this is not a failure or a problem.

A second major goal of the therapy is to overcome drinking problems; this usually means not drinking. A third major goal is to improve the quality of your life. We will work on more specific goals to do this. When your life begins to improve, you will find that drinking is much less of an issue that you might have thought possible. I would not be surprised if you were thinking right this moment that it is impossible to improve the quality of your life. The truth is you can; you are a good candidate for this therapy and there is no reason why you should be any different from all of the other people who have been helped by this therapy. The fact that I am offering you this therapy means that I believe that you have the ability to overcome your difficulties and are capable of making your life more satisfying, comfortable, and enjoyable. You will set your own goals and you will not be expected to try anything that you do not want to try or to do anything that you cannot do.

Cognitive therapy is not a secretive therapy. After all, you are supposed to be learning how to be your own therapist and you cannot do that if you do not know what is going on. If at any time you have any questions or concerns about anything, if you are dissatisfied with the progress you are making or about anything I am doing or not doing, please tell me right away. In fact, it is one of your responsibilities in therapy to ask any questions and raise any concerns that you have. Do you have any questions that you would like to ask now?

After any questions are answered, patients are asked if they would like to participate in cognitive therapy. None have refused to date.

If a patient may need medical detoxification, appropriate care or referral must be made prior to psychotherapy. The need for treatment for other medical (and dental) conditions and physical disabilities (including mobility, visual and auditory limitations) must also be ascertained and appropriate care and/or referral and follow-up provided. In some cases aid with the practical necessities of living is required. Determination of the patients' need for assistance with shelter, food, clothing, rehabilitation services, etc. is also important. Even financially well-situated and practically self-sufficient and highly functional-appearing patients may have concealed needs and problems that must be identified and attended to. Inquiry about proper nutrition, physical or emotional abuse, sexual difficulties, legal or financial problems, untreated dental problems, functional limitations, etc. has on many occasions identified serious problems even among patients whose appearance and presentation belies the need for help in these areas. The therapist must use his or her discretion in regard to how and when to inquire about some potential problems.

This first stage of therapy usually involves one to two sessions. The patients are asked to prepare for the next session by thinking about what they would like to accomplish in therapy, what goals they have, and what problems they would like to overcome.

ESTABLISHING GOALS

Having clearly defined goals is a very important part of cognitive therapy, if not all therapies. While therapists usually have strong opinions about the goals a patient should have, it is important that patients feel that the goals are theirs (cf., Sanchez-Craig, 1990). Therefore the goals must be selected by the patient and developed in a collaborative effort with the therapist. The following process seems to work well for developing goals. Patients are first asked in an open-ended way to list their goals and then to identify a realistic first step toward attaining the goals. Frequently, the goals (and steps) proposed by the patient are very general, vague, and/or impractical. For example, "I want to feel better"; I want my job (or marriage) back"; or "I want friends." Concrete, behaviorally defined practical goals with realistic progressive steps must be worked out. For this exercise, an important goal and at least an initial first step is worked out for each of the following areas: (1) social life and friends; (2) family; (3) intimate or romantic relationship; (4) employment or practical achievement; (5) recreation or avocation; and (6) drinking.

A goal is established for each area unless it is very clear that no improvement in an area is really necessary, an atypical occurrence. Patients often identify additional areas for improvement, for example goals related to health habits or particular problems. If a patient seems to have difficulty with formulating concrete goals and steps to accomplishing them, a formal written "goal ladder" or Goal Attainment Scale may be helpful. Usually most of one session is devoted to developing and discussing goals. One mandatory goal is always to stop drinking, or, at the very least, to achieve a period of abstinence followed by very limited and controlled drinking, (see below).

BETWEEN-SESSIONS WORK OR "HOMEWORK ASSIGNMENTS"

It is important that the patient think about therapy-related issues between sessions and work on developing skills and changing behaviors and circumstances. A 1- or 2-hour per week intervention is inadequate; the attempt to change one's behavior and circumstances must be a major part of the patient's life. Further, working between sessions gives the patient a sense of independence, control, competence, and accomplishment, which is critical for progress. Throughout the therapy, suggestions for between-session work are usually made during each session by the therapist (though proposals often come from the patient, particularly later in the course of treatment). Between-session work may involve preparing for the next session, taking a step toward a goal, working on a problem talked about in the session, trying a thought or behavior experiment (see below), or any other task the therapist believes might be helpful. Patients are asked to decide if they accept the suggestion; if they decline, an alternative is proposed until an acceptable one is found. A patient also has the option to choose not to do any between-session work. The phrase ''homework assignments'' is avoided both to maximize the sense that the patient is choosing to do the work and because many patients feel that ''getting homework is for children.'' Many patients continuously refer to the between-session assignments as ''homework'' or ''assignments.'' When this happens, it is usu-ally a good idea to distinguish the voluntary aspects of the ''suggestions'' from the implicit requirement of a ''homework assignment.'' If a patient repeatedly chooses not to do any between-session work or does not carry out the suggestions he or she has accepted, the implications and consequences of this must be explored and discussed.

At the conclusion of the session in which goals are established, two suggestions for between-sessions work are made. First, the patient is asked to identify and do something that will improve his or her life in some way. He or she is asked to pick something that is easy enough to do before the next session. It can be anything—no matter how minor or trivial—as long as it will make life ''a little bit easier or a little bit better.'' The requirement is for a goal that can be readily and easily accomplished and is usually much easier to do than even the first steps of the goals identified earlier in the session. Its purpose is to demonstrate and begin establishing a mindset and an expectation of taking control of and improving one's life. Examples of such goals that patients have selected are ''buying an electric can opener,'' chosen by a man with arthritis, ''going to a movie,'' chosen by a woman who had not ''seen a movie in years,'' and ''telling my son [with whom he lived] that [he] would not be available to baby-sit'' that Saturday night as he himself would be going out with a friend. This exercise often has a sur-prisingly strong effect on patients who have come to believe that their lives cannot be made better or that doing so would require tremendous effort.

For the second between-sessions work suggestion, the patients are asked to think about how they can ''educate'' the therapist about themselves. It is explained that in order for therapy to be effective, the therapist must know about them as individuals, about their strengths and weaknesses and their history, including the good and bad things in their lives. Patients are asked to be prepared to begin ''educating the therapist'' about themselves starting with the following session. This exercise forms the basis for a more complete history taking and also begins the process of life review, which will be discussed in a later section.

PATIENT HISTORY

In a manner similar to the elicitation of information used in the initial screening, the patient is asked in a very open-ended fashion to present information about him- or herself. During the presentation, questions are primarily for clarification and formal structure is provided only as needed. After about a half hour of the patient's history presentation, more direct questions are asked. One purpose is to fill in the gaps related to the time period or events just described with information that was not covered but that would normally be included in a traditional psychotherapeutic history taking. A second purpose is to help the patient to reconceptualize the times, people, and events so that when needed they develop a more mature, realistic, adaptive, contemporary perspective. An example would be to have the patient consider an experience from childhood involving his or her parents from the point of view of the parents, as opposed to the child's viewpoint which they have maintained. The experience of looking at something from the past from a different more adaptive point of view and coming to even a minor insight or reconceptualization is a powerful one for patients, particularly elderly ones who have held the original sometimes maladaptive one as fact for so many years. Patients typically react by accepting the proposition that if their past might be different than they believed, then so might their future. Helping patients overcome their hopelessness, helplessness, and negative view of the future are major goals of cognitive therapy. The therapist must use every opportunity to reinforce alternatives to these negative views.

There are several other reasons for this nontraditional method of history taking. It is so useful that, in general, the author uses this method for screening and history taking with all adult patients regardless of age or presenting problem. This approach allows the therapist to study the conceptualization system of the patient. It is possible to determine how the individual organizes and processes information; how he or she perceives people and events; the content and applications of his or her attitudes, beliefs, implicit world view, models, and constructs; the structure and patterns and dominant themes of his or her conceptualizations; the relative salience of different experiences and concepts; and his or her maladaptive thoughts, beliefs, and construals. It is also possible to determine the patient's self-image and self-esteem; the extent to which there is a need for (externally imposed) structure; an informal estimate of cognitive, verbal, and memory abilities; and the major role models and formative experiences of the patient's life presented from the patient's own point of view with minimal imposition of the therapist's perspective and beliefs.

Moving from open-ended to structured questions avoids an "inquisition" style, sets the tone for the patient to be an active participant in and responsible for what occurs in therapy, and gives the patient the sense of choosing to inform the therapist about him- or herself, rather than feeling that private matters are being "pried" into by a stranger; this is particularly important for many elderly patients. Choosing to act rather than being passive, reactive, and responsive to various coercions is a recurring theme in cognitive therapy. The attention, thought, and feedback given by the therapist to the patient and his or her history presentation often help the patient feel that the therapist is really interested in and cares about him or her as an individual. In addition, although many people are reluctant and uncomfortable at first, they often enjoy talking about themselves and recounting their past, and they often enjoy having the control and reduced pressure to do so in their own way. Generally speaking, volunteered information is better and more therapeutically useful than elicited information. History taking usually requires four to six sessions.

Presenting one's history also establishes a foundation for "life review" or "reminiscence" therapy (Butler, 1974). Defined as the "taking of an extensive autobiography," this attempted "summation of one's life work" is often very useful. While cognitive therapy encourages a focus on the present and the potential of the future, reviewing and inevitably reconceptualizing one's past is often a necessary step, particularly for elderly patients. Later in the course of therapy, after the history presentation is complete and after he or she has begun to make some progress on their goals, patients are encouraged to engage in a more extensive "autobiography" by writing about themselves and their families, by making tape recordings, and by assembling photographs, souvenirs, and other materials, etc. While all patients are strongly encouraged by the therapist to prepare their own biography or history, if the patient has any family who might be interested, this is a great asset and is usually a powerful incentive. When feasible, patients are encouraged to present their history to the interested relative or friend; if necessary the therapist can also serve as the audience.

ALCOHOL USE

From the first session, it should be made clear that it is the therapist's determination that the patient has an alcohol abuse problem. Based on the information collected during the screening session, the therapist should have clearly identified the patient's alcohol use pattern. In the event of patient resistance to the determination that he or she is an alcoholic or has an alcohol abuse or alcohol dependence problem, the therapist should be able to demonstrate the truth of the assertion that the patient has a serious problem. A patient who does not accept that there is a problem will not attack or overcome it.

Patients are strongly encouraged from the beginning of therapy to stop drinking or at least to significantly curtail it with the stated goal of achieving complete sobriety. Environmental support is recommended. It is often suggested that patients attend Alcoholics Anonymous, (AA). Even for those patients who do not fully participate in the AA program, attending meetings for a time usually has a beneficial effect in terms of changing how they think about drinking and about themselves as drinkers, and it facilitates social association with nondrinkers. Patients are also strongly encouraged to remove all alcohol from their homes and to avoid "drinking environments." It is not uncommon for the relatives of the elderly alcoholic to deny and/or facilitate the problem. The therapist must be prepared to deal with this in the same fashion as they would with the family of a younger alcoholic.

Although a scientific view of substance abuse etiology must be developmental, multidimensional, and fairly complicated (e.g., Zucker & Gomberg, 1986; Glantz, 1992; Glantz, 1987; Tarter, 1983), the most functional applied model of drinking for use with patients is a more simplified and fundamental one. The basic model is that alcoholics' drinking is (maladaptive) coping and/or self-medicating (c.f., Moos et al., 1990). This concept is described to patients and demonstrated through examples of drinking reported by the patient. Occurrences of drinking or wanting to drink that are presented by the patient are analyzed with him or her to determine the maladaptive purpose underlying the alcohol use behavior. Once the patient has assimilated the model, drinking occasions are analyzed and the patient is helped to identify more adaptive alternatives to alcohol use. This is a frequently repeated exercise during and between sessions throughout the course of therapy.

Another important concept presented to patients is that alcohol abuse is a multiply reinforced habit with a long history and that, like most habits, it falls into different patterns with manifestations differing according to personality and circumstance. Patients are assisted to study their patterns of drinking, to identify the purposes that it serves and the circumstances that are most likely to elicit the alcohol urge behaviors. "Warning signals" and "danger points" are identified. A repertoire of rehearsed behaviors, adaptive coping strategies, and skills and behavior alternatives are then developed to avoid or adaptively cope with these high-risk points. Understanding of the patterns of their alcohol abuse and early recognition of the warning signals and danger points are greatly facilitated by the monitoring assignments (described below).

Social or controlled drinking as a goal is not generally recommended and is only accepted from the patient in the cases in which there is some reason to believe that it is not likely to lead to an escalating pattern of alcohol use. The best candidates for controlled drinking are late-onset reactive drinkers with an extensive history of controlled drinking and accomplished changes to their current circumstances and with no severe comorbid psychopathologies. Even in these cases it is recommended that the patient observe an extended period of abstinence before attempting controlled drinking, usually six months or more. A fixed number of drinks per time period—a "danger level"—is established to help the patient recognize whether he or she is escalating to a probable loss of control. A plan is developed for the patient to follow if it is recognized that there is a danger of breaching the warning level. When feasible, at least one close family member or friend is asked by the patient to inform him or her if they think there is a danger of escalating alcohol use.

PROBLEM SOLVING

It is important to balance a focus on the past with a primary focus on improving the present and future. At the beginning of every session the patient is asked about what has happened since the last session, with the clear and stated implication that "things should be happening." The patient is invited to tell the therapist anything that he or she would like to talk about or present a problem that he or she would like to "work on" or "would like help dealing with." Part of every session is spent on "bringing the therapist up to date," and part of most sessions is devoted to working on resolving specific old and new problems; however, an emphasis is placed on current problems. Whenever possible, the therapist helps the patient reconceptualize the problem and then develop for themselves a reasonable resolution with which they are comfortable; the therapist is more active and directive when necessary but becomes less active over time as the patient gains facility. The patient is always expected to take some action on the problem and to inform the therapist about the outcome; reconceptualizing the problem so that it is not a significant concern or actively choosing not to deal with the problem at this time may be considered as acceptable actions. This focus on problem solving is not only intended to help the patient solve particular problems, improve, and become more in control of and hopeful about his or her life, but also is intended to improve, problem analyzing and resolving skills, and thus to increase competence and confidence. As appropriate, the therapist will also track information about goal attainments and discuss overcoming obstacles and formulating new steps and, when needed, new or redefined goals. One of the expectations for progress in the therapy is that during the course of therapy the patient will increasingly develop the skills and accept the responsibility for such tasks as identifying issues and problems to discuss, for carrying out the problem analysis and review of potential resolutions, for the proposal and tracking of goals, etc. This is part of the patient's "becoming his or her own therapist."

Throughout these problem-solving exercises, the patient is directed to use effective analyzing and solving methods. During the discussion of different problems, the patient is asked as needed to define the problem in concrete terms, to identify specific goals, to break the problem down into parts, etc. Developing a more organized approach to problem solving usually makes a major contribution to therapeutic progress for elderly alcoholics. Conceptualizations related to more effective problem solving are also encouraged. For example, self-defeating conceptualizations are discouraged and more objective perspectives are encouraged.

Resolving Major and Long-Standing Issues

Many elderly patients have major long-standing unresolved concerns and problems, which may date from any time in their lives including childhood. The effects of such issues are likely to extend into the present in terms of certain maladaptive themes (e.g., mistrust of others) or specific, tangible problems (e.g., estrangement from family). Major issues may be identified through the history presentation or subsequently in other discussion, and these must be resolved. Standard cognitive therapy approaches are employed.

Maladaptive Thoughts, Styles, and Themes

During the screening and history taking and subsequently during later sessions and through the monitoring assignments (see below), the patient's characteristic thoughts, beliefs, primary constructs, and patterns of conceptualization are observable. This makes it possible to identify maladaptive aspects of the patient's conceptualization and information-processing systems. During discussion and while working on problems, the therapist has the opportunity to help the patient correct these maladaptive construals. The logs and monitoring assignments are also very useful for providing examples to work on. Whenever possible, maladaptive cognitive contents, constructs, conceptualization structures, and information-processing fallacies are identified and discussed with the patient, and an attempt is made to show the ways in which these maladaptive contents and processes lead to problems and facilitate alcohol use. The most common maladaptive conceptualizations and processes observed in alcohol abusers are described in Glantz and McCourt (1983), Glantz (1987), and Ellis et al. (1988).

In terms of maladaptive information processing, for example, a common problem is *dichotomous thinking*, in which events and people are construed in terms of bipolar opposites. When this is the case, the patient is encouraged to "find the shades of gray" and form a less extreme view of the person or occurrence in question. Some patients' conceptualizations are loosely organized and prone to tangents; during discussion these individuals are helped to focus, to structure their thoughts and speech, and to identify the "main point" of what they are thinking or talking about. Some patients' conceptualizations are overly focused on details, and these individuals are helped to think and speak more in terms of summary concepts and general statements, to "think about the forest and not just individual trees"; here the use of metaphors and parallels can also be helpful. Verbal presentations reflect thinking, and shaping the ways in which some-one presents and discusses information can influence the structure of thought processes.

Maladaptive content and perspective are similarly addressed. For example, overly self-focused patients are encouraged to view a situation from the ''other person's point of view''; patients who tend not to focus on their own feelings are helped to do so when describing or analyzing a situation; and patients who typically construe in terms of power or achievement constructs are prodded to also conceptualize in terms of af-fective and affiliative constructs. Specific beliefs and general attitudes that are mal-adaptive or unrealistic are also addressed and more functional alternatives developed with the patient and supported in their use.

In addition to the maladaptive ideas given individuals (including those with particular psychopathologies) may have, different populations tend to have particular themes in-volving maladaptive aspects that are common to that group. Following is a list of general thematic areas related to which the elderly often have maladaptive thoughts and beliefs (an extended description of these areas and the common maladaptive ideas associated with them can be found in Glantz, 1989): (1) Physical illness and disability; (2) death and dying; (3) intimate relationship and social network losses; (4) loss (or lack) of control and power; (5) diminished abilities and dependence; (6) role and accomplish-ment loss; (7) disengagement and reduced pleasure; (8) activity transitions and losses; (9) ageism and low self-image, devaluation; (10) conflicts with family; (11) environ-mental stresses; (12) transitions and other life-stage issues; (13) adapting and problem solving; and (14) starting new endeavors, relationships, romances.

The maladaptive thoughts and beliefs commonly found among elderly alcoholics tend, as a group, to potentially include those associated with the general elderly pop-ulation, the general alcoholic population, and the general populations suffering from the comorbid psychopathologic conditions that the elderly alcoholic might also suffer (e.g., depression, anxiety, etc). However, recurrent themes related to guilt, wanting not to live (though not necessarily wanting to die), and feeling that they deserve the bad things that have happened to them and they do not deserve anything better than they have (though they want better and are bitter at not having it) seem to be additional common specific themes among elderly alcoholics.

A useful paradigm in cognitive therapy is the Thoughts > Feelings > Behavior model $(T > F > B)$, which states that thoughts (and conceptualizations) determine feelings which together determine behavior. This model is explained to patients and illustrated with examples. The use of the model for understanding certain behaviors, including drinking, and the application of the model to the control and self-direction of behavior is discussed and applied to situations and problems raised by the patient. Other cognitive therapy models are discussed as needed.

Skills Training

It is often the case in cognitive therapy that behaviorally based skills are taught to patients, and this has proved useful in the treatment of elderly alcoholics. Training in relaxation techniques is frequently part of the therapy. As appropriate, assertiveness training, a variation of Novaco's (1977) anger control technique, a variation of Mei-chenbaum's (1975) stress inoculation technique, a version of D'Zurilla and Goldfried's (1971) problem-solving strategy, Hoelscher and Edinger's (1988) sleep maintenance improvement approach, and a variety of memory decrement compensation techniques are taught (Wisocki, 1991, is a useful reference for a number of behaviorally based interventions with the elderly).

Behavioral instruction and rehearsal are employed for other areas when it is determined that there is a need; examples include "dating" and "conversation" skills, developing new friendships, and securing employment or volunteer work. Some patients need help with practical problems, for example, assistance in handling financial matters. In these cases the patient is assisted, but the goal is to help the patient get the information and assistance through independent action rather than directly from the therapist. This helps to develop self-reliance, self-confidence, problem solving skills, and a more positive and hopeful and less helpless perspective. Many patients find that self-help books are a useful addition to their between-session work. There are a number of cognitive therapy-oriented or compatible books available on a variety of topics, and these are suggested to patients either at their request or as seems appropriate (e.g., Alberti, & Emmons, 1970; Benson, 1975; Burns, 1980; Emery, 1982; Freeman & DeWolf, 1989).

Logs and Monitoring Assignments

In order to help patients gain insight about and control of their behavior and to help them develop an understanding and amelioration of their conceptualization systems, two between-sessions tasks are recommended. The first is a log or a diary in which the patient records the significant events of the day and his or her related thoughts and feelings. This helps the patient gain some perspective on daily life, provides examples for the various cognitive therapy exercises, and offers a context through which periods of the patient's life can be retrospectively examined with greater objectivity. The comparison of the memory and current construal of an event with a description written at the time is often very helpful, particularly for patients whose perspectives and experience are strongly dominated by affect to the exclusion of more intellective consideration. The log is recommended as an ongoing assignment throughout therapy, and many patients have reported that they continue the practice afterwards.

The second recommended task is the monitoring assignment. Patients are asked to identify a situation involving a strong emotion that they experienced, and to describe the circumstances and the thoughts that preceded the feelings and the behavior that followed. For alcoholic patients, the selected strong emotion is often related to the use or the desire to use alcohol. During the sessions the patient and therapist analyze the report in terms of the $T > F > B$ model and identify maladaptive cognitions and patterns. As the patients gain facility in applying the cognitive therapy perspectives to behaviors, they are asked to include in the log entry their own independently developed analysis of the situations in terms of the determinative roles played by their cognitions. When this level is mastered, patients are asked to include independently devised more adaptive alternatives to the cognitions as well as behavioral alternatives. Patients are also asked to relate the particular situations to more general patterns that apply to themselves. Patients are encouraged to develop the ability and the habit of monitoring their thoughts and feelings and to learn to identify recurrent problematic patterns. Once patients have gained some facility at monitoring and are able to identify maladaptive patterns, they learn to recognize such patterns early enough in the progression to be able to change or curtail the usual sequence.

Social Relationships

In an early article on geriatric alcohol abuse, Droller (1964) stated, "The most important therapy [for elderly alcoholics] is social." The majority of older alcohol abusers have limited (or even nominal), impaired, and/or impoverished friendship and family relationships and social networks. Developing the relevant skills and improving and expanding relationships and activities is critical for these patients. A satisfactory quality of life (and often even sobriety) is likely to be associated with if not contingent upon satisfying affiliative needs (Brown & Chiang, 1983). Starting, improving, and reestablishing relationships is particularly difficult for some elderly patients who either have long histories of disconnection and limited social associations or who have lost important relationships and are fearful of forming and losing new ones. All people also need more intimate interpersonal relationships that provide mutual caring and support. Many elderly adults are afraid of or feel incapable of developing new intimate relationships, yet having some close relationships is also critical to well-being; resistance is often greater still among elderly alcoholics. Patients who do not have both social and intimate relationships must be strongly encouraged and assisted to develop them. Many elderly people would also benefit from romantic and even sexual relationships, and despite the prevalent pessimism among many older adults, romance (and sex) are more possible and satisfying than expected.

Self-Image

Poor self-image and self-esteem are often problems for elderly patients in general and particularly for elderly alcoholics. As a means of eliciting self-esteem for the purposes of discussion, three exercises are used. In the first, patients are asked to prepare a description of themselves to be read in a session. In the second, patients are asked to write the five "most important beliefs" about themselves. When possible, each patient's presentation of his or her self description and list of beliefs is videotaped and shown to the patient. The content and presentation are discussed, focusing on the issues of self-image, self-esteem, and presentation of one's self to others. In the third exercise, the concept of subjective versus chronological age is explained (c.f., Goldsmith & Heiens, 1992) and the patient is asked to state his or her subjective age. The discrepancy and associated reasons form not only a helpful platform for a discussion of self-image and self-respect but are also a good starting point for discussing the patient's own often maladaptive beliefs and prejudices about old age.

Thought and Behavior Experiences and Experiments

Patients learn more from experience than from dialogue or discourse. For this reason, patients are encouraged to explore ideas behaviorally. For example, a man who did not like "anything new," was encouraged to go to a new restaurant and try any dish his wife selected for him. When he found that the meal was "not too bad," he became willing to try a few other new things, which eventually led to a greater openness. Persuasion could not have accomplished what experience did. Abstract and didactic presentation of ideas and cognitive therapy models and ideas are avoided for the most part, and ideas are instead presented in terms of actual situations in the patient's life.

Whenever possible, actions, activities, and behavioral experiments are used to influence reconceptualization and behavior change. For example, an electronics engineer forced into retirement by his firm on the grounds that his expertise was obsolete felt "useless." As an experiment, with assistance he put together a list of professional and volunteer organizations who "just might" want his services and he then contacted them. When he was offered 2 positions (of 11 contacts) he changed his view of himself. As he really was not interested in nor in need of employment, he accepted neither of the offers; however, he later took a volunteer teaching position helping children with learning disabilities "and low opinions of themselves." In some cases, the experiment is carried out as a "thought experiment" done in imagination. For example, a woman who had spent much of her life ambivalently resisting and at the same time trying to win the approval of her family reported that she was afraid to "take her turn doing Thanksgiving" because the family always criticized her efforts. She was encouraged to imagine that she actually did everything possible to make a Thanksgiving meal and evening that would please her relatives. When she realized that she would still be criticized as much as ever, and that she in fact always had done everything she could to win the approval of her family, she decided that she could never please them and perhaps it was "time to stop trying." In other cases role play, role switching, and other exercises are used to convey ideas and to help patients explore possible alternative conceptualizations and behaviors.

The Treatment of Comorbid Conditions

The treatment of comorbid psychiatric conditions is critical to effective intervention with elderly alcoholics. Some patients may even drink as reaction to or consequence of a primary psychiatric disorder (c.f., Schuckit, 1979, 1982). Most patients have at least some degree of anxiety, depression, and/or anhedonia and some, particularly early-onset drinkers, may demonstrate fully active comorbid psychopathologic conditions. Treatment of these conditions is necessary and is usually accomplished through a cognitive therapy intervention that is integrated into the psychotherapy for alcohol abuse. This integration is usually readily accomplished; in fact, there is often so much overlap in terms of foci and methods that few problems occur. However, when extant comorbid conditions are involved, the treatment timeframe must be extended.

Psychoactive Drug Treatment

Psychotherapeutic medications are an important tool in the mental health intervention repertoire, and there are cases where it is appropriate to use these drugs as supplemental or adjunct interventions to cognitive therapy with elderly alcoholics. It is recommended that these drugs be used as conservatively as possible and only in severe cases. Of particular concern are those psychoactives that have a high abuse liability, especially the classes of drugs including sedative-hypnotics and anxiolytics, particularly benzodiazepines. Sedative-hypnotics and anxiolytics are generally not recommended and should be used only in severe cases and with great care. It is recommended that if they are to be used, then the following guidelines should be employed: (1) Prescription should be for the drug with the lowest abuse liability and for as low a dose as will serve the identified purpose; (2) the prescription should be for a short term and then subject to review and, if necessary, represcription rather than refill; (3) prescription should not be on a PRN (''use as needed'') basis but rather on a predetermined schedule; and (4) use of the drug, its effects, side-effects, etc., should be thoroughly discussed with the patient and monitored by the prescribing physician. Occasionally a patient will inquire about the use of disulfiram (Antabuse). Generally this is not recommended as it locates the responsibility for control of alcohol use with an external agent, the drug, rather than with the patient. It has been the experience of this author that only a very small number of patients have expressed interest in using disulfiram; interestingly, more patients have expressed an interest in such interventions as hypnosis.

RELAPSE PREVENTION

Relapse is a common and serious problem for post-treatment alcoholic populations, and successful intervention programs must include relapse prevention components in order to maintain effectiveness over time. Marlatt and his associates have devoted considerable attention to understanding the nature of relapse and have developed effective methods for minimizing recidivism (c.f., Marlatt, 1978; Marlatt & Gordon, 1979; Marlatt & Gordon, 1985; Mackay, Donovan, & Marlatt, 1991). The relapse prevention approaches recommended by Marlatt are incorporated into the approach recommended here for elderly alcohol abusers.

THE THERAPY PLAN

This chapter describes an approach and a number of therapeutic considerations but does not provide a protocol or a specific plan beyond the beginning sessions. An individual plan incorporating the described elements and goals must be developed for each individual patient with constant review and adjustment throughout the course of therapy. A discussion of a few practical issues may be helpful. Sessions last for 50 minutes and are scheduled for once a week at a regular appointment time. However, when the patient first enters treatment, if he or she is actively drinking, sessions are scheduled for twice a week until drinking is either curtailed or stopped; this usually occurs in less than 8 weeks. Toward the end of therapy, sessions are ''tapered off'' with increasing intervals between sessions. At the last session, ''tune up'' (reinforcement) sessions are scheduled for 6 and 12 months post-therapy. For all patients duration of treatment may vary with comorbid condition, practical and health circumstances, family support, etc. Late-onset elderly drinkers are in treatment for an averageof 40 to 55 sessions over a period of 10 to 15 months. Intermittent elderly drinkers are in treatment for an average of 50 to 60 sessions over a period of 12 to 16 months. The range is greatest for early-onset drinkers; the average is 70 to 100 sessions over a period of 18 to 24 months.

ADDITIONAL REFERENCE MATERIALS

Several useful reference materials are cited in relevant parts of the chapter; following are some additional works that may be helpful: Beck, 1976; Beck et al., 1979; Dobson,

1988; Emery, 1981; Freeman et al., 1989; Gallagher et al., 1981; Meichenbaum, 1974; Sanchez-Craig et al., 1984; Sanchez-Craig, Wilkinson, & Walker, 1987; Steuer & Hammen, 1983; Thompson et al., 1986; Thompson et al., 1991; Vallis, 1991; Yost et al., 1986.

References

Abrams, R., & Alexopoulos, G. (1991). Geriatric Addictions. In R. Frances and S. Miller (Eds.)., *Clinical textbook of addictive disorders*. New York: Guilford Press.

Alberti, R., & Emmons, M. (1970). *Your perfect right: A guide to assertive behavior*. San Luis Obispo, California: Impact Press.

Atkinson, J., & Schuckit, M. (1983). Geriatric alcohol and drug misuse and abuse. *Advances in Substance Abuse, Vol. 3*, 195–237.

Atkinson, R., Tolson, R., & Turner, J. (1990). Late versus early onset problem drinking in older men. *Alcoholism: Clinical and Experimental Research, 14*, 574–579.

Beck, A. (1976). *Cognitive therapy and the emotional disorders*. New York: International Universities Press.

Beck, A., Rush, J., Shaw, B., & Emery, G. (1979). *Cognitive therapy of depression*. New York: Guilford Press.

Benson, H. (1975). *The relaxation response*. New York: William Morrow and Company.

Blow, F., Cook, C., Booth, B., Falcon, S., & Freidman, M. (1992). Age-related psychiatric comorbidities and level of functioning in alcoholic veterans seeking outpatient treatment. *Hospital and Community Psychiatry, 43*, 990–995.

Brown, B. B., & Chiang, C. (1983–84). Drug and alcohol abuse among the elderly: Is being alone the key? *International Journal of Aging and Human Development, 18*:1–12.

Burns, D. (1980). *Feeling good: The new mood therapy*. New York: New American Library.

Butler, R. (1974). Successful aging and the role of the life review. *Journal of the American Geriatric Society, 22*, 529–535.

Carruth, B., Williams, E., Mysak, P., & Boudreaux, L. (1975). Community care providers and older problem drinkers. *Grassroots, July Supplement*, 1–5.

Dobson, K. (Ed.). (1988). *Handbook of cognitive-behavioral therapies*. New York: Guilford Press.

Droller, H. (1964). Some aspects of alcoholism in the elderly. *Lancet, 2*, 137–139.

D'Zurilla, T., & Goldfried, M. (1971). Problem solving and behavior modification. *Journal of Abnormal Psychology, 78*, 107–126.

Ellis, A., McInerney, J., DiGiuseppe, R., & Yeager, R. (1988). *Rational-emotive therapy with alcoholics and substance abusers*. New York: Pergamon Press.

Emery, G. (1981). Cognitive therapy with the elderly. In G. Emery, S. Hollon, & R. Bedrosian (Eds.), *New directions in cognitive therapy*. New York: Guilford Press.

Emery, G. (1982). *Own your own life: How the new cognitive therapy can make you feel wonderful*. New York: Signet Press.

Freeman, A., & DeWolf, R. (1989). *Woulda, coulda, shoulda: Overcoming regrets, mistakes, and missed opportunities*. New York: Harper Collins Publishers.

Freeman, A., Simon, K., Beutler, L., & Arkowitz, H. (Eds.). (1989). *A comprehensive handbook of cognitive therapy*. New York: Plenum Press.

Gallagher, D., Thompson, L., Baffa, G., Piatt, C., Ringering, L., & Stone, V. (1981). *Depression in the elderly: A behavioral treatment manual*. Los Angeles: University of Southern California Press.

Glantz, M. D. (1987). Day hospital treatment of alcoholics. In A. Freeman & V. Greenwood (Eds.). *Cognitive therapy: Applications in psychiatric and medical settings*. New York: Human Sciences Press.

Glantz, M. D. (1989). Cognitive therapy with the elderly. In A. Freeman, K. Simon, L. Beutler, & H. Arkowitz (Eds.), *A comprehensive handbook of cognitive therapy*. New York: Plenum Press.

Glantz, M. D. (1992). A developmental psychopathology model of drug abuse vulnerability. In M. Glantz & R. Pickens (Eds.), *Vulnerability to drug abuse*. Washington, DC: American Psychological Association.

Glantz, M. D., & McCourt, W. (1983). Cognitive therapy in groups with alcoholics. In A. Freeman (Ed.), *Cognitive therapy with couples and groups*. New York: Plenum Press.

Glantz, M. D., & Backenheimer, M. (1988). Substance abuse among elderly women. *Clinical Gerontologist, 8*, 3–26.

Glantz, M. D., & Sloboda, Z. (in press). The prevention of drug abuse among the elderly. In R. Coombs & D. Ziedonis (Eds.), *Handbook on drug abuse prevention*. New York: Prentice Hall.

Glatt, M., & Rosin, A. (1964). Aspects of alcoholism in the elderly. *Lancet, 2*, 472–473.

Goldsmith, R., & Heiens, R. (1992). Subjective age: A test of five hypotheses. *Gerontologist, 32*, 312–317.

Gomberg, E. (1980). *Drinking and problem drinking among the elderly*. Ann Arbor: University of Michigan, Institute of Gerontology.

Gomberg, E. (1990). Drugs, alcohol, and aging. In L. T. Kozlowski et al. (Eds.), *Research advances in alcohol and drug problems*, Vol. 10, 171–213.

Hoelscher, T., & Edinger, J. (1988). Treatment of sleep-maintenance insomnia in older adults: Sleep period restriction, sleep education, and modified stimulus control. *Psychology and Aging, 3*, 258–263.

Holzer, C., Robins, L., Myers, J., Weissman, M., Tischler, G., Leaf, P., Anthony, J., & Bednarski, P. (1984). Antecedents and correlates of alcohol abuse and dependence in the elderly. In G. Maddox, L. Robins, & N. Rosenberg (Eds.), *Nature and extent of alcohol problems among the elderly*. Washington, DC: National Institute on Alcohol Abuse and Alcoholism, Government Printing Office.

Liberto, J., Oslin, D., & Ruskin, P. (1992). Alcoholism in older persons: A review of the literature. Hospital and Community Psychiatry, 43, 975–984.

Mackay, P., Donovan, D., & Marlatt, G. A. (1991). Cognitive and behavioral approaches to alcohol abuse. In R. Frances and S. Miller (Eds.), *Clinical textbook of addictive disorders*. New York: Plenum Press.

Marlatt, G. A. (1978). Craving for alcohol, loss of control, and relapse: A cognitive-behavioral analysis. In P. Nathan, G. A. Marlatt, & T. Loberg (Eds.), *Alcoholism: New directions in behavioral research and treatment*. New York: Plenum Press.

Marlatt, G. A., & Gordon, J. (1979). Determinants of relapse: Implications for the maintenance of behavior change. In P. Davidson (Ed.), *Behavioral medicine: Changing health lifestyles*. New York: Brunner/Mazel Publishers.

Marlatt, G. A., & Gordon, J. (Eds.). (1985). *Relapse prevention: Maintenance strategies in the treatment of addictive behaviors*. New York: Guilford Press.

Meichenbaum, D. (1974). Self-instructional strategy training: A cognitive prosthesis for the aged. *Human Development, 17*, 273–280.

Meichenbaum, D. (1975). A self-instructional approach to stress management: A proposal for stress inoculation training. In C. Spielberger & I. Sarason (Eds.), *Stress and anxiety*, Vol. 2. New York: Wiley Press.

Monti, P., Abrams, D., Binkoff, J., Zwick, W., Liepman, M., Nirenberg, T., & Rohsenow, D. (1990). Communication skills training, communication skills training with family, and cognitive behavioral mood management training for alcoholics. *Journal of Studies on Alcohol, 51*, 263–270.

Moos, R., Brennan, P., Fondacaro, M., & Moos, B. (1990). Approach and avoidance coping responses among older problem and nonproblem drinkers. *Psychology and Aging, 5*, 31–40.

Novaco, R. (1977). A cognitive therapy for anger and its application to a case of depression. *Journal of Consulting and Clinical Psychology, 45*, 600–608.

Oei, T., Lim, A., & Young, R. (1991). Cognitive processes and cognitive behavior therapy in the treatment of problem drinking. *Journal of Addictive Diseases, 10*, 63–80.

Rechtschaffen, A. (1959). Psychotherapy with geriatric patients: A review of the literature. *Journal of Gerontology, 14*, 73–84.

Rosin, A., & Glatt, M. (1971). Alcohol excess in the elderly. *Quarterly Journal of Studies on Alcohol, 32*, 53–59.

Sanchez-Craig, M. (1975). A self-control strategy for drinking tendencies. *Ontario Psychology, 7*, 25–29.

Sanchez-Craig, M. (1990). Brief didactic treatment of alcohol and drug-related problems: An approach based on client choice. *British Journal of Addiction, 85*, 169–177.

Sanchez-Craig, M., Annis, H., Bornet, A., & MacDonald, D. (1984). Random assignment to abstinence and controlled drinking: Evaluation of a cognitive-behavioral program for problem drinkers. *Journal of Consulting and Clinical Psychology, 52*, 390–403.

Sanchez-Craig, M., Wilkinson, D., & Walker, K. (1987). Theory and methods for secondary prevention of alcohol problems: A cognitively based approach. In W. Cox (Ed.), *Treatment and prevention of alcohol problems*. Orlando, Florida: Academic Press.

Schuckit, M. (1979). *Drug and alcohol abuse: A clinical guide to diagnosis and treatment*. New York: Plenum Press.

Schuckit, M. (1982). A clinical review of alcohol, alcoholism, and the elderly patient. *Journal of Clinical Psychiatry, 43*, 396–399.

Schuckit, M. A., Morrissey, E. M., & O'Leary, M. R. (1978). Alcohol problems in elderly men and women. *Addictive Diseases, 3*, 405–416.

Smart, R., & Adlaf, E. (1988). Alcohol and drug use among the elderly: Trends in use and characteristics of users. *Canadian Journal of Public Health, 79*, 236–242.

Steuer, J., & Hammen, C. (1983). Cognitive-behavioral group therapy for the depressed elderly: Issues and adaptions. *Cognitive Therapy and Research, 7*, 285–296.

Tarter, R. (1983). The causes of alcoholism: A biopsychological analysis. In E. Gottheil, K. Druley, T. Skoloda, & H. Waxman (Eds.), *Etiological aspects of alcohol and drug abuse*. Springfield, Illinois: Charles Thomas Publisher.

Thompson, L., Davies, R., Gallagher, D., & Krantz, S. (1986). Cognitive therapy with older adults. *Clinical Gerontologist, 5*, 245–279.

Thompson, L., Gantz, F., Florsheim, M., DelMaestro, S., Rodman, J., Gallagher-Thompson, D., & Bryan, H. (1991). Cognitive-behavioral therapy for affective disorders in the elderly. In W. Myers (Ed.), *New techniques in the psychotherapy of older patients*. Washington, DC: American Psychiatric Press.

Vallis, T. M. (1991). Theoretical and conceptual bases of cognitive therapy. In T. M. Vallis, J. Howes, & P. Miller (Eds.), *The challenge of cognitive therapy: Applications to nontraditional populations*. New York: Plenum Press.

Wisocki, P. (Ed.). (1991). *Handbook of clinical behavior therapy with the elderly client*. New York: Plenum Press.

Yost, E., Beutler, L., Corbishley, A., & Allender, J. (1986). *Group cognitive therapy: A treatment method for the depressed elderly*. New York: Pergamon.

Zucker, R., & Gomberg, E. (1986). Etiology of alcoholism reconsidered: The case for a biopsychosocial process. *American Psychologist, 41*, 783–793.

15

Life Context, Coping Responses, and Adaptive Outcomes: A Stress and Coping Perspective on Late-Life Problem Drinking

PENNY L. BRENNAN AND RUDOLF H. MOOS

Late-life problem drinking is an important health and social concern. Recent research in this area has generated considerable information about the prevalence and personal characteristics of late-life problem drinkers (for reviews see Finney & Moos, 1984; Liberto, Oslin, & Ruskin, 1992). By contrast, relatively little is known about the life contexts and adaptive efforts of these individuals and how these factors influence older problem drinkers' alcohol abuse and health-related functioning. Accordingly, we have applied a stress and coping perspective to the study of late-life problem drinking.

A STRESS AND COPING PERSPECTIVE ON LATE-LIFE DRINKING PROBLEMS

Our examination of late-life drinking problems is part of a broader program of research that emphasizes the importance of life context and coping responses for predicting adaptational outcomes (Moos, 1992). The stress and coping perspective that guides our work is shown in Figure 15.1. We assume that the environmental system (Panel I) consists of ongoing stressors and social resources in several life domains. The personal system (Panel II) includes an individual's demographic characteristics and such personal resources as cognitive ability and prior experience coping with stressful life circumstances. Panel III includes negative life events, such as age-related loss events and other acute stressors. The model suggests that these factors influence how individuals appraise, cope with, and seek formal help to alleviate stressful life circumstances (Panel IV). All four sets of factors influence individuals' adaptive outcomes—their substance use, health-related functioning, and stressor resolution (Panel V). The bidirectional paths in the model show that the stress and coping process involves multiple causal paths and encompasses both short-term processes of adjustment (e.g., heightened stres-

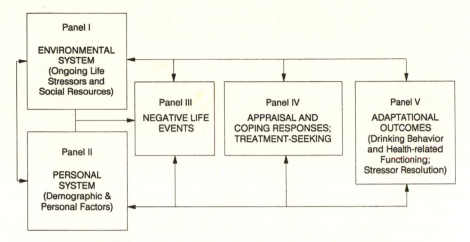

Figure 15.1. A conceptual model of the stress and coping process.

sors promote problem drinking and treatment seeking) and longer-range adaptational outcomes (e.g., treatment results in subsequent remission and stressor reduction).

This stress and coping framework raises many issues about late-life problem drinking; we address several of them in this chapter. First, the framework implies that older adults' drinking behavior is associated with their life contexts and coping efforts. Accordingly, we examine whether the life stressors, social resources, and coping responses of late-life problem drinkers differ from those of non-problem drinkers.

Second, this framework suggests a need to focus more closely on each of the links in problem drinkers' stress and coping process. Thus, we examine connections between life context and functioning among older problem drinkers, with special attention to the relative importance of certain types (acute versus chronic) and domains (e.g., spouse versus friends) of stressors for predicting alcohol use and health-related functioning. In addition, we focus on the associations of coping strategies and treatment-seeking with adaptational outcomes. We then examine whether older problem drinkers' stressors and social resources influence their choice of coping strategies and their efforts to seek formal care for alcohol-related problems.

Third, the framework implies that features of alcohol use, such as the severity and duration of drinking problems, affect individuals' health and life contexts. Hence, we compare the functioning and life contexts of older adults who have recently begun to have drinking problems (late-onset problem drinkers) with those of individuals whose problems with alcohol are longstanding (early-onset problem drinkers).

Finally, the stress and coping perspective implies that contextual factors may predict critical changes in drinking behavior, such as remission and abstention from alcohol, and that life context is subsequently affected by such changes. Hence, we describe the extent and predictors of short-term (1-year) remission among older problem drinkers, and examine whether the correlates of remission differ among late and early-onset problem drinkers. We also examine whether drinking status over the 1-year interval (continued problem drinking versus remission) has different implications for men and women. Where appropriate, we point out treatment and evaluation implications of our results and conclude by highlighting directions for future research.

CHARACTERISTICS OF PROBLEM
AND NON-PROBLEM DRINKERS

We used information from an initial screening survey and from a second, more detailed assessment of drinking problems (Drinking Problems Index; Finney, Moos, & Brennan, 1991) to select and classify a large group of individuals between the ages of 55 and 65 into three groups: *remitted problem drinkers*, individuals who had no current drinking problems, but had experienced such problems in the past; *problem drinkers*, individuals who had current alcohol-related problems; and *non-problem drinkers*, individuals who consumed alcohol but had no current or past drinking problems. The overall project involved an initial assessment of these individuals' life contexts, coping and treatment-seeking, alcohol use, and other aspects of health-related functioning. One year later we conducted a follow-up on 95% of the surviving individuals, and a 4-year follow-up has just been completed. We focus in this chapter on the initial and 1-year follow-up of the problem and non-problem drinkers. (For sampling details, see Brennan & Moos, 1990; Moos, Brennan, Fondacaro, & Moos, 1990.)

At initial assessment, the demographic characteristics of the problem drinkers were similar to those of the non-problem drinkers. On average, the individuals in each group were 61 years old and had two or more years of vocational or college education. Most of them were Caucasian and were Protestant or Catholic. However, compared with the problem drinkers, the non-problem drinkers were more likely to be married (62% versus 77%).

By definition, non-problem drinkers were individuals who experienced no negative consequences associated with their use of alcohol. In contrast, problem drinkers reported an average of five current drinking problems. These problems ranged from symptoms indicative of dependence on alcohol (such as skipping meals because of drinking) to negative psychological consequences of drinking (for instance, feeling confused after drinking) and adverse social consequences (such as complaints about drinking from family members). Problem drinkers consumed more ethanol than non-problem drinkers did, on both typical drinking occasions (3.4 ounces versus 1.6 ounces) and heavier drinking occasions (5.7 ounces versus 2.5 ounces).

LIFE CONTEXT, COPING RESPONSES,
AND TREATMENT SEEKING

Acute and Chronic Life Stressors

It is often suggested that life stressors are associated with problem drinking in late adulthood, but evidence in support of this view is equivocal. Ekerdt and his colleagues (1989) found a moderate association between retirement and onset of periodic heavy drinking and new drinking problems. Older adults arrested for driving under the influence reported more recent negative life events than controls did (Wells-Parker et al., 1983). However, a prospective study by Hermos and associates (1984) showed that men who experienced a serious negative health event—the development of heart disease or hypertension—subsequently *reduced* their alcohol consumption.

However, most studies of older adults have found no relationship between stressors and drinking outcomes, perhaps because they have indexed life stressors with a single traumatic event, such as widowhood or relocation (e.g., Barnes, 1979; Kivela et al., 1988), or have assessed stressors using a life event checklist (e.g., LaGreca, Akers, & Dwyer, 1988). This approach taps a limited number and range of the stressors that older adults experience (Chiriboga & Cutler, 1980) and overlooks the importance of chronic stressors for predicting negative health outcomes (Avison & Turner, 1988; Moos, Fenn, Billings, & Moos, 1989; Rutter, 1986).

To examine whether late-life problem drinkers experience more stressful life contexts than non-problem drinkers do, we assessed each group using the Life Stressors and Social Resources Inventory (LISRES; Moos & Moos, 1994). The life stressors indices in this measure cover the number of acute negative events that respondents have experienced in the past year and their chronic stressors in each of eight life domains (physical health, finances, home and neighborhood, work, spouse, children, extended family, and friends, for scoring and psychometric details, see Moos & Moos, 1992).

Problem drinkers experienced somewhat more negative life events than non-problem drinkers did. As shown in Figure 15.2, they also reported more chronic stressors, including more ongoing adversity involving home and neighborhood (such as lack of quiet and safety), financial problems (such as inability to pay bills), and persistent

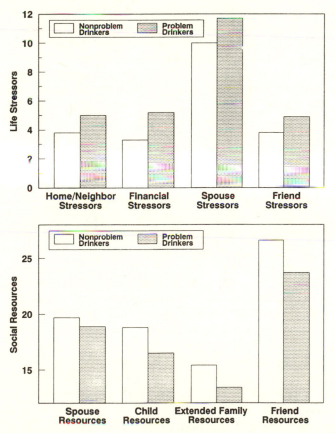

Figure 15.2. Selected life stressors and social resources of non-problem and problem drinkers.

interpersonal conflicts with spouses and friends. In addition, men with drinking problems reported more ongoing stressors involving children, and women with drinking problems reported more ongoing stressors with extended family members (Brennan & Moos, 1990). These results support the idea that short-term negative events, such as accidents, job loss, and marital separation, are experienced more frequently by older adults with alcohol problems, as is ongoing adversity across a variety of life domains.

Social Resources

Considerable research shows that older adults who lack social resources are at risk for adverse health outcomes, including increased physical symptoms and depression (Antonucci, 1990). However, comparatively little attention has been paid to the relationship between social resource deficits and late-life problem drinking. To address this issue, we used the social resources indices of the LISRES to assess the financial resources and social support available to older problem drinkers. These indices assess respondents total annual income as well as the degree of empathy and emotional support available from coworkers, spouse, children, extended family, and friends.

As expected, problem drinkers had fewer financial resources than did non-problem drinkers. As shown in Figure 15.2, they also had less support from their spouses, children, extended family, and friends (Brennan & Moos, 1990). The life contexts of problem drinkers are thus not only more stressful than those of non-problem drinkers, but also deficient in both material and interpersonal support. This may reflect a relationship in which ongoing stressors and a lack of interpersonal resources place individuals at risk for continued alcohol abuse. Moreover, late-life alcohol abuse may generate stressors that have a cumulative negative effect on financial well-being and social relationships.

Coping Responses

The way in which older adults appraise and manage life stressors may influence their drinking practices, health-related functioning, and ability to resolve stressful life circumstances effectively. In general, use of approach coping strategies is associated with better adaptive outcomes, whereas avoidance coping predicts poorer adaptation (Holahan & Moos, 1987; Moos, Finney, & Cronkite, 1990).

To compare the coping responses of older problem and non-problem drinkers, we asked respondents in each group to complete the Coping Responses Inventory (CRI; Moos, 1993). This measure asks respondents to identify their most important stressor of the past year (focal stressor) and to respond to items concerning their appraisal of that stressor and efforts to cope with it (for scoring and psychometric details, see Moos, 1993).

Problem and non-problem drinkers reported similar kinds of focal stressors and used comparable levels of approach strategies to manage their stressors. For example, as shown in Figure 15.3, problem and non-problem drinkers alike frequently used coping strategies such as logical analysis and support-seeking to deal with stressors. However, problem drinkers more frequently managed stressors with avoidance coping strategies. Figure 15.3 shows that problem drinkers reacted to stressors with more resigned acceptance (e.g., "I accepted it; nothing could be done") and cognitive avoidance (e.g.,

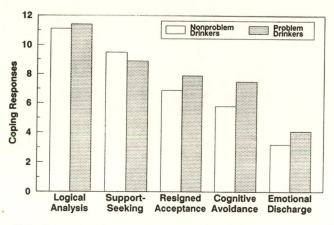

Figure 15.3. Selected coping responses of non-problem and problem drinkers.

"I tried to forget the whole thing") than non-problem drinkers did. Problem drinkers also used more emotional discharge coping responses, such as crying or shouting to release tension (Moos, Brennan, Fondacaro, & Moos, 1990).

These results suggest that, compared with non-problem drinkers of the same age, late-life problem drinkers are more passive and avoidant in response to stressors, and more likely to express negative emotion openly. Passivity, avoidance, and emotion-focused coping may hinder problem drinkers' ability to anticipate and prevent stressors and may interfere with their efforts to alleviate stressors that do occur. These problem drinkers' overall coping style may help explain their more stressful, less supportive life contexts. For example, problem drinkers' use of emotional discharge coping responses may place ongoing strain on their relationships with friends and family members

Treatment Seeking

Consistent with their relative lack of approach coping, less than 10% of the problem drinkers sought help specifically for their drinking problems; a somewhat higher percentage sought assistance with a personal problem from a mental health professional (about 25%) or physician (about 50%) (Moos, Brennan, & Moos, 1991). These results support concerns that late-life problem drinkers remain hidden from and receive insufficient attention from health care providers (Beresford et al., 1988; Dunham, 1986). The fact that they seek help primarily form mental health care providers and physicians suggest that older patients may present their difficulties as global emotional distress or as a physical complaint rather than as alcohol-related. Care providers may also fail to recognize or respond adequately to substance abuse in older patients. In this regard, older substance abuse patients receive less specialized treatment for their alcohol and drug problems than do younger substance abuse patients (Moos, Mertens, & Brennan, 1993).

Overall, these comparisons show that the life circumstances of older problem drinkers are more stressful and less supportive than those of non-problem drinkers and that late-life problem drinkers are somewhat deficient in their ability actively and effectively to manage the stressors they identify as the most salient in their lives. Furthermore, they indicate that the majority of late-life problem drinkers do not receive formal treatment for their drinking problems.

THE STRESS AND COPING PROCESS
AMONG OLDER PROBLEM DRINKERS

The group differences we have described suggest that the stress and coping process is involved in the maintenance of older problem drinkers' alcohol-related problems. We next focus more closely on connections in this process, in part to highlight relationships that might have implications for the prevention and treatment of late-life drinking problems.

We address three specific questions about the stress and coping process among late-life problem drinkers. What are the associations of different types of stressors (acute versus chronic) and different domains of stressors and social resources with adaptational outcomes? How are coping responses and treatment-seeking related to outcomes? Do stressor characteristics and social resources influence problem drinkers' choice of coping responses and their treatment seeking? The findings described here are based on our initial assessment of the problem drinkers.

Life Stressors, Social Resources and Adaptational Outcomes

Overall, problem drinkers who experienced more stressful life contexts and more deficits in social resources functioned more poorly than did problem drinkers in more benign circumstances. Individuals who reported more negative life events had more alcohol-related problems and were more depressed. Problem drinkers with more ongoing stressors and less interpersonal support also showed poorer adaptational outcomes. For example, Figure 15.4 shows that spouse stressors were associated with more

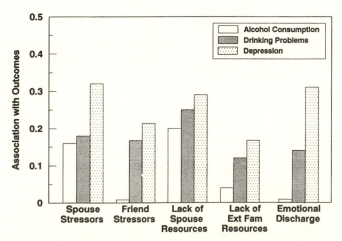

Figure 15.4. Associations of selected stressors, social resources, and coping responses with adaptational outcomes.

alcohol consumption, drinking problems, and depression. Similarly, individuals who reported more conflicts with friends and a lack of support from spouses and extended family members tended to report more alcohol consumption, drinking problems, and depression. These findings correspond to previous research with older adults that shows a link between more stressful, unsupportive contexts, and poorer health-related outcomes (Antonucci, 1990; Krause, 1986).

As noted earlier, studies of the relationship between life context and health outcomes typically employ global measures of acute stressors. However, acute stressors may affect individuals differently than ongoing adversity (Avison & Turner, 1988; Moos, Fenn, Billings, & Moos, 1989; Rutter, 1986). Moreover, some domains of stressors may be more salient than others for predicting health-related outcomes (Brennan & Moos, 1990; Swindle & Moos, 1992).

In fact, our results highlight the importance of separately assessing negative life events and chronic stressors: the latter accounted for a significant proportion of the variance in drinking behavior and health-related functioning even after acute life events were considered (Brennan & Moos, 1990). Studies that use a single transitional event or a count of negative life events typically show little or no association between stressors and late-life drinking problems. A broader assessment procedure may increase the likelihood of identifying a relationship between stressful life circumstances and drinking behavior.

The results also underscore the importance of assessing individual domains of stressors and social resources, and their relationships to functioning outcomes. For instance, independent of other stressors, marital conflicts were associated with more alcohol consumption and drinking problems. Independent of other social resources, less support from friends and spouses predicted more alcohol-related problems. These findings indicate that for older problem drinkers, conflicts and a lack of support within significant interpersonal relationships have especially strong links to alcohol abuse. Global stresor assessments cannot identify these domain-specific relationships.

Coping Responses, Treatment Seeking and Adaptational Outcomes

We focus next on the associations of older problem drinkers' coping responses and treatment seeking with their adaptive outcomes, including drinking behavior, health-related outcomes, and stressor resolution. Even after demographic factors, stressor characteristics, appraisal, and social resources were considered, coping responses were predictably related to the functioning criteria. In general, problem drinkers who used more avoidance coping were functioning more poorly. For example, individuals who relied more heavily on cognitive avoidance reported more physical symptoms and depression. As shown in Figure 15.4, those who used more emotional discharge strategies also tended to report more alcohol consumption, drinking problems, and depression (Moos, Brennan, Fondacaro, & Moos, 1990).

In contrast, individuals who managed their stressors with more positive reappraisal and less cognitive avoidance had more self-confidence. Yet, active coping efforts did not always alleviate distress: Individuals who sought more guidance and support tended to experience more depression and physical symptoms. Similarly, problem drinkers who sought formal treatment for their drinking and personal problems functioned more poorly, as indicated by heavier alcohol consumption and higher levels of drinking problems, depression, and physical symptoms (Brennan & Moos, 1991). In part, this reflects the fact that more distressed individuals are likely to seek help. Nonetheless, other factors may contribute to the fact that seeking help is related to poorer adjustment, at least in the short run.

Seeking guidance may result in poorer outcomes because it prolongs problem resolution. "Supportive" family members and friends may minimize the magnitude of stressors, encourage excessive rumination about a problem, or otherwise inhibit an individual's efforts to resolve stressors. Moreover, seeking support is not the same as receiving it; distressed individuals may request help from individuals who cannot or will not assist them. Seeking support in conjunction with other active approach responses, such as positive reappraisal or problem solving, may be a more effective way to alleviate stressors. In support of this idea, we found that problem drinkers who relied less heavily on support seeking and cognitive avoidance, and who used more positive reappraisal strategies, were more likely to report successful resolution of their stressors (Moos, Brennan, Fondacaro, & Moos, 1990).

Life Stressors and Social Resources as Determinants of Coping Responses and Treatment Seeking

We have seen that life stressors, social resources, and coping responses are related to problem drinkers' adaptational outcomes. In addition to their direct link to outcomes, stressors and resources may affect outcomes by providing a context that influences individuals' choice of specific coping responses. Accordingly, we examined contextual predictors of coping strategies and help-seeking (Moos, Brennan, Fondacaro, & Moos, 1990).

People's coping responses vary with the type of stressful situations they encounter (Lazarus & Folkman, 1984; McCrae, 1984). We found that older problem drinkers who coped with financial- and work-related stressors relied heavily on logical analysis and problem solving, and less on cognitive avoidance and resigned acceptance. In contrast, those who identified personal illness as their focal stressor used both more approach and more avoidance coping responses, especially support seeking and cognitive avoidance.

Problem drinkers who experienced more negative life events in the past year also used both more approach strategies (especially support seeking and problem solving) and more avoidance strategies (especially emotional discharge). This reflects the fact that when individuals initially experience severe stressors, they tend to alternate between approach and avoidance coping strategies in the effort to manage their circumstances and emotions. In addition, longitudinal research suggests that persistent, severe stressors curtail individuals' efforts to pursue active ways of resolving their problems and encourage increased reliance on avoidance coping (Fondacaro & Moos, 1989).

In general, social resource deficits influenced problem drinkers to adopt avoidance coping strategies: Individuals who lacked support from spouse and friends used fewer positive reappraisal and guidance-seeking strategies; they also tended to rely more on cognitive avoidance and emotional discharge strategies. Are individuals who lack personal resources and reliable sources of informal assistance more likely to seek formal treatment for their drinking and related problems? As noted, more severely impaired individuals sought help for drinking and personal problems (Brennan & Moos, 1991). Moreover, problem drinkers who lacked financial resources and support from spouses, children, extended family, and friends were more likely to seek formal treatment for drinking and personal problems, as were those who had more financial, spouse, and child stressors (Brennan & Moos, 1991). These findings support the idea that problem drinkers who have depleted their sources of informal assistance turn to formal treatment sources for support.

In summary, our initial analyses of the stress and coping process among older problem drinkers confirms that individuals in more stressful and less supportive life contexts tend to choose more avoidance coping strategies. This choice tends to result in negative outcomes (e.g., Billings & Moos, 1984; Cooper, Russell, & George, 1988; Haley et al., 1987); here, it was associated with worse drinking outcomes, poorer health-related functioning, and less effective stressor resolution. Thus, the process of stress and coping among older problem drinkers is characterized by mutual interrelationships among poorer quality of life, less effective coping responses, need for formal treatment, more severe drinking problems, and poorer health-related outcomes.

On a positive note, these linkages are amenable to change. Our results indicate that coping efforts are relatively flexible responses that are affected by stressor characteristics and availability of social support. Similarly, treatment seeking is not a fixed characteristic of individuals but stems in part from stressor severity and a lack of alternative, informal sources of assistance. Thus, the adaptive efforts of older problem drinkers can be improved through interventions that target either problem drinkers (e.g., reduction of reliance on avoidance coping) or their life contexts (e.g., augmentation of available social support).

LATE-ONSET AND EARLY-ONSET PROBLEM DRINKERS

Early descriptions of late-life problem drinking (e.g., Droller, 1964; Rosin & Glatt, 1971), distinguished between two types of older problem drinkers: early onset problem drinkers, whose alcohol abuse begins in younger adulthood and continues into later life, and *late-onset* problem drinkers, whose alcohol misuse first begins during late adulthood, presumably in response to age-related loss events. Subsequent research has confirmed that a significant proportion of older adults with alcohol-related difficulties are late-onset problem drinkers (Atkinson et al., 1985; Atkinson et al., 1990; Hurt et al., 1988). Consistent with this, about one-third of the problem drinkers in our sample were late-onset problem drinkers (Brennan & Moos, 1991).

Also consistent with prior research (Atkinson et al., 1985; Atkinson et al., 1990; Schonfeld & Dupree, 1991), the late-onset problem drinkers in our sample had less severe problems with alcohol than did the early-onset problem drinkers. Late-onset problem drinkers consumed somewhat less ethanol on both typical and heavier drinking occasions and reported fewer drinking problems. In addition, each of the individual items that indexed negative consequences of drinking was endorsed less frequently by late-onset than by early-onset problem drinkers. For instance, late-onset problem drinkers were less likely to endorse items indicative of physical dependence on alcohol: 14% of late-onset problem drinkers skipped meals because of drinking compared with 35% of early-onset problem drinkers. In addition, fewer late-onset problem drinkers reported negative social consequences associated with alcohol use. For example, 36% of late-onset problem drinkers reported that a family member had complained about their drinking in the past year; 52% of early-onset problem drinkers did so (Brennan & Moos, 1991).

Our stress and coping perspective implies a bidirectional relationship between life context and time of onset of alcohol problems, wherein stressors initially trigger drinking problems and ongoing alcohol problems adversely affect functioning and life context. Age-related loss events are often touted as critical determinants of late-onset drinking problems. Thus, we examined whether late-onset problem drinkers experienced more recent loss events than either early-onset or non-problem drinkers. Because of the recency of their alcohol-related difficulties, we expected late-onset problem drinkers to report a level of chronic stressors intermediate between that of early-onset and non-problem drinkers.

In support of the idea that acute life events prompt drinking problems among older adults, Finlayson and his associates (1988) noted that, compared with early-onset problem drinkers, late-onset individuals experienced more stressful life events antecedent to their alcohol problems. In contrast, we found no difference in the frequency with which late-onset, early-onset, and non-problem drinkers experienced recent loss events, including undesirable relocation, retirement, or death of a spouse, family member, or friend.

Consistent with the idea that time of onset affects life context, we found an overall pattern in which late-onset problem drinkers tended to report more chronic stressors than non-problem drinkers, but fewer than those of early-onset problem drinkers. We found a similar pattern with respect to health-related functioning. For example, late-onset problem drinkers reported a level of physical symptoms intermediate between that of non-problem drinkers and early-onset problem drinkers (Brennan & Moos, 1991). This is consistent with prior research that shows fewer symptoms of depression and anxiety, less overall psychopathology, and more life satisfaction among late-onset compared with early-onset problem drinkers (Atkinson et al., 1990; Schonfeld & Dupree, 1991).

Does drinking problem chronicity influence social resources? Although Schonfeld and Dupree (1991) showed that late- and early-onset problem drinkers do not differ in perceived social support, indirect evidence suggests that late-onset individuals have more social resources than early-onset individuals: Late-onset problem drinkers are more likely to be women, married, and better educated (Atkinson et al., 1985; Atkinson et al., 1990; Hurt et al., 1988). We found the same demographic pattern. Moreover, although the late-onset problem drinkers in our sample reported fewer financial, spouse, and extended family resources than did non-problem drinkers, they had more support from children and friends than did early-onset problem drinkers.

Taken together, these results do not support the idea that age-related loss events are primary risk factors for the development of late-onset alcohol problems. However, drinking problem chronicity does appear to influence the quality of health-related functioning and life contexts of older problem drinkers. Chronic drinking problems may take a cumulative toll on individuals' health and their relationships with family members and friends. Alternatively, supportive relationships may protect some individuals from developing drinking problems until late in adulthood.

These results have several potential treatment implications. First, they suggest that older adults with late-onset drinking problems may be relatively difficult to recognize.

Recent age-related losses are not good indicators of risk for late onset of drinking problems, and the relatively mild drinking problems and intact physical and social functioning of these individuals may diminish the chances that health care providers will recognize them as problem drinkers. This implies a need for more sensitive screening methods. Second, time of onset may be an important factor to consider in the formulation of treatment plans. For example, it may be easier to incorporate support of children and friends in the treatment plans of late-onset problem drinkers than in those of early-onset individuals.

Finally, chronicity and severity of drinking problems should be considered in efforts to evaluate the success of treatment programs for older problem drinkers. For instance, measures of group outcome may be affected by the proportion of patients who have more recent or less severe alcohol problems. In support of this concern, several studies show that early-onset problem drinkers have poorer prognoses than late-onset problem drinkers (Atkinson et al., 1985; Atkinson et al., 1990; Schonfeld & Dupree, 1992). In a related vein, older problem drinkers who have more complex substance abuse diagnoses and/or concomitant psychiatric disorders require more treatment and are more likely to be readmitted than those with only alcohol dependence diagnoses (Moos, Brennan, & Mertens, 1994).

PROCESS OF REMISSION AMONG LATE-LIFE PROBLEM DRINKERS

Our stress and coping framework suggests that individual characteristics and contextual factors influence critical changes in drinking behavior, such as remission from drinking problems and abstention from alcohol. In turn, such changes may lead to improved functioning and life context. Accordingly, we conducted a 1-year follow-up of these problem drinkers (Moos, Brennan, & Moos, 1991) and addressed the following questions. At initial assessment, are to-be-remitted drinkers at an advantage relative to individuals who will continue to be problem drinkers with regard to functioning, life stressors, and social resources? At follow-up, do remitted problem drinkers function better and have more supportive life contexts than continuing problem drinkers do? Do they attain levels of functioning and support comparable to those of non-problem drinkers? What factors predict remission over a 1-year interval? Do these factors vary according to time of onset of drinking problems?

To address these questions, we obtained follow-up information from 96% of the surviving individuals we had originally classified as problem drinkers. These respondents were categorized as *remitted problem drinkers* if they reported that they had experienced no drinking problems during the past 12 months, and *non-remitted problem drinkers* if they had experienced one or more drinking problems during the past year. We also followed 95% of the surviving non-problem drinkers; individuals who still had no drinking problems at follow-up comprised a comparison group.

Advantages of To-Be-Remitted Problem Drinkers

Like other researchers (Glynn, Bouchard, LoCastro, & Laird, 1985; Fillmore, 1987a, 1987b; Wilsnack, Wilsnack, & Klassen, 1984), we found a relatively high rate of short-term remission (29%). At initial assessment, to-be-remitted individuals differed from those who would continue to have drinking problems. There were more women in the to-be-remitted group, and to-be-remitted individuals reported fewer drinking problems and less alcohol consumption. They also reported different social relationships: To-be-remitted individuals had somewhat poorer relationships with their spouses, had fewer friends who approved of drinking, and were more likely to have sought help from a mental health professional. Three aspects of life context may thus facilitate the short-term remission process: marital strains that motivate drinking behavior change; reduced contact with individuals who approve of drinking; and assistance from formal care providers.

Remitted versus Non-Remitted Problem Drinkers at Follow-Up

At follow-up, remitted problem drinkers generally continued to function poorly. They had about the same physical symptoms, depression, and stressors as non-remitted drinkers, and they reported an ongoing lack of financial resources and support from spouses and friends. In most respects, remitted problem drinkers also remained at a disadvantage relative to non-problem drinkers. However, whereas individuals who continued to have drinking problems had lost social resources from spouses and friends over the follow-up interval, remitted individuals had not. Moreover, remitted problem drinkers reported a significant decline in their friends' approval of drinking, but this did not occur among individuals who continued to have drinking problems.

These results indicate that short-term remission does not have an immediate or dramatic impact on older problem drinkers' functioning and life contexts. This may reflect the fact that these remitted drinkers had had relatively little time to gain mastery over their substance abuse. While remission is being consolidated, difficulties associated with alcohol abuse, such as physical symptoms and depression, may persist. Even after stable remission is attained, it may take longer than one year to eliminate life stressors exacerbated by alcohol abuse and to regain the emotional support of family members. Nonetheless, short-term remission appears to prevent further deterioration of marital quality and relationships with friends. Furthermore, remitted problem drinkers appear to avoid friends who might encourage excessive alcohol consumption. This strategy may increase the likelihood of continued remission.

Predicting Remission and Abstention

Our earlier analyses highlighted the fact that late- and early-onset problem drinkers differ in their functioning and life contexts. We wanted to know whether the predictors of remission and abstention also differed in these groups. In both groups, lighter drinking and financial stressors predicted remission and abstention. However, health and social factors were more closely linked to remission among late-onset problem drinkers. They were also associated with abstention in this group (see Figure 15.5). Specifically, having more health stressors, a hospitalization in the past year, less support from one's spouse, and fewer friends who approved of drinking predicted abstention among the late-onset drinkers. In contrast, the most salient correlate of remission and abstention among early-onset drinkers was seeking help from both informal sources and professional care providers (Moos et al., 1991).

These results imply that individuals whose problems with alcohol have begun more

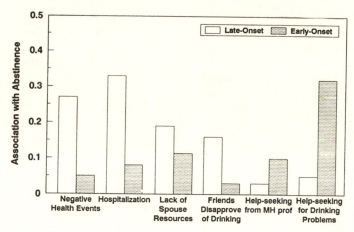

Figure 15.5. Associations of selected life context factors with abstinence among late-onset and early-onset problem drinkers.

recently may be more reactive to health problems and social influences than are individuals with long-standing drinking problems. Health-related problems and social control from informal sources may be sufficient to motivate changes in the drinking habits of late-onset individuals, whereas early-onset individuals may need more dramatic health challenges and structured help to assist them with remission.

To summarize, we found moderate rates of remission among older problem drinkers. The correlates of remission differed for late-onset and early-onset problem drinkers, highlighting again the importance of distinguishing between these groups when formulating treatment and evaluation plans. Although remission appears to prevent further deterioration of interpersonal relationships, it does not immediately result in improved health-related functioning and other aspects of life context. Longer-term follow-ups are needed to determine connections between life context and continued remission, and to determine whether contextual factors influence subsequent relapse.

Consequences of Drinking Status: Gender Differences in Life Context and Functioning

A growing literature shows that problem-drinking women differ from their male counterparts. We therefore compared the life contexts and functioning of older problem-drinking men and women at initial assessment and analyzed follow-up data to see whether drinking status over a 1-year interval (continued problem drinking versus remission) has different implications for men and women.

At initial assessment, the life contexts and functioning of men and women with late-life drinking problems differed. Briefly, women reported fewer financial but more family-related stressors than men did. However, they also had more support from friends and family. Compared with men, women also consumed less alcohol and had less severe drinking problems, but used more psychoactive medications and were more depressed (Brennan & Moos, 1990; Brennan, Moos, & Kim, 1993).

Ongoing drinking problems may have a cumulative negative effect on life context, especially in areas where alcohol abuse interferes with traditional role functioning.

Thus, we predicted that, relative to their male counterparts, women who continued to have drinking problems over the 1-year interval would experience increased interpersonal stressors and a withdrawal of interpersonal support. In fact, whereas the social resources of women with ongoing drinking problems remained relatively stable over the 1-year interval, men with ongoing drinking problems lost support from their children. This indicates that a father's drinking problems can adversely affect his relationships with children well into the later stages of family life.

The stability of these women's social support suggests a need to obtain more information about the role of social resources in women's problem drinking. Social relationships can function as liabilities as well as assets (Rock, 1990). Does some of the "support" that family members give these women encourage them to rely on alcohol and to avoid treatment? Perhaps some characteristics of social resources (such as availability of instrumental help) protect against substance abuse, whereas others (such as unconditional empathy) help sustain it.

Contrary to expectation, men with ongoing drinking problems reported a decline in conflicts with friends, and women with ongoing drinking problems experienced a decline in spouse stressors; women were no more depressed at follow-up than were their male counterparts. By facilitating social interactions, excessive alcohol use may serve a short-term adaptive function. Steinglass and his colleagues (1987) have noted that abusive alcohol patterns are often maintained because they temporarily enhance family communication and functioning, thereby preserving equilibrium in the family system.

We predicted that remission from drinking problems would be associated with improved life contexts for women, in part because it would improve their ability to fulfill traditional roles. In fact, women who remitted experienced a loss of support from extended family members over the 1-year interval. They also reported more family stressors and considerably more depression than did remitted men. Thus, the families of women undergoing short-term remission appear to be less supportive than those of remitted men. The relative severity of men's drinking problems may help account for this finding. Relief from these problems may elicit more favorable reactions from men's families. Another possibility is that the heightened negative effect women experience during remission is associated with a short-term increase in interpersonal problems. Overall and his colleagues (1985) reported a link between depression and ongoing interpersonal conflicts among alcoholics in remission. Together, these results indicate that the consequences of ongoing drinking problems and remission differ for men and women. Women with late-life drinking problems may therefore benefit from treatment approaches that are more closely tailored to their life circumstances.

FUTURE DIRECTIONS

A stress and coping perspective can be used to enhance our understanding of late-life problem drinking. Our research has confirmed that there are connections among older problem drinkers' life contexts, their efforts to adapt to these contexts, and outcomes such as drinking behavior, health-related functioning, and stressor resolution. But it has also raised new questions about these connections.

Our measures of life context and coping responses permit a more integrated and comprehensive assessment of the stress and coping process among older problem drinkers. The Life Stressors and Social Resources Inventory (Moos & Moos, 1994) and Coping Responses Inventory (Moos, 1993) allow us simultaneously to examine the independent effects of stressors, social resources, and coping responses on drinking outcomes, and to determine how various features of stressors—such as their severity, chronicity, and source—influence these outcomes. However, the information we have obtained challenges us to specify in more detail the complex relationships among life context, coping responses, and late-life problem drinking. For example, more work is needed to describe the direction of causality in the stress and coping process of older problem drinkers. How much do life context factors promote or inhibit late-life drinking? How much does maladaptive drinking behavior generate new stressors and erode social resources? What are the causal relationships among stressors, social resources, and coping responses? Can interactions among these factors help predict adaptive outcomes? In addition, we need to develop models that acknowledge both the immediate effects of stressors, social resources, and coping responses, and their role in longer-term adaptational outcomes.

Our results imply several avenues for future research on the course of remission among older problem drinkers. There was a moderate prevalence of short-term remission among these individuals. Longer-term follow-ups can help clarify what contextual factors and coping strategies foreshadow continued remission. A first step is to examine how factors associated with short-term remission—such as spouse and health stressors, friends' approval of drinking, and treatment seeking—affect longer-term remission and abstinence. In addition, our analyses point to several factors that may play a role in relapse. For example, early-onset problem drinkers may be particularly vulnerable to a lack of continuous, structured care; depression and a lack of family support may place remitted women at risk for relapse. Another factor to examine is the relatively slow improvement in life context and functioning experienced by remitted individuals. We plan to examine these issues using our 4-year follow-up information on this sample.

The findings indicate that very few late-life problem drinkers seek treatment. One challenge is to find out why: What individual, life context, and care setting characteristics deter older adults from seeking assistance with their alcohol-related problems? Another challenge is to devise screening methods to identify late-life problem drinkers more accurately, especially those with recent onset of drinking problems. Moreover, we need to know what individual characteristics and contextual factors enhance treatment compliance and successful outcomes among older problem drinkers. In this regard, our research suggests that both life context (e.g., social support) and individual characteristics (e.g., reliance on avoidance coping) may be fruitful areas for intervention.

These results underscore the importance of treatment approaches that address the varied needs of late-life problem drinkers. For example, our results suggest that late-onset problem drinkers may be sensitive to alcohol-related changes in their health status; they may therefore benefit from health care providers' warnings about risks of excessive alcohol consumption. Similarly, these drinkers may be relatively responsive to significant others' objections to their alcohol abuse. In contrast, early-onset individuals—especially those with more complex substance abuse disorders and concomitant psychiatric disorders—may require more structured health care resources to recover successfully from drinking problems. The heterogeneity of older problem drinkers is important to recognize in evaluations of treatment programs for them.

In conclusion, use of a stress and coping framework has helped us begin to describe connections among older problem drinkers' life contexts, coping efforts, and adaptive outcomes. More work is needed to provide richer details about these connections and to determine the usefulness of prevention and treatment efforts based on a stress and coping perspective on late-life problem drinking.

Acknowledgments

Preparation of the manuscript was supported in part by the Department of Veterans Affairs Health Services Research and Development Service research funds, and by NIAAA Grants AA06699 and AA02863. We thank Kristina Kelly for data reanalyses and Debbie Davis for assistance with graphics. Mark Greenbaum and Kathleen Schutte made valuable comments on an earlier version of the manuscript.

References

Antonucci, T. C. (1990). Social supports and social relationships. In R. H. Binstock and L. K. George (Eds.). *Handbook of aging and the social sciences* 3rd ed. (pp. 205–226). New York: Academic Press.

Atkinson, R. M., Turner, J.A., Kofoed, L. L., & Tolson, R. L. (1985). Early versus late onset alcoholism in older persons: Preliminary findings. *Alcoholism: Clinical and Experimental Research, 9*, 513–515.

Atkinson, R. M., Tolson, R. L., Turner, J. A. (1990). Late versus early onset problem drinking in older men. *Alcoholism: Clinical and Experimental Research, 14*, 574–579.

Avison, W. R., & Turner, R. J. (1988). Stressful life events and depressive symptoms: Disaggregating the affects of acute stressors and chronic strains. *Journal of Health and Social Behavior, 29*, 253–264

Barnes, G. M. (1979). Alcohol use among older persons: Findings from a Western New York general population survey. *Journal of the American Geriatrics Society, 27*, 244–250.

Beresford, T. P., Blow, F. C., Brower, K. J., Adams, K. M., & Hall, R. C. W. (1988). Alcoholism and aging in the general hospital. *Psychosomatics, 29*, 61–72.

Billings, A., & Moos, R. (1984). Coping, stress, and social resources among adults with unipolar depression. *Journal of Personality and Social Psychology, 46*, 877–891.

Brennan, P. L., & Moos, R. H. (1991). Functioning, life context, and help-seeking among late-onset problem drinkers: Comparisons with nonproblem and early-onset problem drinkers. *British Journal of Addiction, 86*, 1139–1150.

Brennan, P. L., & Moos, R. H. (1990). Life stressors, social resources, and late-life problem drinking. *Psychology and Aging, 5*, 491–501.

Brennan, P. L., Moos, R. H., & Kim, J. Y. (1993). Gender differences in the individual characteristics and life contexts of late-middle-aged and older problem drinkers. *British Journal of Addiction, 88*, 781–790.

Chiriboga, D. A., & Cutler, L. (1980). Stress and adaptation: Life span perspectives. In L. W. Poon (Ed.), *Aging in the 80s* (pp. 347–362). Washington, DC: American Psychological Association.

Cooper, M. L., Russell, M., & George, W. H. (1988). Coping expectancies and alcohol abuse: A test of social learning formulations. *Journal of Abnormal Psychology, 97*, 218–320.

Droller, H. (1964). Some aspects of alcoholism in the elderly. *The Lancet*, 137–139.

Dunham, R. G. (1986). Noticing alcoholism in the elderly and women: A nationwide examination of referral behavior. *Journal of Drug Issues, 16*, 397–406.

Ekerdt D. J., DeLabry, L. O., Glynn, R. J., & Davis, R. W. (1989). Changes in drinking behaviors with retirement: Findings from the Normative Aging Study. *Journal of Studies on Alcohol, 50,* 347–353.

Fillmore, K. M. (1987a). Prevalence, incidence and chronicity of drinking patterns and problems among men as a function of age: A longitudinal and cohort analysis. *British Journal of Addiction, 82,* 801–811.

Finlayson, R. E., Hurt, R. D., Davis, L. J., & Morse, R. M. (1988). Alcoholism in elderly persons: A study of the psychiatric and psychosocial features of 216 patients. *Mayo Clinic Proceedings, 63,* 761–768.

Finney, J. W., & Moos, R. H. (1984). Life stressors and problem drinking among older adults. In M. Galanter (Ed.), *Recent developments in alcoholism,* Vol. 2, (pp. 267–288). New York: Plenum Press.

Finney, J. W., Moos, R. H., & Brennan, P. L. (1991). The Drinking Problems Index: A measure to assess alcohol-related problems among older adults. *Journal of Substance Abuse, 3,* 395–404.

Fondacaro, M., & Moos, R. (1989). Life stressors and coping: A longitudinal analysis among depressed and nondepressed adults. *Journal of Community Psychology, 17,* 330–340.

Glynn, R. J., Bouchard, G. R., LoCastro, J. S., & Laird, N. M. (1985). Aging and generational effects on drinking behaviors in men: Results from the Normative Aging Study. *American Journal of Public Health, 75,* 1413–1419.

Haley, W. E., Levine, E. G., Brown, S. L., & Bartolucci, A. A. (1987). Stress, appraisal, coping, and social support as predictors of adaptational outcome among dementia caregivers. *Psychology and Aging, 2,* 323–330.

Hermos, J. A., LoCastro, J. S., Bouchard, G. R., glynn, R. J. (1984). Influence of cardiovascular disease on alcohol consumption among men in the Normative Aging Study. In G. Maddox, L. N. Robins, & N. Rosenberg (Eds.), *The nature and extent of alcohol problems among the elderly* (pp. 117–132). New York: Springer.

Holahan, C. J., & Moos, R. (1987). The personal and contextual determinants of coping strategies. *Journal of Personality and Social Psychology, 52,* 946–955.

Hurt, R. D., Finlayson, R. E., Morse, R. M., Davis, L. J. (1988). Alcoholism in elderly persons: Medical aspects and prognosis of 216 patients. *Mayo Clinic Proceedings, 63,* 753–760.

Kivela, S., Nissinen, A., Ketola, A., Punsar, S., Puska, P., & Karvonen, M. (1988). Changes in alcohol consumption during a ten-year follow-up among Finnish men aged 55–74 years. *Functional Neurology, 3, 167–178.*

Krause, N. (1986). Life stress as a correlate of depression among older adults. *Psychiatry Research, 18,* 227–237.

LaGreca, A. J., Akers, R. L., & Dwyer, J. W. (1988). Life events and alcohol behavior among older adults. *The Gerontologist, 28,* 552–558.

Lazarus, R.. S., & Folkman, S. (1984). *Stress, appraisal, and coping.* New York: Springer Publishing.

Liberto, J. G., Oslin, D. W., Ruskin, P. E. (1992). Alcoholism in older persons: A review of the literature. *Hospital and Community Psychiatry, 43,* 975–984.

McCrae, R. R. (1984). Situational determinants of coping responses: Loss, threat, and challenge. *Journal of Personality and Social Psychology, 46,* 919–928.

Moos, R. (1993). *The Coping Responses Inventory Adult Form manual.* Odessa, FL: Psychological Assessment Resources.

Moos, R. H. (1992). Understanding individuals' life contexts: Implications for stress reduction and prevention. In M. Kessler, S. E. Goldston, & Joffe (Eds.), *The present and future of prevention research* (pp. 196–213). Newbury Park, CA: Sage.

Moos, R. H., Brennan P. L., Fondacaro, M. R., & Moos, B. S. (1990). Approach and avoidance coping among older problem and nonproblem drinkers. *Psychology and Aging, 5,* 31–40.

Moos, R. H., Brennan P. L., & Mertens, J. R. Diagnostic subgroups and predictors of one-year readmission among late-middle-aged and older substance abuse patients. *Journal of Studies on Alcohol.*

Moos, R. H., Brennan, P. L., & Moos, B. S. (191). Short-term processes of remission and non-remission among late-life problem drinkers. *Alcoholism: Clinical and Experimental Research, 15,* 948–955.

Moos, R., Fenn, C., Billings, A., & Moos, B. (1989). Assessing life stressors and social resources: Applications to alcoholic patients. *Journal of Substance Abuse, 1,* 135–152.

Moos, R., Finney, J., & Cronkite, R. (1990). *Alcoholism treatment: Context, process, and outcome.* New York: Oxford University Press.

Moos, R. H., Mertens, J. R., & Brennan, P. L. (1993). Patterns of diagnosis and treatment among late-middle-aged and older substance abuse patients. *Journal of Studies on Alcohol, 54,* 479–487.

Moos, R., & Moos, B. (1994). *Life Stressors and Social Resources Inventory: Preliminary manual.*

Overall, J. E., Reilly, E. L., Kelley, J. T., Hollister, L. E. (1985). Persistence of depression in detoxified adults. Alcoholism: Clinical and Experimental Research, 9, 331–333.

Rook, K. S. (1990). Parallels in the study of social support and social strain. *Journal of Social and Clinical Psychology, 9,* 118–132.

Rosin, A. J., & Glatt, M. M. (1971). Alcohol excess in the elderly. *Quarterly Journal of Studies on Alcohol, 32,* 53–59.

Rutter, M. (1986). Meyerian psychobiology, personality development, and the role of life experiences. *American Journal of Psychiatry, 143,* 1077–1087.

Schonfeld, L. & Dupree, L. W. (1991). Antecedents of drinking for early- and late-onset elderly alcohol abusers. *Journal of Studies on Alcohol, 52,* 587–592.

Steinglass, P., Bennett, L., Wolin, S. J., & Reiss, D. (1987). *The alcoholic family.* New York: Basic Books.

Swindle, R. W., & Moos, R. H. (1992). Life domains in stressors, coping, and adjustment. In W. B. Walsh, K. H. Craik, & R. H. Price (Eds.), *Person-environment psychology: Models and perspectives* (pp. 1–33). New York: Erlbaum.

Wells-Parker, E., Miles, S., & Spencer, B. (1983). Stress experiences and drinking histories of elderly drunken-driving offenders. *Journal of Studies on Alcohol, 44,* 429–437.

Wilsnack, R. W., Wilsnack, S. C., & Klassen, A. D. (1984). Women's drinking and drinking problems: Patterns from a 1981 national survey. *American Journal of Public Health, 74,* 1231–1238.

16

Treatment of Medically Ill Alcoholics in the Primary-Care Setting

MARK L. WILLENBRING, DOUGLAS OLSON, JOHN BIELINSKI, AND JOHN LYNCH

Alcohol dependence causes a great deal of premature medical morbidity and mortality. The U.S. Department of Health and Human Services has reported that in 1985, at least 4% of short hospital stays in nongovernment hospitals were related to alcohol abuse, and in 1986, alcoholic cirrhosis of the liver was the ninth leading cause of death in the United States. One-quarter of patients in general medical-surgical hospital beds are thought to have a drinking problem (U.S. Department of Health and Human Services, 1990, McIntosh, 1982).

Current treatments for alcohol dependence are only partially effective, they appear to be most effective early in its course and in relatively mild cases (Moos et al., 1990). A substantial proportion of alcoholics show little, if any, response to treatment (Vaillant, 1983). Many of those with alcohol dependence refractory to treatment eventually die of its medical complications (Finney & Moos, 1991; Bullock et al., 1992). Recently, efforts have begun to focus on developing more specific treatments matched for specific subpopulations of alcoholics, such as the elderly, adolescents, and persons with both mental illness and substance use disorders.

Persons with serious medical complications of alcohol dependence are highly visible and needy consumers of health and social services. While not previously identified as such, these medically ill alcoholics (MIAs) may be a subpopulation that requires a specific treatment approach. A preliminary study at the Minneapolis VA Medical Center recently examined the characteristics of MIAs. Willenbring and colleagues (1993) compared medical patients referred to treatment with an ambulatory population requesting treatment. Compared to the ambulatory patients, medically ill alcoholics were older and were likely to present with health and family concerns. They were more likely than ambulatory patients to have depression and anxiety, and many had cognitive impairment. Most were unable to work or were retired, and many lived alone. In contrast, the younger ambulatory patients typically had legal and vocational concerns. They were more likely to demonstrate impulsivity and character disorder, and more of them had abused drugs other than alcohol.

These data are consistent with studies examining differences between younger and older alcoholics in general. However, the study also examined differences between referred medical patients accepting transfer to the treatment program and those who refused. Compared to those accepting transfer, MIAs refusing treatment had more exposure to previous treatment and to Alcoholics Anonymous (AA), and greater elevations in liver function tests and mean corpuscular volume of red cells. This suggests that they had more severe medical illness, and perhaps more severe or refractory alcohol dependence. They were also less likely to return for follow-up clinic visits: While 80% of those accepting transfer followed up at future medical clinic appointments, only 25% of refusers did.

This study confirmed subjective impressions that those MIAs least likely to accept and respond to traditional treatment or AA nevertheless continue to receive general medical services. Unfortunately, the study also validated some of the frustration physicians and other professional staff may experience in attempting to treat MIAs. For the sickest and most needy group of MIAs, referral to a treatment program did not provide any benefit.

On a more positive note, the study provided some useful data concerning the particular needs and issues of MIAs. Awareness of these needs, coupled with the knowledge that conventional treatments are generally ineffective, may offer some guidance in developing a more effective intervention. We know that MIAs continue to seek medical care, yet often resist referral to conventional treatment. Therefore, an intervention might be more effectively delivered in the primary medical care setting, ideally by medical personnel. Since many MIAs have substantial social service needs, these should be included as part of the intervention. Further, MIAs use multiple services, are difficult to engage in treatment, and often fail to attend follow-up clinic appointments, which suggests that case management with active outreach and follow-up components may be appropriate. Finally, since many MIAs live alone and do not work, estranged family members should be helped to reconnect with patients in a healthy way so that they can lend support to the treatment plan.

In order to develop an intervention, one would have to confront the pessimism engendered by practitioners' experience with MIAs. Perhaps the most central issue is the standard against which success is measured. While permanent abstinence from alcohol is obviously a worthwhile goal, it may not be the only one, or even the most important one in some circumstances. For example, in very advanced liver disease, whether the patient drinks or not may not greatly affect life expectancy. In that circumstance, making patients comfortable and helping them put their affairs in order may be important goals. More generally, something less than total and permanent abstinence could result in substantial improvements in well-being, morbidity, and survival. In that case, goals of reduction of drinking frequency or quantity may be worthwhile.

The issue of goals is a critical one. Traditionally, a goal of complete and permanent abstinence has been accepted as the only goal worth setting. Unfortunately, this all-or-none thinking discourages efforts that could be helpful, even if they only result in partial or temporary improvement. Whereas in most other diseases we seem to be able to accept partial ortemporary improvements as important, it seems difficult to do for alcohol dependence. It is likely this has something to do with a belief that drinking is a ''voluntary'' activity, whereas having diabetes is ''not their fault.'' Whatever one believes, research has demonstrated that treatment outcomes intermediate between permanent remission of drinking and no response are the rule, not the exception (Moos et al.,

1990). Changing our notions of what constitutes a reasonable expectation of outcomes for MIAs is therefore critical to planning a clinical intervention. For example, while five-year survival rates of 40 to 60% are commonly reported for MIAs (Finney & Moos, 1991; Bullock et al., 1992), the same can be said of many chronic illnesses. This range of outcomes is better than many other common illnesses that we continue to treat. It should not be too large a leap for physicians to think of MIAs as they do cancer, heart disease, or diabetes patients.

Furthermore, some data suggest that the prognosis of MIAs may be better than clinical experience would indicate. Hermos (1984), in a review of published studies, found that improvement was relatively common, especially if one considered improvement that fell short of indefinite abstinence. It is notable that participation in a formal treatment program was usually not necessary for such improvement to occur, as Vaillant also found for alcoholism in general (Vaillant, 1983). In our own experience, we have noted that such patients frequently do make use of general medical care, even if they are not willing to engage in an alcoholism treatment program. In the study of medical patients referred to alcoholism treatment noted above (Willenbring et al., 1993), even 25% of the less compliant alcoholics followed up at medical clinic appointments. With more active follow-up, it is likely this figure could be improved. These facts suggest that an approach that brings alcohol treatment principles into the general medical setting may prove beneficial for this group.

Over the past 6 years, a model of treatment has been developed specifically for MIAs at the Minneapolis Veterans Affairs Medical Center. Based upon the above analysis, it has the following characteristics: (1) Comprehensive medical treatment is the central component and patients are engaged through their medical concerns, (2) alcohol treatment interventions are delivered in the primary-care setting by primary-care personnel (physicians and nurse practitioners) and are seemlessly integrated with medical care, (3) coordination of care with assertive outreach and follow-up are provided, and (4) social and family concerns are addressed within the clinic. This chapter will describe the clinic and present some preliminary outcome data from a case-control study that suggest that this approach may improve the outcome of MIAs while reducing hospital use.

SETTING AND CLINICAL METHOD

The Alcohol Related Disorders (ARD) clinic is an outpatient primary-care clinic at the Minneapolis VA Medical Center, a 650-bed tertiary care hospital located in south Minneapolis. The hospital serves a large catchment area that includes both urban and rural residents of Minnesota, as well as parts of northwestern Wisconsin, northern Iowa, and eastern North and South Dakota.

The ARD Clinic began 6 years ago as a demonstration project specifically for developing and testing innovative treatment approaches for patients with serious alcohol-related medical disorders. The target population includes actively drinking, severely dependent alcoholics who require ongoing medical care for serious alcohol-related diseases, such as alcoholic liver disease, alcoholic pancreatitis, gastrointestinal bleeding resulting from gastritis or esophageal varices, and alcoholic cardiomyopathy. Patients typically have little social support; most have already gone through one or more alcohol treatments; and some have required civil commitment to alcoholism treatment in the past. Excluded from the clinic are those with a history of serious mental illness other than depression, current dependence on other drugs, severe dementia, a terminal illness (unrelated to alcohol use) with a life expectancy of less than 12 months, refusal to participate, or residence more than 100 miles from the medical center. Patients are referred to the clinic from either inpatient or outpatient physicians, though most are referred during hospitalization. Patients are screened at an outpatient appointment following discharge.

Techniques for addressing excessive drinking and psychosocial problems are integrated with primary medical care. Primary-care professionals, including physicians and nurse practitioners, are the principal caregivers (as opposed to alcoholism counselors or mental health professionals), and care is provided within the general outpatient medical care setting. All patients receive a 2-day inpatient evaluation by a multidisciplinary team composed of an internist, a part-time psychiatrist, three nurse practitioners, a registered nurse, a psychologist, a social worker, and clerical personnel. After discharge, a treatment plan is developed and presented to the patient and to any family members who are involved. In general, the goal of the ARD Clinic is to induce remission of drinking and related medical conditions whenever possible, to reduce the number, length, and severity of relapses, and to extend life for our patients. Specific treatment goals, therefore, include those that fall short of the traditional ideal of permanent abstinence. For example, engagement of the patient and family may be the primary goal for the first 6 months. Over a period of 1 year, a 20% change in any specific index, such as drinks per day, drinking days per month, or liver function tests, is usually set as a minimum indication of positive change.

Once they have accepted the treatment plan, patients are seen monthly at outpatient clinic visits with either a nurse practitioner or a physician (or both). Visit frequency is increased as needed. Mental health and social services are available when needed and are also provided within the primary care setting. At each clinic visit, a recent drinking history is taken, medical problems are reviewed, and the relationship between the two is discussed. A specific set of follow-up questions are asked by any staff member at a clinic visit. Special progress notes with these items are used, so that quantity and frequency of drinking and staff ratings of severity of drinking and medical problems can be monitored closely.

Biological indicators of heavy drinking, such as the gamma-glutamyl transferase, amylase and lipase, or blood pressure, are monitored at each visit, and patients are given graphic as well as verbal feedback regarding their progress using these indicators. Patients are encouraged and supported in their efforts to stop or cut down on drinking. Case management, aggressive follow-up, and family involvement constitute important facets of the overall care provided. While patients are encouraged to attend Alcoholics Anonymous, few actually do. Instead, two support groups of medically ill alcoholics meet weekly at the hospital, and they are facilitated by recovering alcoholic volunteers. Clinic staff members oversee these groups and provide training and supervision for the volunteers.

Any kind of alcohol intervention that may reduce drinking and its effects is used when appropriate. For example, families may provide critical support by refusing to facilitate the purchase of alcohol, encouraging the acceptance of sober housing, or alerting ARD Clinic staff members about a relapse. Asset management, both voluntary and involuntary, has emerged as a powerful tool for improving motivation of patients and acts to directly reduce the amount of money available to purchase alcohol. At times, emergency involuntary hospitalization, civil commitment, and convervatorships have been used to intervene. While care is taken to protect the rights and dignity of the patient at all times, these patients often have life-threatening complications that require immediate intervention. All such interventions have due process safeguards that protect patients' rights and provide oversight of clinic efforts and their outcome. Nevertheless, decisions to take such drastic action can never be taken lightly and are never easy. They frequently require considerable discussion and consultation within the team as well as with other professionals, including attorneys. A study of the efficacy of coercive interventions and their ethical implications is currently underway.

It typically takes 18 to 36 months to implement a treatment plan fully, and improvement is often seen only after 12 to 18 months of treatment. Patients' treatment within the ARD Clinic continues indefinitely, and patients are only discharged when they have achieved 2 years of stable abstinence, or when they repeatedly request discharge and resist all efforts to help them (an infrequent occurrence). The general experience in the clinic is that about two-thirds of patients show significant improvement, and a substantial portion eventually achieve stable remission of alcoholism. Additional details about the clinic's operations, forms, policies, and procedures are available from the senior author.

Conceptually, the ARD Clinic approach differs from conventional treatment in that the drinking problem in this particular population is viewed as a chronic, recurring one, where many or most patients may not become permanently abstinent. Intermediate goals are pursued, including decreased drinking per episode, longer periods of abstinence, reduced hospital use, and improved quality of life. In addition, care is seen as being needed for relatively long periods, and in an outpatient setting. While the program differs conceptually and practically from conventional treatment programs, many patients in the ARD Clinic have participated in such treatment in the past, and occasionally the ARD team will recommend admission to the inpatient program at the hospital for one of our patients. Staff members of the inpatient and outpatient treatment programs also refer patients to the ARD Clinic after discharge. Additionally, halfway houses, nursing homes, and board-and-lodging care are used when needed.

EVALUATION

Subjects

Several studies are underway to examine the effectiveness of all or part of the ARD Clinic intervention. This report details the preliminary results of an ongoing quasi-experimental study.

Fifty-six white male veterans referred to the ARD clinic were included in this study. The ARD group consisted of 30 patients screened and accepted into the ARD clinic. The control (CTL) group included 26 patients who were referred to the ARD Clinic and who met criteria for ARD Clinic admission but were not accepted in the clinic because it was full at the time. CTL patients were referred to other appropriate medical clinics within the medical center for follow-up care. There were also other medical centers within the metropolitan area where patients could seek follow-up care. CTL patients were all offered conventional alcoholism treatment, though none of them opted for this at the time of screening. Conventional treatment continued to be available to all patients throughout the period examined. Since this was a retrospective study, prior informed consent was not obtained.

To be eligible for the ARD clinic a patient must be actively drinking or at imminent risk of relapse (pathological drinking within the last six months). In addition, the patient must be suffering from one or more symptomatic alcohol-related illnesses. Most patients were referred during an acute medical hospitalization for their alcohol-related disorder and had been drinking immediately prior to that hospitalization. Other inclusion and exclusion criteria are as noted above

An ARD Clinic staff member (e.g., nurse practitioner, social worker, or psychologist) conducted the initial screening interviews. They gathered information regarding general health, history of problems with alcohol, and recent drinking behavior. A DSM-III-R criteria checklist (Helzer & Janca, 1988) was used to assess the number of symptoms of alcohol dependence. Patients were asked about frequency and quantity of alcoholic beverages consumed in standard drinks. A standard drink was defined as 1.5 oz. distilled beverage, 12 oz. beer, 5 oz. table wine, or 3 oz. fortified wine.

Data Collection and Analysis

Two research assistants collected data from a period 1 year prior to the screening interview, to 13 months following it. Demographic data, drinking histories, medical diagnoses, and hospital visits were collected on all subjects by examining medical records and data available on the hospital computer system. Data available on the hospital computer system included laboratory results, hospitalizations (including admitting diagnosis), and clinic enrollments. Number of DSM-III-R criteria positive for alcohol dependence was determined from the checklist filled out by the clinic staff member at the screening interview. Death of a patient was determined by the Veterans Affairs Decedent Affairs Office, which maintains a very complete database on beneficiaries.

Data analysis consisted of t-tests or analysis of variance for continuous variables, and chi-square analysis for categorical variables. Logarithmic transformation was performed for positively skewed variables. Where this was not appropriate or still did not result in a satisfactory distribution, or when Bartlett's test for homogeneity of variances was significant, nonparametric analyses such as the Kruskal-Wallace analysis of variances were used. Results were considered significant at the $p < .05$ level.

Results

Table 16.1 shows baseline characteristics for both groups. Subjects in general were unemployed older white males with severe alcohol dependence and 3 to 4 medical diagnoses, the most common of which were alcoholic liver disease and pancreatitis. The groups were generally well matched, the only differences being that the ARD Clinic group showed a trend towards more medical diagnoses and also contained more widowers. Outcome results are shown in Figure 16.1.

Table 16.1 Baseline Characteristics of ARD Clinic and Control Groups. All Values Represent Mean ± Standard Deviation. Values in Parentheses Represent Percentages. U = Mann-Whitney Statistic.

Variable	ARD	Control	Statistical Test
Age (years)	61.5 ± 9.9	58.7 ± 11.0	t = 1.0, df = 54, p = .31
Education (years)	11.7 ± 2.1	11.6 ± 2.3	t = .17, df = 31, p = .86
Never Married	3 (11)	5 (18)	χ^2 = 6.66, df = 3, p = .06
Married	6 (21)	8 (29)	
Divorced	9 (32)	12 (43)	
Widowed	8 (29)	1 (4)	
Number of medical diagnoses	4.3 ± 4.3	3.5 ± 1.5	t = 2.1, df = 51, p = .05
Number of past detoxification center admissions	2.1 ± 4.1	8.2 ± 19.2	U = 426, df = 1, p = .52
Number of driving under the influence convictions	1.0 ± 1.1	0.8 ± 1.4	U = 436, df = 1, p = .42
Number of previous alcohol treatments	2.3 ± 2.6	3.3 ± 4.2	U = 362, df = 1, p = .64
Number of positive DSM III-R criteria for alcohol dependence	7.6 ± 2.0	7.2 ± 2.0	U = 380, df = 1, p = .87
Drinking days per week	5.8 ± 1.9	6.8 ± 0.7	U = 337, df = 1, p = .29
Standard drinks per day	17.0 ± 11.0	18.5 ± 12.9	t = −.45, df = 47, p = .66
Number of hospital admissions year prior to screen	1.2 ± 1.0	1.1 ± 0.8	t = .34, df = 54, p = .73
Number of hospital days year prior to screen	17.7 ± 14.5	13.8 ± 13.6	t = 1.0, df = 54, p = .30
Number of ER & urgent care visits year prior to screen	1.9 ± 1.7	2.2 ± 2.4	t = −.48 df = 54, p = .64
Number of outpatient clinic visits year prior to screen	4.3 ± 4.3	4.4 ± 5.1	t = −.09, df = 43, p = .93

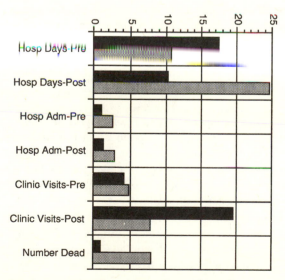

Figure 16.1. Comparison of ARD Clinic (black columns) patients and control patients (gray columns) referred elsewhere for care. All data represent findings at 12 months, except for number dead, which includes 13 months. Group differences for clinic visits and deaths during follow-up were significant at the p = .01 level. Hosp Days = hospital days; Hosp Adm = hospital admissions.

Hospital Use

The relationship between groups on hospital days reversed, with ARD days decreasing and control days increasing (t = .14, df = 54, p = .89). The lack of statistical significance may be due to large standard deviations and a small sample size. However, a paired-sample t-test comparing hospital days before and after screen date was significant for the ARD group (t = 2.33, df = 29, p = .027), but not for the controls (= 1.66, df = 22, p = .11). The number of hospital admissions rose in each group and were not significantly different.

Clinic Visits

Clinic visits increased significantly in the ARD group in the post-screen period (t = −8.03, df = 28, p < .001), while remaining unchanged in the controls (t = −1.63, df = 14, p = .126). Difference between groups on post-screen clinic visits was significant (t = 6.4, df = 51, p < .001).

Mortality

Only one of 30 (3%) ARD Clinic patients died in the 13-month follow-up period, whereas 8 of 26 (31%) control patients died during the same period (χ^2 = 8.19, df = 1, p = .004).

DISCUSSION

Medically ill alcoholics constitute a subpopulation of older alcoholics whose care disproportionately falls to medical and general social services professionals. Multiple studies have documented substantial morbidity and mortality in this group. Until now little effort has been specifically directed toward developing interventions to improve the outcome of MIAs. The Alcohol Related Disorders (ARD) Clinic model discussed in this chapter appears to show promise as an intervention that may improve this outcome.

It is not entirely surprising that this intervention may be more effective than standard care. Many complex chronic conditions respond better to coordinated care specific to their needs that is delivered in a flexible fashion with active follow-up (Willenbring et al., 1991). In fact, this happens to be so with older alcoholics in general, whether medically ill or not (see Atkinson's discussion in chapter in volume). What remains to be seen is how best to constitute and administer it.

As presently constituted, this is an expensive intervention, and one that may not be easy to duplicate in other settings because of limitations of staffing, bureaucratic barriers, and lack of funding. On the other hand, what has been developed is a prototype, not the definitive or refined model. It is likely that there are critical elements of this intervention that might be maintained in a streamlined version, and other elements that may be dropped. Some elements of this intervention could be included in everyday medical and nursing practice, even without formation of a special clinic. For example, the specific set of questions concerning alcohol use could be used routinely, as could regular use of biological indicators of drinking and feedback of results to patients. Gastroenterology departments may already have many MIAs in their clinics. Adding some of these interventions would not necessarily involve any increase in staffing, and yet might yield improvement in outcome. The same could be said about general medical clinics.

There are barriers that may be encountered when importing these treatment principles to other sites. Medical and nursing staff may have negative reactions to treating these patients, or they may feel that it is hopeless. Both services providers and service administrators may have difficulty understanding the need for a different intervention for this group, since conventional treatment is already widely available. Providing information for these staff members may be essential. Initially, the most effective way to influence opinions and attitudes is through experience. One patient who does well may turn a skeptic into a believer. As the new clinic develops, information concerning outcome of patients in general can be provided.

Most complex systems include multiple services delivered by separate programs, departments, or divisions. Services are often delivered in an uncoordinated fashion, resulting in a variety of administrative barriers. Programs may have policies excluding alcoholics, or staff members may informally screen them out before admission. Most programs operate according to their own internal policies and procedures, which usually do not stress coordination with other agencies or programs. Thus, program staff may not recognize a care coordinator as having any authority, which may hinder integration of services considerably. Another administrative barrier is funding. Third-party payers may not reimburse certain activities, especially those provided by nurses.

There may also be ideological barriers and ignorance of the specific needs of the population. In particular, most providers and insurers think of traditional treatment when dealing with alcoholism. The problem of ideology is especially acute when trying to work with traditional alcoholism treatment programs. In our facility, there was overt resistance to implementation of the ARD Clinic by some treatment program staff. They felt that what we were doing amounted to enabling, and that the proper way to treat these patients was to continue to recommend treatment and AA attendance. While these fears are understandable, they are not supportable. Traditional treatment simply does not work with most MIAs. Continuing to recommend an ineffective treatment, or one that patients will not participate in, seems futile. The fears expressed by treatment program staff appear to be based primarily in ideology, although fears about competition for resources may also play a role. In contrast, our method has been pragmatic rather than ideological, and we use whatever methods improve outcome the most. Quality improvement approaches are used to maximize impact overall. Evaluation of individual and program goals is facilitated by use of specific quantity-frequency measures at each visit, measurable indicators of improvement, and specific, measurable goals for each patient.

Critics may question whether setting immediate goals short of complete abstinence means we are giving up on patients. This argument assumes that there is a method available that effectively results in abstinence. Since there is no such method known, this argument also fails. The ARD Clinic accepts patients that everyone else, including other alcoholism treatment programs, has given up on, and provides care indefinitely, whether patients improve, stay the same, or deteriorate.

Caring for patients who continue to deteriorate is one of the most difficult tasks for staff members. There is a constant tendency either to get too involved or to reject the patient angrily. One must maintain the focus on providing comfort care, and treating that which is treatable, in order to be helpful to such patients. Patients die from alcohol dependence as surely as they do from other chronic disorders. It is important that staff members have an opportunity to ventilate their feelings about this and other aspects of care and that team members support each other. Families and patients also need to be educated about the natural history of alcoholism and helped to deal with feelings of guilt and remorse. They need opportunities to air their feelings, and empathy and understanding by staff members can provide substantial relief in themselves. Patients must be helped to perform age-appropriate tasks, such as reviewing their life and its meaning. They may need to express remorse, especially to family members, to clear their conscience for perceived wrongs they committed. Sometimes, patients set a goal of dying sober, and accomplishing this can be very meaningful for them and their families.

It is evident that changing the way one views this group of patients is a critical part of treating them more effectively. Many of the methods used in the ARD Clinic are techniques that are already a standard part of the armamentarium of general medical, nursing, and social services professionals. However, conceptual change must happen before these techniques are used with MIAs. Once this occurs, it can be very satisfying to provide effective treatment that is appreciated by patients, families, and colleagues. The essence of this attitudinal change is to approach alcoholism as a chronic, incurable, but treatable illness. In the end, one can always treat the patient, even when the disease is incurable.

Acknowledgments

This research was supported by grants from the Veterans Affairs Research Service to Drs. Willenbring and Olson. The authors thank Richard Lofgren, M.D., Pat Kappas-Larson, R.N., M.P.H., and Mary Gales-Wenz, M.S.W., for their contributions to this project, and thank Richard Magraw, M.D., and Robert Petzel, M.D., for their support.

References

Bullock, K. D., Reed, R. J., & Grant, I. (1992). Reduced mortality risk in alcoholics who achieve long-term abstinence. *Journal of the American Medical Association, 267*, 668–672.

Finney, J. W., & Moos, R. H. (1991). The long-term course of treated alcoholism: I. Mortality, relapse and remission rates and comparisons with community controls. *Journal of Studies on Alcohol, 52*, 44–54.

Hermos, J. A. (1984). Drinking by cirrhotic patients under medical care: A literature survey. *Alcoholism: Clinical and Experimental Research, 8*, 314–318.

McIntosh, I. D. (1982). Alcohol-related disabilities in general hospital patients: A critical assessment of the evidence. *International Journal of Addictions, 17*, 609–639.

Moss, R. H., Cronkhite, R. C., & Finney, J. W. (1990). *Alcoholism treatment: Context, process, and outcome.* New York: Oxford University Press.

U.S. Department of Health and Human Services. (1990). Seventh Special Report to the U.S. Congress on Alcohol and Health. Rockville, MD.

Vaillant, G. E. (1983). The natural history of alcoholism. Cambridge, Massachusetts: Harvard University Press.

Willenbring, M. L., Johnson, S., & Tan, E. (1994). Characteristics of male medical patients referred to alcoholism treatment. *Journal of Substance Abuse Treatment, 11*, 259–265.

Willenbring, M. L., Ridgely, M. S., Stinchfield, R., & Rose, M. (1991). *Application of case management in alcohol and drug dependence: Matching treatments and populations.* National Institute on Alcohol Abuse and Alcoholism, DHHS Pub. No. (ADM) 91-1766, Washington, DC: Supt. of Docs., U.S. Govt. Print. Off.

IV

SPECIAL GROUPS

17

Drinking and Problem Drinking in Older Women

SHARON C. WILSNACK,
NANCY D. VOGELTANZ, LOUISE E. DIERS,
AND RICHARD W. WILSNACK

In a comprehensive review of research on alcohol, drugs, and aging in 1990, Gomberg observed that "information about elderly female alcoholics is sparse" (p. 197). Since that review, research on *women's drinking* and on *elderly alcohol problems* in general has increased substantially. However, although a few recent studies have specifically addressed older women's problem drinking, such studies remain rare. This chapter reviews·major findings from studies specifically about older women's alcohol or drug use, and attempts to glean information on older women's drinking from general research on women and on aging. After reviewing recent findings about patterns and trends in older women's drinking, drinking problems, and multiple substance abuse, the chapter discusses demographic, personal, interpersonal, and social-environmental factors that may increase older women's risks of problem drinking. The final sections describe two recent treatment programs for older women with drinking problems and offer some suggestions for future research and practice.

Because longitudinal data on older women's drinking are scarce, the chapter makes extensive use of published and unpublished findings from our national longitudinal study of women's drinking. Our initial survey in 1981 interviewed a probability sample of 914 women, stratified to include 500 women who drank four or more drinks per week. A follow-up survey in 1986 reinterviewed 143 women who in 1981 had reported at least two of three indicators·of potential problem drinking (average daily consumption of one ounce or more of ethanol, one or more drinking-related problems in the past 12 months, and one or more alcohol dependence symptoms in the past 12 months), plus 157 women who drank more than once a month in 1981 but reported none of the three problem drinking indicators. In 1991 a 10 year follow-up survey interviewed 696 women from the 1981 sample (85% of those not deceased or incapacitated), plus a new stratified sample of 403 women aged 21 to 30. Additional information about sample design, methods, and analysis of the 1981, 1986, and 1991 surveys can be found in R. Wilsnack, S. Wilsnack, & Klassen (1984); S. Wilsnack, Klassen, Schur, & R. Wilsnack (1991); and R. Wilsnack, Harris, & S. Wilsnack (1993).

EPIDEMIOLOGY OF DRINKING AND PROBLEM DRINKING
IN OLDER WOMEN

Some Methodological Issues

Older women in the general population report low levels of drinking, heavy drinking, and adverse drinking consequences. In fact, in all available surveys, women over age 60 or 65 report the lowest levels of alcohol use and alcohol-related problems of any age-gender group. This consistent pattern might lead some observers to conclude that alcohol is not a problem for older women.

That conclusion is unwarranted, for several reasons. Because the proportion of body fat increases with age, and the volume of body fluids declines, the same amount of alcohol produces higher blood alcohol concentrations in older than in younger drinkers (e.g., Dufour, Archer, & Gordis, 1992). Also, of all age-gender groups, older women are the largest users of prescription psychoactive medications, many of which interact with alcohol in undesired ways (Gomberg, 1990; Graham, Carver, & Brett, in press). Higher blood alcohol concentrations and increased risks of alcohol-drug interactions can make even relatively low levels of alcohol consumption hazardous for older women.

Alcohol-related problems and alcohol disorders may be poorly detected among the elderly in general due to the youth-oriented bias of current measurement instruments (Caracci & Miller, 1991; Finney, Moos, & Brennan, 1991; Graham, 1986). In addition, older women specifically may under-report the alcohol problems they do have, perhaps in response to the "triple stigma" of being female, elderly, and alcoholic (Rathbone-McCuan & Triegaardt, 1979). Heightened effects of alcohol in the elderly, increased risks of alcohol-drug interactions, and inadequate measurement and possible underreporting of older women's drinking problems all suggest that the epidemiological data presented in the sections that follow are likely to indicate *lower limits* of the prevalence of drinking and related problems among older women.

Age, Gender, and Drinking in Cross-National Perspective

Data from 39 longitudinal surveys in 15 countries (Fillmore, Golding, Leino et al., in press; Fillmore, Hartka, Johnstone et al., 1991) show that in every country and time period represented, levels of alcohol consumption and alcohol-related problems were lowest in the oldest age groups of respondents. Within the oldest age groups, in every country and time period, women reported less drinking and fewer drinking problems than men. For a more detailed understanding of these broad patterns in North America, this review focuses on recent studies in the United States and Canada, with emphasis on larger community surveys and national surveys where available.

Cross-Sectional Surveys of U. S./Canadian Samples

Drinking and Heavy Drinking

Recent national surveys in the United States and Canada show how sharply women's drinking declines as women age, particularly after age 60. Table 17.1 summarizes rates of drinking and heavy drinking (14 or more standard drinks per week) among women

Table 17.1 Percentages of Women Who Are Drinkers and Heavy Drinkers, by Age Group, 1971–1991

Age Group	HP 1971	HP 1972	HP 1973	HP 1973	HP 1974	ORC 1975	RAC 1976	SRG 1979	UND 1981	NHIS 1983	ARG 1984	NHIS 1988	ARG 1990	NHIS 1990	UND 1991
21–34															
Drinkers	71	67	72	65	71	68	71	77	70	79	73	71	73	76	74
Heavy drinkers	6	4	5	3	6	5	4	5	6	4	7	3	3	2	4
35–49															
Drinkers	64	56	63	55	55	57	73	65	72	74	64	68	64	74	65
Heavy drinkers	5	4	8	5	6	3	3	8	9	5	6	4	2	2	3
50–64															
Drinkers	47	44	43	50	49	48	50	49	52	67	62	59	57	66	52
Heavy drinkers	5	4	5	4	4	1	3	3	4	4	4	4	2	2	2
65 and over															
Drinkers	26	42	29	28	36	32	37	40	33	53	44	45	32	52	29
Heavy drinkers	0	5	2	2	2	1	0	2	2	3	2	2	1	2	1

Sources: Johnson et al. (1977), R. W. Wilsnack et al. (1984), Williams & DeBakey (1992) (reanalyzed by S. F. DeBakey), Hilton (1988), Midanik & Room (1992) (reanalyzed by L. T. Midanik), Williams et al. (1993) (reanalyzed by S. F. DeBakey).

HP = Harris Poll; ORC = Opinion Research Corporation; RAC = Response Analysis Corporation; SRG = Social Research Group (later Alcohol Research Group); UND = University of North Dakota; NHIS = National Health Interview Survey; ARG = Alcohol Research Group.

in four age groups in 15 U. S. surveys from 1971 to 1991. In the 1984 U. S. survey conducted by the Alcohol Research Group, drinkers declined from a majority of women aged 21 to 34 (73%) to a minority of women aged 65 and older (44%); heavy drinking declined from 7% to 2% of the same age groups. In our 1991 U. S. survey, drinking declined from 74% of women aged 21 to 34 to 29% of women aged 65 and older, while heavy drinking dropped from 4% to 1% of the same age groups. A 1989 Canadian national survey not included in the table (Graham, Carver, & Brett, in press) found drinking by 77% of women aged 20 to 64 but only 46% of women aged 65 and older; 5% of the younger women and 1% of the older women reported consuming five or more drinks on one occasion at least once per month. The increase of abstinence with age seems greater than the decline of heavy drinking, but that may be only because relatively few women drink heavily even at younger ages. The consistency of higher abstinence rates among older women across 20 years of surveys makes it unlikely that this pattern resulted from historical or cohort changes rather than from effects of aging.

Alcohol-Related Problems and Alcohol Disorders

Rates of drinking-related problems and alcohol dependence symptoms in general population surveys show the same general pattern of age-related decline. In the large St. Louis, New Haven, and Baltimore samples of the Epidemiological Catchment Area (ECA) Study (Holzer, Robins, Myers et al., 1984), the six-month prevalence of DSM-III alcohol abuse or dependence was only 0.1% to 0.7% in women aged 60 and older, compared with a range of 1.4% to 3.3% among women aged 18 to 39. The 1988 National Health Interview Survey (NHIS) found a similar age-related pattern, with the 12-month prevalence of DSM-III-R alcohol abuse and dependence at 10.1% among women aged 18 to 29 but only 0.37% among women aged 65 and older (Grant, Harford, Chou et al., 1991).

Among women in our 1991 U. S. national survey, women aged 65 and older were the least likely to report drinking-related problems or symptoms of alcohol dependence. Only 2.5% of the oldest women reported one or more drinking-related problem in the past 12 months, compared with 24.8% of women aged 21 to 34, 10.8% of women aged 35 to 49, and 7.5% of women aged 50 to 64. One or more symptoms of alcohol dependence in the past 12 months were reported by only 1.1% of women aged 65 and older, compared with 17.7% of women aged 21 to 34, 10.5% of women aged 35 to 49, and 3.9% of women aged 50 to 64.

Rates of adverse drinking consequences among *all* women in specific age groups are clearly affected by age-related differences in rates of drinking versus abstention. Even when only women who *drink* are considered, older women typically report low rates of drinking problems and dependence symptoms. This pattern, for 10-year age groups in our 1981 and 1991 U. S. national surveys, can be seen in Table 17.2, which we discuss in more detail later. In both the 1981 and 1991 surveys, women drinkers aged 61 to 70 had lower rates of drinking problems and alcohol dependence symptoms than did women drinkers in any other age group.

Lifetime Prevalence of Alcohol Disorders

Older persons not only report fewer *current* alcohol disorders; in several recent studies they have reported less *lifetime* experience of alcohol abuse or dependence than younger

Table 17.2. National Longitudinal Study of Women's Drinking: Comparing 1981 and 1991 Drinking Patterns among Women of the Same Age, in Percent (Weighted)

Age	Year	Abstainers (%)	Heavier Drinkers (%)	Frequency > 1/Mo.[a]	Quantity > 1 Drink[a]	Days of ≥ 6 Drinks ≥ 1[a]	Days Felt Drunk > 1[a]	Problem Consequences ≥ 1[a]	Dependence Symptoms ≥ 1[a]	N	(N)
21–30	1981	24.3	6.8 (9.0)	39.9 (52.7)	56.1 (74.2)	40.7 (51.7)	38.1 (48.1)	32.8 (42.7)	23.6 (30.2)	275	(238)
	1991	27.1	4.4 (6.0)	36.7b (50.0)	49.4c (67.4)c	27.5b (37.5)d	40.9 (55.8)f	26.5c (35.0)c	22.1 (29.7)	405	(305)
31–40	1981	29.8	4.2 (6.0)	35.0 (49.5)	41.5 (58.7)	24.0 (30.5)	21.2 (24.3)	13.8 (19.7)	9.5 (13.3)	194	(162)
	1991	31.1	3.5 (5.1)	26.3b (38.0)	42.5 (61.9)	17.1c (24.7)c	34.6f (50.0)f	17.3 (25.0)	10.5 (14.9)	235	(182)
41–50	1981	32.8	9.9 (15.0)	37.9 (57.3)	37.1 (55.2)	22.5 (29.9)	16.7 (21.2)	13.2 (19.5)	10.8 (16.0)	147	(116)
	1991	33.6	2.3b (3.5)c	22.6c (33.8)d	25.6c (38.5)d	9.5d (14.2)d	13.1 (19.7)	9.9 (13.2)b	8.7 (11.4)	162	(124)
51–60	1981	44.5	5.2 (8.7)	29.2 (52.3)	29.4 (52.6)	14.3 (16.6)	9.5 (14.2)	7.6 (11.3)	4.0 (7.1)	132	(91)
	1991	49.1	1.4 (2.7)b	22.6b (44.3)	24.6b (49.1)	10.4b (20.5)	12.3 (24.1)	6.8 (13.4)	3.7 (7.2)	122	(78)
61–70	1981	64.0	4.1 (11.3)	23.5 (60.5)	18.4 (47.7)	11.8 (22.6)	6.1 (8.9)	3.3 (9.0)	1.7 (4.7)	104	(58)
	1991	60.1	1.1 (2.7)b	11.2 (27.5)e	14.4 (36.2)b	5.8c (14.5)b	3.6 (9.1)	3.1 (7.5)	1.1 (2.6)	99	(55)

Note: Percentages are given first for all women, then in parentheses for current drinkers (women who drank in the past 12 months). N's are weighted but adjusted to equal actual sample sizes. Percentages for respondents in their seventies and eighties are not presented here because N's for these age groups are too small for reliable estimates.

[a] In past 12 months. [b] $p < .10$, [c] $p < .05$, [d] $p < .01$, [e] $p < .001$, one-tailed, Kendall's Tau$_c$ for the full range of drinking measures.

[f] $p < .05$, two-tailed, Kendall's Tau$_c$ for the full range of reported days that respondents felt drunk.

persons. In all five ECA sites, persons under age 45 reported higher lifetime rates of alcohol abuse/dependence than did older persons, with these age differences most pronounced in women in four of the five sites (Holzer et al., 1984; Robins, Helzer, Przybeck, & Regier, 1988). In the 1989 Canadian national survey (Graham, Carver, & Brett, in press), women aged 20 to 64 were more than twice as likely as women aged 65 and older (18% versus 7%) to recall at least one alcohol-related problem during their lifetime; corresponding rates for younger versus older *men* were 36% and 23%. These patterns may suggest that alcohol disorders are becoming more prevalent in the general U. S. population (Robins, et al., 1988), since rates are higher among newer drinkers with shorter periods at risk. However, problem rates among the aged could also have been reduced by differential mortality (heavy drinkers dying earlier), age-related declines in recall (alcohol problems more distant in time may be more easily forgotten), and changing awareness of alcohol effects (with young women drinkers today more alert to drinking-related impairment and hazards than women drinkers might have been decades ago) (see Holzer et al., 1984; S. Wilsnack & R. Wilsnack, 1993).

Drinking Patterns among Older Women

In contrast to measures of heavy drinking and adverse drinking consequences, the *frequency* of drinking does not decline as clearly with advancing age among older women who continue to drink. Among all women in the 1984 U. S. national survey, daily drinking was as common at ages 60 and older (5%) as at ages 30 to 49, and more common than in women aged 18 to 29 (2%) or 50 to 59 (3%) (Hilton, 1991). In the 1989 Canadian national survey, women aged 65 and older were just as likely (5%) as women aged 20 to 64 (4%) to drink four or more times per week; among current drinkers, older women were *more* likely (10%) than women aged 20 to 64 (6%) to report drinking four or more times per week (Graham, Carver, & Brett, in press). Earlier Canadian data, from a 1985 telephone survey in St. John's, Newfoundland (McKim & Quinlan, 1991), found that age-related declines in drinking were primarily due to a steady decline in the quantity of alcohol consumed on an occasion, whereas frequency of consumption showed little association with age for either women or men.

Cross-sectional correlations between age and drinking measures in both our 1981 and 1991 national samples (R. Wilsnack et al., 1993) showed that age was a poor predictor of drinking frequency and of average volume of consumption (quantity $\times$ frequency) among women who were current drinkers. On the other hand, greater age among drinkers was significantly associated with having fewer drinks per drinking day, fewer occasions of heavy episodic drinking (six or more drinks on a drinking day) or intoxication, and fewer drinking problems and alcohol dependence symptoms. The irrelevance of age to drinking frequency and volume among women who continue to drink may reflect a tendency for women either to develop stable drinking patterns or to stop drinking. Together with additional longitudinal data presented below, these patterns may identify a subgroup of older women who continue to engage in relatively frequent light or moderate drinking, with few apparent problem consequences.

Trends in Older Women's Drinking, 1971–1991

The 15 surveys in Table 17.1 not only show how drinking and heavy drinking become rarer among older women, but should also reveal any historical trends in women's drinking from 1971 to 1991. Historical changes are neither obvious nor powerful in the data, but segmented regression analyses suggest that any change in the proportion of women who were drinkers was upward through the 1970s and downward beginning in the early 1980s (R. Wilsnack et al., 1993). A decline in the prevalence of drinking during the 1980s was detectible in all age groups, including women aged 65 and older. For rates of heavier drinking (14 or more drinks per week), no decline was detectible in the 1980s for women over 50, possibly because of the consistently low prevalence of heavier drinking among older women (ranging only from 0 to 5% over the 20 years). Trend analyses were hampered by variations in definitions of drinking and heavy drinking in the 15 surveys compared. For example, rates of drinking in the 1983 and 1990 NHIS surveys may have been increased by questions sensitive to very infrequent drinking. Nonetheless, a conclusion that drinking *per se* declined among women in the 1980s is consistent with studies comparing pairs of surveys conducted during the 1980s (Caetano & Kaskutas, 1993; Midanik & Clark, 1992; Williams & DeBakey, 1992), and it is also consistent with evidence of a decline in per capita alcohol sales during that decade (Williams, Stinson, Clem, & Noble, 1992).

Longitudinal Surveys of Older Women

Longitudinal drinking surveys of adult women are few, but they have some important advantages over the cross-sectional studies summarized above. In particular, longitudinal studies avoid the problems of noncomparable drinking measures across surveys, and they may allow effects of aging on drinking to be distinguished from general historical changes and/or influences affecting a particular age cohort.

Data from several longitudinal studies support the patterns noted in the cross-sectional studies reviewed above: age-related declines in women's rates of drinking, heavier drinking, and adverse drinking consequences but not necessarily in the frequency or overall volume of drinking among women who continue to drink. In Fillmore et al.'s (1991) longitudinal data on drinkers in the United States, women in their sixties drank as much per drinking occasion as women in their twenties, and women drinkers drank *more* frequently after age 40 than before. However, these analyses do not show the incidence and chronicity of abstinence as people age. A 1980–1987 longitudinal community survey of healthy elderly persons (Adams, Garry, Rhyne, Hunt, & Goodwin, 1990) found a significant drop in the percentage of elderly persons who drank but no change in mean alcohol intake over time among those who continued to drink. When women in the 1971–1974 National Health and Nutrition Examination Survey (NHANES I) were reinterviewed in the 1982–1984 Epidemiologic Follow-up Study (NHEFS), a large majority of older women were abstainers or light drinkers at both times (82% of women aged 55 to 64 and 89% of women aged 65 to 74 in 1971–1974) (Dufour, Colliver, Grigson, & Stinson, 1990). Among the women aged 55 to 64 in 1971–1974, 6% continued moderate or heavy drinking and 6% shifted down to light drinking or abstinence; among the women aged 65 to 74, 4% continued moderate or heavy drinking and 4% shifted to light drinking or abstinence.

A striking finding in our 1981–1991 national longitudinal survey was women's tendency to become and remain abstinent as they aged. As shown in Table 17.3, 43% of women aged 50 to 64 in 1981 were abstainers in both 1981 and 1991, and a further 20% drank at least occasionally in 1981 but had stopped drinking by 1991. Among

Table 17.3. Women's Changes in Abstention vs. Drinking between 1981 and 1991 Surveys, by Age in 1981

	Drinking Status in 1991	
Drinking Status in 1981	Abstainer (%)	Drinker (%)
Age 21–34 (N = 312)[a]		
Abstainer	17.9	8.9
Drinker	13.2	60.0
Age 35–49 (N = 197)		
Abstainer	24.3	3.2
Drinker	15.7	56.8
Age 50–64 (N = 143)		
Abstainer	43.3	6.8
Drinker	19.7	30.2
Age 65+ (N = 44)		
Abstainer	63.5	—
Drinker	17.4	19.0

[a]Ns given here are weighted cell frequencies rounded to integer values.

women aged 65 and older in 1981, 64% abstained from alcohol in both 1981 and 1991, while 17% reported at least some drinking in 1981 but none in 1991.

Other analyses of the 1981–1991 longitudinal data show that the frequency, quantity per occasion, and total volume of alcohol consumption declined among all women drinkers as they aged 10 years. After women drinkers had reached their thirties, adverse drinking consequences became increasingly infrequent and rarely increased over the 10 years between surveys, and nonproblematic drinking patterns became more stable and predictable (R. Wilsnack et al., 1993). These patterns are consistent with earlier findings that women's drinking patterns are more variable in youth and become steadier or more chronic as women age (e.g., Fillmore et al., 1991; S. Wilsnack et al., 1991).

The idea of chronicity may suggest that among older women who continue to drink, heavy or problematic drinking patterns will persist. Our data on women who were drinkers both in 1981 and in 1991 indicate that among the continuing drinkers after age 50, a majority of women who were daily drinkers in 1981 still drank several times a week 10 years later, and a majority of women who had more than one drink per occasion in 1981 still had at least two per occasion 10 years later. However, the numbers of frequent multiple-drink consumers among these women (now 60 or older) were too small for statistically reliable inferences. Furthermore, over a 10-year period there was no evidence of any continuity of becoming intoxicated or having other adverse drinking consequences among these older continuing drinkers. Therefore, chronicity may be a term that describes lower levels of elderly women's drinking better than abusive drinking patterns. This interpretation is consistent with longitudinal data from older men (Fillmore, 1987; Stall, 1986) and from one sample that included older women (Adams et al., 1990), indicating greater stability of light and moderate drinking patterns than of heavier drinking patterns among older persons who continue to drink.

Post-Prohibition Era Drinking among Older Women: A Possible Cohort Effect?

Although rates of heavy drinking and drinking problems are now low among elderly women, concern has been expressed that these rates may increase as cohorts of women who grew up during the Prohibition era are replaced by cohorts who grew up after Prohibition was repealed (see Glantz & Backenheimer, 1988; Gomberg, 1990). Some findings from cross-sectional analyses might indicate increased drinking among older women who learned to drink after the 1920s. Using retrospective data on lifetime drinking patterns from the NHANES I Epidemiologic Follow-up Study (NHEFS), Dufour et al. (1990) compared respondents aged 65 to 74 and respondents aged 75 to 84. Members of the older cohort, who were all in their early twenties during Prohibition, were more likely than members of the younger cohort to report that they had been abstainers at age 25, possibly reflecting an effect of Prohibition in deterring young people from starting to drink. In addition, retrospectively reported lifetime drinking levels for 10-year age intervals showed that the younger cohort, who spent most of their twenties in the period after repeal of Prohibition, had a higher prevalence of heavy drinking at each age interval. Other evidence comes from the 1989 Canadian national survey (Graham, Carver, & Brett, in press), in which women aged 65 or older were more likely to report being lifelong abstainers (21%) than women aged 20 to 64 (7%), men aged 65 and older (7%), or men aged 20 to 64 (2%). Graham et al. interpret this pattern as a cohort effect that predicts increased rates of drinking among future cohorts of older women. In contrast, Holzer et al. (1984) failed to find evidence of a post-Prohibition effect in their analyses of data from three ECA sites. They predicted that their oldest cohort, born before 1905, should have pre-Prohibition rates of alcohol abuse or dependence (retrospectively reported) similar to those in the youngest (post-Prohibition) cohort, with cohorts reaching maturity during Prohibition falling below the other two groups. The ECA data did not support this prediction; rather, rates of alcohol abuse/dependence were lower the earlier respondents were born, with no special effect of Prohibition.

Some of our national survey findings may help reveal how older women's drinking has been influenced by growing up after Prohibition. The 1971–1991 trend analyses (Table 17.1) show no recent increase in rates of drinking or heavy drinking among women aged 65 or older. Table 17.2 includes detailed comparisons of women drinkers in their sixties in 1981 (born in 1911–1920, with childhood or adolescent exposure to Prohibition earlier in childhood). The post-repeal cohort (1991) shows *declines* rather than increases in most measures of drinking behavior, with a sharp drop in the percentage of women drinkers who drink more than once a month. The trend analyses and longitudinal analyses together suggest that any tendencies toward increased drinking and drinking problems among older women who learned to drink after the repeal of Prohibition have been outweighed by more recent historical influences that seem to be leading women to drink more conservatively.

Problem Drinking Prevalence in General Population Samples: Additional Caveats

As discussed earlier, the relatively low rates of drinking and drinking problems reported by older women in general population surveys probably under-represents the true extent of the alcohol problem within this population, for several reasons: the increased toxicity of alcohol and alcohol-drug interactions with age, age and gender bias in survey questions about drinking-related problems, and possible underreporting by older persons in general, and perhaps by older women in particular. In addition, most general population surveys fail to sample institutionalized persons, including hospitalized patients and nursing home residents. Because of the increased medical and psychiatric pathology asso-ciated with heavy alcohol use, the prevalence of problem drinking in medical and institutional-care settings is usually higher than in the general population (Curtis, Geller, Stokes, Levine, & Moore, 1989; Liberto, Oslin, & Ruskin, 1992; Schuckit, 1982). Although hospitals and nursing homes provide a valuable setting for identification and treatment of older women problem drinkers, evidence suggests that health care profes-sionals do a poor job of detecting alcohol problems of older patients, especially older women (Lichtenberg, Gibbons, Nanna, & Blumenthal, 1993; Moore, Bone, Geller, et al., 1989).

MULTIPLE SUBSTANCE USE IN OLDER WOMEN

One reason for concern about drinking among elderly women is that effects of alcohol may interact with effects of other substances that older women use. Older women's multiple substance use may be overlooked because the other substances used are often legally obtained medications (over-the-counter or prescribed), not the illicit drugs that attract the attention of the criminal justice system to younger multiple drug users.

Clinical studies have found elevated rates of other substance use, abuse, and depen-dence among women in treatment for alcohol problems. Several studies suggest that abuse of licit psychoactive prescription drugs such as minor tranquilizers and sedatives may be more common among middle-aged and older alcoholic women (Celentano & McQueen, 1984; Mulford, 1977; Rathbone-McCuan & Roberds, 1980), while younger women may be increasingly likely to combine alcohol use with use of illicit drugs such as cocaine and marijuana (Association of Junior Leagues, 1988; Lex, 1993). Clinical studies (Finlayson, Hurt, Davis, & Morse, 1988; Gomberg, 1992; Schuckit, Morrissey, & O'Leary, 1978) and community studies (Brennan, Moos, & Kim, 1993) comparing elderly female and male problem drinkers have found that the women are more likely than the men to report use of or dependence on prescription psychoactive drugs such as tranquilizers.

The most detailed data on use of alcohol and prescribed psychoactive drugs by older women in the general population come from the 1989 Canadian Alcohol and Drug Survey (Carver, Graham, & Lundy, 1991; Graham, Carver, & Brett, in press). In this national telephone survey, 1,118 female respondents age 65 and older reported the lowest rates of drinking and smoking of any age-gender group in the survey, but the highest rates of using prescription drugs (psychoactive or otherwise). Data analyses revealed three general patterns of substance use among the older women: (1) Religiosity was associated with less drinking and smoking, but more use of sleeping pills; (2) use of prescribed psychoactive drugs was associated with poorer health and higher levels of stress; and (3) drinking was more prevalent among healthier, higher socioeconomic status, unwidowed, less elderly women. These patterns suggest the hypothesis that, although alcohol and other drugs may be used *concurrently* by older problem-drinking women in clinical samples, in the general population psychoactive medications may more often be *alternatives* to alcohol. However, even if alcohol turns out to be more an alternative than a supplement for older women's other drugs, there are still good reasons for concern about alcohol-drug interactions in older women.

ANTECENDENTS AND CORRELATES OF PROBLEM DRINKING IN OLDER WOMEN

Although older women in the general population may have low *rates* of alcohol problems, the *numbers* of older women with alcohol problems are large. There are currently about 19 million women aged 65 and older in the United States (U. S. Bureau of the Census, 1992), with a projected 25 to 30 million by the year 2020 (Liberto et al., 1992). Grant et al.'s (1991) estimated 0.37% 12-month prevalence of DSM-III-R alcohol abuse or dependence among women aged 65 and older in 1988, and our finding that approximately 1% of women in this age group reported at least one alcohol dependence symptom in 1991, suggest that roughly 70,000 to 190,000 women aged 65 and older are currently experiencing symptoms of alcohol dependence. If the same prevalence rates continue, the larger population of older women by the year 2020 will include between 90,000 and 300,000 women aged 65 or older with at least some symptoms of alcohol dependence. These estimates are conservative. They omit older women who suffer adverse effects of drinking (such as accidents) without symptoms of alcohol dependence, or who do not report alcohol-related symptoms and problems actually experienced. The estimates also omit women who drink moderately but risk adverse effects from alcohol-drug interactions or from increased biological sensitivity to alcohol associated with age and gender.

If drinking has hazards for small percentages but large numbers of older women, what personal or social-environmental factors can help predict *which* older women who drink will develop problems related to their alcohol use? Predictors of problem drinking in older women are hard to identify because of the scarcity of relevant research. On the one hand, research on antecedents and correlates of problem drinking in women has often not given special attention to *older* women as a distinct subgroup (see, e.g., NIAAA, 1980, 1986; S. Wilsnack et al., 1991). On the other hand, studies of drinking and problem drinking among the *elderly* have often been based on clinical samples (see Gomberg, 1990) or on samples of men (e.g., Atkinson, Tolson, & Turner, 1990; Glynn, Bouchard, LoCastro et al., 1986; Temple & Leino, 1989). The lack of data on older problem-drinking women in the general population forces this review of risk factors to extrapolate sometimes from findings on women that are not age-specific, and from findings about elderly drinking that are not gender-specific. In this review, *problem drinking* refers to any use of alcohol that creates specific adverse consequences; *older women* refers to women aged 65 and older, unless otherwise indicated.

Demographic Correlates and Partner Drinking

Marital Status

Research has found repeatedly that never-married, divorced or separated, and cohabiting women have higher rates of problem drinking, while married and widowed women have lower rates (Cahalan, Cisin, & Crossley, 1969; Clark & Midanik, 1982; Holzer et al., 1984; S. Wilsnack, R. Wilsnack, & Klassen, 1986). Because most widows are older women, the apparent protective effects of widowhood might result from or contribute to the observed effects of aging described earlier. To resolve this uncertainty of causes, it is important to compare older married and widowed women.

Results of such comparisons thus far have not always found reduced risks among widows. In the 1989 Canadian national survey, Graham, Carver, and Brett (in press) found that widowed women aged 65 and older drank less than married women and were much more likely to be abstainers. In the ECA study (Holzer et al., 1984), alcohol disorders were more prevalent in older married women than widows, only in the St. Louis sample. In the 1985 National Household Survey on Drug Abuse (Robbins, 1991), none of four measures of alcohol abuse were related to the marital status of older women (aged 55 and older, $N=601$). Both the ECA study and the NIDA household survey found that rates of alcohol abuse were particularly low among *men* who were married rather than widowers. Possible gender differences in how marriage affects drinking among the elderly need to be examined more closely.

Partner Drinking

Although marital disruption may contribute to older men's problem drinking (because of increased stress, loneliness, or reduced social control), Gomberg (1990) suggests that drinking husbands may help explain why more older wives than widows have problems with alcohol. Among problem drinkers, women are generally more likely to have heavy or problem drinking partners/spouses than men are. This asymmetry occurs partly because more men than women have drinking problems, but also perhaps because men may influence how women drink more than vice versa (Haavio-Mannila, 1991; R. Wilsnack & S. Wilsnack, 1990). Gomberg and Lisansky (1984) cite clinical evidence suggesting that women may become involved in heavy or problem drinking because of the "transmission of symptomatic drinking behavior" from problem-drinking husbands/partners (p. 254), and they conclude that the presence of a heavy drinker in a woman's life may be a critical antecedent or risk factor for her own problem drinking. Strong associations between women's drinking and that of their partners have been reported not only in the United States but also throughout the Nordic countries (Dahlgren, 1979; Haavio-Mannila, 1991; Hammer & Vaglum, 1989; Seppa, Koivula, & Sillanaukee, 1992).

Other possible evidence for partner influences on older women's problem drinking emerged in analyses of our 1981 national survey (R. Wilsnack & Cheloha, 1987). Most of the women aged 65 or older who reported any indicators of problem drinking also had two other characteristics: They relied on other people to help them make difficult decisions, and their closest companions were drinkers. Among older women reporting signs of problem drinking, from 55% to 100% of the risk of several problem-drinking behaviors could be attributed to having an advisor who was a drinker (Kahn & Sempos, 1989), *if* the relationship preceded the problem behaviors. Caution is necessary in interpreting the cross-sectional analyses, because older women who are already abusing alcohol might prefer the company and counsel of other drinkers.

Although many older women with drinking problems may drink in part in response to the social circumstances of marriage (including their partner's drinking), clinical evidence suggests that the psychological distress and isolation of widowhood can also aggravate alcohol abuse among some women drinkers. In a study of 250 widows and 100 widowers (mean age = 61 years), significant increases in alcohol consumption occurred over the 13-month period following the spouse's death (Zisook, Shuchter, & Mulvihill, 1990). At the end of the first year of bereavement, 30% of the widows and widowers had increased the number of days they drank each month, and the mean number of drinks per drinking day also increased significantly. Unfortunately, gender-specific analyses are not reported, although a summary of demographic factors analyzed indicates that men are more likely than women to show both increased frequency and increased quantity of drinking. Heavy drinking prior to the spouse's death was most predictive of significant increases in drinking after the spouse's death, with a history of depression and current dissatisfaction with emotional supports also predicting increased drinking. If widowhood is most likely to produce detectable problem drinking among women with histories of drinking and depression, one possible explanation is that loss of a partner removes both important social controls over one's drinking and important protection from drinking consequences. This hypothesized consequence fits the findings of a small clinical study of elderly problem drinkers (Hubbard, Santos, & Santos, 1979) in which five widowed women problem drinkers were all described as "team alcoholics." In these marriages, both marital partners had abused alcohol for years, with the wife's problem drinking becoming visible only after her husband's death.

To summarize, one way to synthesize what little is known about marriage and older women's drinking is to hypothesize that marriage is a major contributor and widowhood a minor contributor to problem drinking by these women. Older women are more likely to have drinking problems if they have male partners who drink and who may facilitate their spouse's alcohol abuse or dependence. Loss of a drinking partner may take away drinking opportunities and motives for many women, but may also lead some older drinkers to use alcohol in more medicative, less controlled, and less protected ways, making their alcohol abuse more severe or more overt.

Education and Income

The limited information about the socioeconomic status of older women drinkers suggests that higher education or income may make older women, like younger women, more likely to use alcohol, but may have little impact on drinking consequences. Several studies have found that the better educated elderly are more likely to use alcohol (Borgatta, Montgomery, & Borgatta, 1982; LaGreca, Akers, & Dwyer, 1988); and Graham, Carver, and Brett (in press) in Canada found specifically that older women who were more educated and had higher household incomes were more likely to drink. Our 1981 survey data showed that after controlling for effects of age, income (and to a lesser extent education) increased the probability that women would drink. However, neither income nor education had any significant effect on risks of adverse consequences or alcohol dependence among women drinkers (R. Wilsnack, S. Wilsnack, & Klassen, 1987). Furthermore, although Holzer et al. (1984) found that alcohol disorders were more prevalent in poorer households, this pattern was neither strong nor consistent for older women. Thus far, there is little to suggest that socioeconomic status has any powerful influence on the likelihood of problem consequences among older women who do drink.

Employment Status

Employment and Nontraditional Employment. The percentage of employed older women in general population surveys is generally quite low. In the Canadian national survey (Graham, Carver, & Brett, in press), for example, 95% of the older women were homemakers. In our 1991 U. S. survey, only 4% of women aged 65 and older were employed full-time outside the home, with another 9% reporting part-time employment. Although the small numbers of employed older women make statistical analyses unreliable, it would seem logical to assume that older women who continue to work will show the same small increases in consumption that younger women do (R. Wilsnack & S. Wilsnack, 1992). This may be particularly true for older women employed in managerial/professional occupations or in other occupations typically dominated by men, which have been associated with heavier and/or more frequent drinking by women in several studies (Haavio-Mannila, 1991; Kubicka, Csemy, & Kozeny, 1991; LaRosa, 1990; R. Wilsnack & Wright, 1991).

Available survey data do not identify any strong associations between employment status of older women and *problem* drinking. There was no apparent relationship between employment status and problem drinking either across the total ECA study sample, or for older women specifically (Holzer et al., 1984). Older women's (aged 55 and older) problem drinking was not related to employment status in the 1985 NIDA Household Survey, although full-time employment was negatively related to problem drinking in older men (Robbins, 1991). Unfortunately, analyses of the NIDA survey data included homemakers in the "unemployed" category (Robbins, 1991), thus combining a category that may be at higher risk for problem drinking (unemployed women seeking work) with a group that may be at lower risk (homemakers) (see R. Wilsnack & S. Wilsnack, 1992). Although not statistically significant, older women working part-time in the 1985 NIDA survey reported the most frequent intoxication (an average of 7 days drunk in the past year, as compared with 0.2 to 1.0 days in other employment categories). Women employed part-time also had elevated rates of heavier drinking and drinking problems in our 1981 and 1986 surveys (R. Wilsnack et al., 1984; S. Wilsnack et al., 1991), perhaps reflecting distinctive drinking opportunities and/or stresses associated with less than full-time paid employment.

Unemployment and Retirement. Although time-order and causality are often uncertain, several studies (e.g., Borgatta et al., 1982) report increased drinking and/or drinking problems among unemployed persons in the general population, and a similar relationship might be hypothesized for older women who want to work but are unable to find or hold paid employment. Although *retirement* appears in most lists of age-related stressors believed to increase risks of late-onset problem drinking (see below), we are not aware of any literature specifically addressing the effects of retirement on the drinking behavior of older women. Future cohorts of older women will include larger numbers of women with long-term employment and career histories outside the home, for whom retirement may pose major transitions in social networks, marital and family relationships, and identity and self-esteem. Future research on alcohol use and alcohol problems in older women should include attention to retirement, perhaps particularly among women with primary career identifications, as a potentially new risk factor for problem drinking in later life.

Ethnicity

Most studies of older women's drinking have used predominantly white samples, and several studies that have looked for ethnic variations in elderly drinking patterns have failed to find them (Borgatta et al., 1982; Holzer et al., 1984). A 1984 national survey that oversampled ethnic minority respondents found lower rates of drinking and drinking problems among African-American and Hispanic women than among white women, including the small samples of women aged 60 and older (Caetano, 1991; Herd, 1991). Given the strong associations between acculturation and heavier drinking among younger Hispanic women (Gilbert & Collins, in press), one question for future research is whether successive cohorts of older Hispanic women will show increased drinking and drinking problems over time. Additional research is also needed on drinking behavior of older women in smaller ethnic minority groups, including Asian-American and American Indian women.

Genetic/Biologic, Psychological, and Social Antecedents

Early-Onset Antecedents

While almost nothing is known about what causes chronicity of problem drinking throughout women's adult lives, it is possible that some factors that cause women to become problem drinkers when they are young might also help perpetuate problem drinking into old age. One such factor might be genetic predisposition for alcohol dependence. Genetic vulnerability is believed to have a significant influence on the development of alcohol dependence, particularly if such dependence is severe and develops early in life (e.g., Bohman, Sigvardsson, & Cloninger, 1981; Goodwin, 1976; Kendler, Heath, Neale, Kessler, & Eaves, 1992). What is not as clear is whether the available studies do (McGue & Slutske, 1993) or do not (Heath, Slutske, & Madden, in press; Hill, 1993) support a relatively greater contribution of genetic factors to alcohol disorders in men than in women. Genetic vulnerability almost certainly contributes to lifelong drinking problems of some women. However, the low prevalence of drinking problems among older women suggests that unless genetic or early influences are rare or fatal (i.e., resulting in early mortality), such influences appear to have relatively little power to impel heavy or poorly controlled drinking by the time women reach old age.

Late-Onset Problem Drinking

Gender Differences in Late-Onset Problem Drinking. A further complication of explaining older women's problem drinking is that some women do not even begin to abuse alcohol until they are middle-aged or older—the so-called "late-onset" or "recent-onset" problem drinkers. Identifying factors that predict late-onset problem drinking may be particularly important for understanding older women's problem drinking, since a later onset of alcohol problems may be more characteristic of women than of men (Atkinson, 1992). Although definitions of "late onset" vary in terms of age and recency criteria, most studies of gender differences among problem drinkers have found that older women are more likely than older men to report recent onset of alcohol problems. For example, a comparison of 41 older female and 83 older male alcoholics in treatment (mean ages in mid-sixties) showed that 38% of the women but only 4% of the men reported the onset of problem drinking within the last 10 years (Gomberg, 1992). In a study of 151 older men and 65 older women admitted for treatment of alcohol-related problems (Hurt, Finlayson, Morse, & Davis, 1988), 46% of the women and 39% of the men reported that their problem drinking began after age 60. In the

ECA data on persons with lifetime alcohol disorders (Holzer et al., 1984), 50% of the 50 older women (aged 60 and older) but only 27% of the 237 older men reported the onset of alcohol problems at age 40 or later. In a community survey by Moos, Brennan, and colleagues of persons aged 55 to 65, 704 men and women (37% of those surveyed) reported one or more current alcohol-related problems (Finney et al., 1991; Moos, Brennan, & Moos, 1991). Of these problem drinkers, 46% of the women but only 28% of the men reported alcohol problem onset in the past two years (percentages derived from Brennan & Moos, 1991, Table 1).

Age-Related Stressors and Late-Onset Problem Drinking. Late-onset problem drinking is sometimes viewed as a response to negative and stressful life changes that occur with aging: loss of spouse and friends, change of residence, chronic difficulties with health and finances, and dwindling social support (see Rosin & Glatt, 1971; Zimberg, 1974). There is remarkably little evidence that clearly supports this idea. Although some clinical studies have found associations between life stressors and late-life alcohol problems (Finlayson et al., 1988), surveys of general population samples generally have not (Borgatta et al., 1982; Brennan & Moos, 1991; La Greca et al., 1988).

Other Explanations of Late-Onset Problem Drinking. The life-stressors model implies that late-onset problem drinking among older women is a qualitative change in drinking behavior driven by some sudden, special need for alcohol. An alternative theoretical perspective is that some women's drinking problems may evolve gradually, belatedly, and almost accidentally because of changes in the circumstances in which they normally drink. In later life some older women may have more time that they can afford to spend drinking (Busby, Campbell, Borrie, & Spears, 1988), fewer role responsibilities that might inhibit drinking (R. Wilsnack & Cheloha, 1987), and more occasions of social interaction for pleasure that may seem more enjoyable with the effects of alcohol (Alexander & Duff, 1988). Older women in these circumstances may be particularly influenced by the drinking norms and opportunities created by their companionship and social interaction.

This perspective has been most relevant to the findings of Akers and colleagues (e.g., Akers, LaGreca, Cochran, & Sellers, 1989) in their studies of drinking in retirement communities. These authors postulate that "drinking among the elderly is related to the norms and behavior of one's primary groups . . . and the balance of reinforcement for drinking" (p. 625). In their sample of 1,410 older respondents, much of the variance in drinking behavior could be accounted for by social learning variables, particularly by differential reinforcement of drinking behavior. However, it is not clear to what extent social norms and reinforcers would facilitate older women's drinking relative to men's, and to what extent companions and neighbors would influence the drinking of older women who do not live in communities of their agemates.

Depression and Problem Drinking in Older Women

Problem drinking and depression are associated in both clinical and general population studies, with the associations tending to be stronger among women than among men. Clinical studies of psychiatric comorbidity consistently find depression more common in alcoholic women, and antisocial personality disorder and other substance use disorders more common in alcoholic men (e.g., Hesselbrock & Hesselbrock, in press; Hesselbrock, Meyer, & Keener, 1985). Several general population surveys have also linked depression and women's drinking (Hartka et al., 1991; Midanik, 1983).

It is more difficult to discern the implications of comorbidity research for *older* women. Brennan, Moos, and colleagues' community survey of older problem drinkers found that women reported more depression than men, even when problem drinking was in remission (Brennan et al., 1993). If longitudinal findings from all women in our 1981 and 1986 surveys also apply to older women specifically, depression may predict the chronicity of problem drinking among older women already experiencing alcohol-related problems better than it predicts the onset of such problems (S. Wilsnack et al., 1991). Despite disagreement about the clinical and prognostic significance of comorbid alcohol abuse and depression (e.g., Hesselbrock & Hesselbrock, in press; Rounsaville, Dolinsky, Babor, & Meyer, 1987; Schuckit, 1985), assessing and treating depression may be an important aspect of treating problem drinking in some older women (Rathbone-McCuan & Roberds, 1980).

Characteristics of Older Women's Primary Relationships

For older women who are married or involved in an intimate nonmarital relationship, drinking may be influenced not merely by how their partners drink, but also by how they get along with their partners. Although effects of marital distress and conflict on women's problem drinking have received some attention in the general literature on women and alcohol (e.g., McCrady, 1990; Olenick & Chambers, 1991; Williams & Klerman, 1984), there has been remarkably little research on how older women drinkers relate to partners in ongoing relationships, and very little is known about problems in these relationships.

In a study discussed earlier of 250 widows and 100 widowers (Zisook et al., 1990), 26% of the widows and widowers *decreased* the frequency of their drinking after their spouse died. Although gender-specific findings were not reported, the authors noted that men were more likely than women to *increase* their drinking following their spouse's death. One possible cause for a decline in drinking for some widows might be the loss of a heavier drinking partner who had created opportunities and incentives for the woman to drink. Another possible cause might be the release from troubled or conflicted marriages in which marital distress led women to use alcohol to medicate their negative feelings. Research is not yet available that could evaluate the relative importance of these two potential effects of widowhood.

Whether or not older women's problem drinking arises from relationship problems, their drinking may be reinforced if it seems to reduce relationship problems. In Brennan and Moos's community study of late-life problem drinkers, 183 female problem drinkers (aged 55 to 65) initially reported higher levels of stress and lower levels of support in relationships with spouses than 476 male problem drinkers did. One year later, 38% of the women and 26% of the men reported no drinking-related problems. Among these "remitted" problem drinkers, women still reported higher levels of spousal stress and significantly lower levels of spousal support (as well as more depression and extended family stress) than did men. But women whose drinking problems continued over the one-year follow-up interval reported reduced levels of spousal stress. Among older problem drinkers, women may be more distressed by spouses than men are, even when their own drinking problems abate, perhaps because more of the women have problem-drinking spouses who are unable to be supportive for their wives (Brennan et al., 1993), or perhaps because husbands may be more intolerant of wives with drinking problems than vice versa (see also Beckman & Amaro, 1984; S. Wilsnack, 1991a). The reduced spousal stress experienced by older women who continued problem drinking may be a sign that drinking can help women maintain communication and reduce conflict within the marital system, perhaps particularly if the husband is also a heavy or problem drinker. The possibility that some older women drink in part to enhance marital harmony is consistent with recent feminist formulations of women's use of alcohol as an attempt to maintain important interpersonal relationships (Covington & Surrey, in press). Such use of alcohol may also explain why a relatively large proportion of older women drinkers report positive expectancies about the effects of alcohol on interpersonal intimacy: Among women drinkers age 65 and older in our 1991 national survey, 35% indicated that drinking made them feel closer to the person they shared drinks with, and 48% said that it was easier to be open with other people when they were drinking.

Sexuality and Problem Drinking in Older Women

One way that older women may use alcohol to improve relationships is to make sexual activity more pleasurable or less distressing. However, despite growing recent attention to links between drinking behavior and sexual activity (e.g., NIAAA, 1991; Norris, 1993), apparently no one has studied such links specifically in *older* women. This neglect may reflect a cultural stereotype that sexuality declines or disappears at older ages (e.g., Zeiss, 1982), perhaps particularly among older women. As Edith Gomberg has noted, "Twenty years ago . . . researchers thought that only *men* drank and were sexual; today it seems that researchers believe that only *young* people drink and are sexual" (Gomberg, 1993).

Most older persons have active sexual lives (subject to limitations created by loss of sexual partners, health problems, or other age-related influences), so there is no reason to assume that drinking behavior of older women is *not* related to their sexual experience. It is true, judging from our 1981 and 1991 surveys, that older women drinkers are somewhat less likely than younger women drinkers to report positive expectancies about the effects of drinking on sexuality, perhaps because the older drinkers grew up during a time of more conservative norms about women's drinking and sexuality. Nonetheless, in 1991 40% of the women drinkers aged 65 and older indicated that they sometimes or usually felt less sexually inhibited after drinking, and 30% of older women drinkers reported that sexual activity was more pleasurable after drinking. Because such a large minority of older women drinkers has positive beliefs about effects of drinking on sexual experience, it is likely that some of them use alcohol in part to reduce sexual inhibition or to enhance sexual pleasure.

Another related reason for older women to seek the effects of alcohol may be experiences of sexual dysfunction. In addition to sexual difficulties arising from her own physiology or psychology (see Mooradian & Greiff, 1990), an older woman's sexual well-being may be affected by age-related or other sexual problems originating with her husband or partner, perhaps especially if he is physically ill and/or a heavy drinker (e.g., O'Farrell, 1990; S. Wilsnack, 1984). The loss or absence of a sexual partner can be an additional source of distress for many older women. Our 1981 and 1991 surveys included an index of sexual problems that asked about lifetime lack of sexual interest, lifetime lack of orgasm, low frequency of orgasm, and vaginismus (Klassen & Wilsnack, 1986; S. Wilsnack, 1991b). In both the 1981 and 1991 surveys, women aged 65 and older had higher scores on this index than did younger women; in 1991, 54% of women aged 65 and older reported at least one of these sexual problems. Because older women may experience a range of problems related to sexual expression and sexual satisfaction, and because sexual problems have been linked to heavier drinking and to chronicity of problem drinking among women in the general population (S. Wilsnack et al., 1991), it is reasonable to hypothesize that sexual dysfunction is a risk factor for problem drinking in some older women. It is further possible that early experiences of childhood sexual abuse may contribute both to sexual dysfunction and to self-medicative alcohol use in some older women, as they appear to do in age-undifferentiated samples of women in several recent studies (Miller, Downs, & Testa, 1993; S. Wilsnack, Klassen, Vogeltanz, & Harris, 1994).

Older Women's Drinking Contexts

Little information is available about the physical and social contexts in which older women's drinking occurs. One possibly high-risk environment for both older women and older men is retirement communities. Alexander and Duff (1988) found that rates of nonabstention and weekly drinking were considerably higher among residents of three middle-class retirement communities in California and Oregon than among older persons in the general population. Of the 260 residents interviewed (median age 76 years), 46% reported drinking at least once a week. Although gender-specific rates are not provided, 68% of the sample was female. Alcohol consumption levels were also related to community context in a large study of 1,410 persons aged 60 or older living in two retirement communities and two age-heterogeneous communities in Florida and New Jersey (Akers et al., 1989).

Higher rates of drinking and heavier drinking in retirement communities may be related to the availability of drinking partners and social reinforcements for drinking. Consistent with this idea is Alexander and Duff's finding that retirees' level of social interaction was significantly related to their alcohol consumption. Hurt et al.'s (1988) finding that late-onset problem drinkers entering treatment were significantly more likely than early-onset problem drinkers to have lived in a retirement complex suggests the possible role of one living context in promoting the late-life onset of problem drinking.

REMISSION OF ALCOHOL PROBLEMS IN OLDER WOMEN

Longitudinal data on older problem drinkers show considerable fluctuation and spontaneous remission in drinking-related problems, particularly among late-onset problem drinkers (Atkinson, 1992; Schuckit, Atkinson, Miller, & Berman, 1980). The limited data on older *women* suggest that spontaneous remission may be relatively common, perhaps even more common among older women than among their male counterparts. In longitudinal analyses of our 1981 and 1986 survey data for women aged 50 and older, 26% of the women who reported at least two of three problem-drinking indicators in 1981 reported none of the three indicators in 1986; an additional 38% reported only one indicator in 1986 (S. Wilsnack et al., 1991). In their community sample of older problem drinkers, Brennan et al. (1993) found that, among persons reporting one or more drinking problems at initial assessment, a larger proportion of women (38%) than men (26%) reported no drinking problems at a 1-year follow-up.

There are several reasons why remission from problem drinking may be more likely for older women than for older men. Remission is more common if problems are newer, fewer, and milder (Atkinson, 1992; Moos et al., 1991), as older women's drinking problems tend to be. Older women's drinking opportunities and drinking partners. More speculatively, older women's social environments may become less "masculine" with age, for example, with retirement from a male-dominated work environment or with the death of a heavier drinking husband, which may in turn encourage more moderate drinking or even abstention. Finally, for some older women (e.g., those whose marriages were not happy, or who experienced stressful caretaking responsibilities for an ill spouse) widowhood may have some positive aspects that reduce the need for alcohol. Further research on predictors of spontaneous remission of late-life problem drinking may reveal how those predictors can be used or reinforced to reduce risks of alcohol abuse among older women drinkers.

SPECIAL TREATMENT NEEDS OF OLDER WOMEN: SOME PRELIMINARY FINDINGS

Empirical research dealing specifically with the treatment experiences and needs of older women problem drinkers is scarce. However, the existing literature suggests that older women may have unique treatment needs distinctive from those of younger persons and men. One program designed to meet the special treatment needs of older women is the North of Market Older Women's Alcohol Program (Fredriksen, 1992). This program provides specialized outreach and treatment services for older women problem drinkers in an impoverished, high-crime area of San Francisco. Findings from the program suggest that nontraditional techniques designed to "build up" older women's independent living skills and self-esteem are superior to traditional confrontational tactics for "breaking down" women's defenses. Although complete abstinence was not the goal for most clients in the program, approximately 60% of the women attained complete sobriety for at least 3 months during the year following entry into the program.

Similarly, the Community Older Persons Alcohol (COPA) Program (Graham, Saunders, Flower et al., in press) was designed to provide outreach and treatment services for older persons with alcohol and drug problems in Toronto. The program's philosophy was built upon the assumptions (1) that older problem drinkers are not likely to self-refer for treatment but rather need to be reached out to; (2) that the older person's admitting to having a drinking problem is not a primary prerequisite for treatment; and (3) that acquiring skills necessary for the older person's independent living in the community is a paramount goal of treatment. Preliminary research indicates that the older persons in the program reported greater impairments in cognitive functioning and daily living skills than younger problem drinkers, and that reduced alcohol consumption was beneficial in helping to recover or maintain independent living skills. Graham et al.

reported that approximately 75% of COPA clients achieved at least some improvement that was stable over time.

CONCLUSIONS: SOME DIRECTIONS FOR FUTURE RESEARCH AND PRACTICE

Patterns and Trends

Non-Problem Drinking in Older Women: Lessons for Prevention?

Although the bulk of this review focuses on older women who do develop problems with alcohol, perhaps the most striking epidemiological finding is the relatively low rates of heavy drinking and drinking problems reported by this population subgroup. An important task for future research is to determine how valid these low prevalence rates are, and to what extent they may be artifacts of (1) age- and gender-biased measures; (2) under-reporting specific to (or more common in) older women; and (3) the absence of the most at-risk or impaired women from surveys of the noninstitutionalized elderly.

To the extent that older women *do* have fewer problems with alcohol, better research on what leads older women to abstain or drink moderately may have implications for more general prevention of problem drinking. Graham, Carver, and Brett (in press) describe the ''well off'' elderly woman drinker—healthier, better educated, and more likely to be economically comfortable. Gomberg (1990) speculates that older women may be more ''viable'' than older men—in better health, with more social support and more social roles. Adlaf, Smart, and Jansen (1989) found that older women in senior citizen housing were happier, less lonely, and better connected to family and friends than were older men. Even among older persons with drinking problems, older women may experience more support from children, extended family members, and friends (Brennan et al., 1993). It is important not only to understand what causes some older women to develop problems with alcohol, but also to understand what protects the large majority of older women from adverse drinking consequences.

What About the Future: Will Younger Women Carry "Bad Habits" into Old Age?

Although recent trend analyses and longitudinal analyses do not show any major rise in alcohol consumption among older women who learned to drink after Prohibition, it is possible that other cohort experiences at younger ages may have lasting effects on older women's drinking. One can speculate about delayed effects from the normalization of women's drinking after World War II, or from experimentation with intoxicating drugs by the adolescents of the 1970s, although the limited epidemiological evidence to date does not indicate any major effects of these historical changes on women's drinking in 1991 (R. Wilsnack et al., 1993). The possibility that older women's drinking may surge in future cohorts is a major theme in the geriatric alcohol literature, and it deserves careful evaluation in ongoing epidemiological research. Such evaluation will also need to give close scrutiny to the prevalence of multiple substance abuse, in the sense that older women may knowingly use alcohol as part of self-medication in combination with prescription and over-the-counter drugs and/or may show some rise in use of illicit drugs as a cohort effect of the more permissive alcohol and drug use norms of the 1960s and 1970s.

Antecedents and Risk Factors

Better Models for Late-Onset Problem Drinking: What about Life Stressors?

In research thus far on older women's drinking, there is a notable lack of empirical support for the assumption that age-related stressors are important as causes or conditions for late-onset problem drinking. Future research needs to evaluate not only why this assumption has been so widespread, but also why it has not been confirmed. At least two possible reasons for the negative findings can be suggested for further study. (1) What is reported as late-onset problem drinking may actually have a much earlier onset, disguised either because older women are ashamed to admit how long they have been having drinking problems, or because protective relationships with drinking partners and companions mask alcohol abuse and buffer its social consequences until those relationships end (e.g., in widowhood). (2) Stressful life events may not cause older women to abuse alcohol simply because of the nature or the acute severity of the events; however, older women's drinking may increase in response to how chronic the effects of stressful events become and how helpless a woman feels to reduce or escape those effects (R. Wilsnack, 1992).

Partner Drinking: A Powerful Risk (or Remission) Factor?

If support for a life-stressor model of late-onset problem drinking is equivocal at best, there is almost universal support for the influence on women's drinking of the drinking behavior of their husbands or partners. Future research needs to study the processes by which male partners may increase older women's drinking and drinking problems; for example, creation of opportunities and reinforcements for drinking; intensification of marital stress created by a partner's drinking; development of sexual problems related to a partner's drinking; and encouragement of women's use of companionate drinking to make it easier to get help from, communicate with, or get along with a heavy-drinking partner. Longitudinal research may learn how the *loss* of a heavy- or problem-drinking partner affects older women's drinking, perhaps by making a woman's own long-standing problem drinking more visible, or perhaps by allowing improvement or remission of a woman's heavy or problem drinking when the relationship stresses and/or drinking opportunities that maintained her drinking are gone.

Identification and Treatment

There is clearly a need for more age- and gender-sensitive diagnostic and research instruments to help identify problem drinking in older women. Investigators proposing new measures of alcohol problems among older drinkers (e.g., Blow, 1991; Finney et al., 1991) should be encouraged to include older women in studies evaluating the instruments, and to analyze and report gender similarities and differences in the measures' sensitivity. There is an equally great need for more research on gender- and age-specific treatment models. Evaluation of treatment outcomes for same-sex/mixed-age, same-age/mixed-sex, and age- and sex-specific treatment is essential to plan for anticipated increases in the need for geriatric alcohol services. Because older persons appear to do as well as younger persons even in mixed-age treatment programs (Fitzgerald & Mulford, 1992; Janik & Dunham, 1983), and women appear to do as well as or better than men in mixed-sex treatment programs (McCrady & Raytek, 1993; Vannicelli, 1984), it is possible that older women might have greatly superior treatment outcomes relative to other age-gender groups if they were treated in settings sensitive to special issues of *both* age and gender.

The blindness of health professionals to problem drinking in older women patients (e.g., Curtis et al., 1989; Lichtenberg et al., 1993) suggests an urgent need for professional reeducation about drinking in older women, to improve the ability of physicians and others to see the signs of alcohol abuse in elderly female patients. Some health professionals may feel reluctant to identify or confront problems when they are uncertain what treatment will work. However, the only treatment strategy for older women that is sure *not* to work is the one that is currently widely used: pretending that older women have no drinking problems.

Ageist/Sexist Stereotypes: Blind Spots and Neglected Issues

Age and gender stereotypes have helped to create and maintain blind spots in what is known about problem drinking in older women. Reluctance to pay attention to negative aspects of elderly marriages (perhaps from a wish to believe that all long marriages are happy) may have led to failures to detect or study how marital conflict and stress affect older women's drinking, including how older women may use alcohol to get along better with drinking spouses. An assumption that all "losses" in old age are purely negative may have led clinicians and researchers to ignore potentially positive aspects of late-life transitions such as retirement or widowhood. An assumption that aging women become asexual may help explain the total lack of information about how sexual experience and sexual dysfunction may be related to alcohol use among older women. And stereotypes about feminine values and priorities may explain why the sparse literature on older women's drinking pays so much attention to widowhood and bereavement, and so little attention to ways that retirement could be a major late-life stressor to an older woman highly devoted to her job or career.

Stereotypes simplify and homogenize groups of people. Therefore, the greatest damage from age and gender stereotypes, in research on older women's problem drinking, may have been to minimize the heterogeneity of older women in general, and older women problem drinkers in particular. Older women, like older men and other drinkers of all ages, use alcohol for a variety of reasons and develop alcohol problems for an equally wide range of reasons. One 75-year-old woman may experience depression and self-medicative drinking in response to loss of a lifelong happy marriage, while another may experience remission of problem drinking due to relief from marital stress and support for drinking from a heavy-drinking partner. A more differentiated view of older women's lives, and the role of alcohol in them, may encourage the development of more complex models for understanding how older women use and abuse alcohol, and may encourage approaches to treatment and prevention that deal with the individualized as well as the shared characteristics of women with drinking problems late in life.

Acknowledgments

The 1981–1991 U. S. national longitudinal survey reported in this chapter was supported by Research Grant No. 5 R37 AA04610 from the National Institute on Alcohol Abuse and Alcoholism. The authors appreciate the collaboration of project director Albert D. Klassen, statistical advisor T. Robert Harris, computer specialist Perry Benson, and staff of the National Opinion Research Center which conducted the survey fieldwork. Expert assistance with manuscript preparation was provided by Loraine Olson and Michelle Schumacher. We are grateful to Dr. Kathryn Graham and colleagues of the Addiction Research Foundation for providing unpublished reports and manuscripts from their pioneering work on problem drinking in older women and men.

References

Adams, W. L., Garry, P. H., Rhyne, R., Hunt, W. C., & Goodwin, J. S. (1990). Alcohol intake in the healthy elderly. *Journal of the American Geriatrics Society, 38*, 211–216.

Adlaf, E. M., Smart, R. G., & Jansen, V. A. (1989). *Alcohol use, drug use, and well-being among a sample of older adults in Toronto.* Toronto: Addiction Research Foundation. Cited in Carver et al., 1991.

Akers, R. L., LaGreca, A. J., Cochran, J., & Sellers, C. (1989). Social learning theory and alcohol behavior among the elderly. *The Sociological Quarterly, 30*, 625–638.

Alexander, F., & Duff, R. W. (1988). Social interaction and alcohol use in retirement communities. *The Geronotologist, 28*, 632–636.

Association of Junior Leagues (1988). *Summary of findings: WOMAN-TO-WOMAN Community Services Survey.* New York: Association of Junior Leagues.

Atkinson, R. M. (June, 1992). *Epidemiology of late onset problem drinking in older adults.* Paper presented at the Annual Meeting, Research Society on Alcoholism, San Diego, CA.

Atkinson, R. M., Tolson, R. L., & Turner, J. A. (1990). Late versus early onset problem drinking in older men. *Alcoholism: Clinical and Experimental Research, 14*, 574–579.

Beckman, L. J., & Amaro, H. (1984). Patterns of women's use of alcohol treatment agencies. In S. C. Wilsnack & L. J. Beckman (Eds.), *Alcohol problems in women: Antecedents, consequences, and intervention* (pp. 319–348). New York: Guilford.

Blow, F. (1991). *Michigan Alcoholism Screening Test—Geriatric Version (MAST-G).* Ann Arbor: University of Michigan Alcohol Research Center.

Bohman, M., Sigvardsson, S., & Cloninger, C. R. (1981). Maternal inheritance of alcohol abuse: Cross-fostering analysis of adopted women. *Archives of General Psychiatry, 38*, 965–969.

Borgatta, E. F., Montgomery, R. J. V., & Borgatta, M. L. (1982). Alcohol use and abuse, life crisis events, and the elderly. *Research on Aging, 4*, 378–408.

Brennan, P. L., & Moos, R. H. (1991). Functioning, life context, and help-seeking among late-onset problem drinkers: Comparisons with nonproblem and early-onset problem drinkers. *British Journal of Addiction, 86*, 1139–1150.

Brennan, P. L., Moos, R. H., & Kim, J. Y. (1993). Gender differences in the individual characteristics and life contexts of late-middle-aged and older problem drinkers. *Addiction, 88*, 781–790.

Busby, W. J., Campbell, A. J., Borrie, M. J., & Spears, G. F. S. (1988). Alcohol use in a community-based sample of subjects aged 70 years and older. *Journal of the American Geriatrics Society, 36*, 301–305.

Caetano, R. (1991). Findings from the 1984 National Survey of Alcohol Use among U.S. Hispanics. In W. B. Clark & M. E. Hilton (Eds.), *Alcohol in America: Drinking practices and problems* (pp. 293–307). Albany: State University of New York Press.

Caetano, R., & Kaskutas, L. A. (June, 1993). *Longitudinal changes in drinking patterns among whites, blacks, and Hispanics: 1984–1992*. Paper presented at the Annual Meeting, Research Society on Alcoholism, San Antonio, Texas.

Cahalan, D., Cisin, I. H., & Crossley, H. M. (1969). *American drinking practices: A national study of drinking behavior and attitudes*. New Brunswick, NJ: Rutgers Center of Alcohol Studies.

Caracci, G., & Miller, N. S. (1991). Epidemiology and diagnosis of alcoholism in the elderly (a review). *International Journal of Geriatric Psychiatry, 6*, 511–515.

Carver, V., Graham, K., & Lundy, C. (February, 1991). *Older women: Their use of alcohol and other substances*. Working paper prepared for Health and Welfare Canada. London (Ontario) and Toronto: Addiction Research Foundation.

Celentano, D. D., & McQueen, D. V. (1984). Multiple substance abuse among women with alcohol-related problems. In S. C. Wilsnack & L. J. Beckman (Eds.), *Alcohol problems in women: Antecedents, consequences, and intervention* (pp. 97–116). New York: Guilford.

Clark, W. B., & Midanik, L. (1982). Alcohol use and alcohol problems among U.S. adults: Results of the 1979 national survey. In National Institute on Alcohol Abuse and Alcoholism, *Alcohol consumption and related problems* (Alcohol and Health Monograph No. 1, Department of Health and Human Services Publication No. ADM 82-1190) (pp. 3–52). Washington, DC: U.S. Government Printing Office.

Covington, S. S., & Surrey, J. L. (in press). The relational model of women's psychological development: Implications for substance abuse. In R. W. Wilsnack & S. C. Wilsnack (Eds.), *Gender and alcohol*. New Brunswick, NJ: Rutgers Center of Alcohol Studies.

Curtis, J. R., Geller, G., Stokes, E. J., Levine, D. M., & Moore, R. D. (1989). Characteristics, diagnosis, and treatment of alcoholism in elderly patients. *Journal of the American Geriatrics Society, 37*, 310–316.

Dahlgren, L. (1979). *Female alcoholics: A psychiatric and social study*. Stockholm: Karolinska Institute.

Dufour, M. C., Archer, L., & Gordis, E. (1992). Alcohol and the elderly. *Clinics in Geriatric Medicine, 8*, 1, 127–141.

Dufour, M., Colliver, J., Grigson, M. B., & Stinson, F. (1990). Use of alcohol and tobacco. In J. C. Cornoni-Huntley, R. R. Huntley, & J. J. Feldman (Eds.), *Health status and well-being of the elderly* (pp. 172–183). New York: Oxford University Press.

Fillmore, K. M. (1987). Prevalence, incidence, and chronicity of drinking patterns and problems among men as a function of age: A longitudinal and cohort analysis. *British Journal of Addiction, 82*, 77–83.

Fillmore, K. M., Golding, J. M., Leino, E. V., Motoyoshi, M., Shoemaker, C., Terry, H., Ager, C. R., & Ferrer, H. P. (in press). Patterns and trends in women's and men's drinking. In R. W. Wilsnack & S. C. Wilsnack (Eds.), *Gender and alcohol*. New Brunswick, N. J.: Rutgers Center of Alcohol Studies.

Fillmore, K. M., Hartka, E., Johnstone, B. M., Leino, E. V., Motoyoshi, M., & Temple, M. T. (1991). A meta-analysis of life course variation in drinking. *British Journal of Addiction, 86*, 1221–1268.

Finlayson, R. E., Hurt, R. D., Davis, L. J., & Morse, R. M. (1988). Alcoholism in elderly persons: A study of the psychiatric and psychosocial features of 216 inpatients. *Mayo Clinic Proceedings, 63*, 761–768.

Finney, J. W., Moos, R. H., & Brennan, P. L. (1991). The Drinking Problems Index: A measure to assess alcohol-related problems among older adults. *Journal of Substance Abuse, 3*, 395–404.

Fitzgerald, J. L., & Mulford, H. A. (1992). Elderly vs. younger problem drinker "treatment" and recovery experiences. *British Journal of Addiction, 87*, 1281–1291.

Fredriksen, K. I. (1992). North of Market: Older women's alcohol outreach program. *The Gerontologist, 32*, 270–272.

Gilbert, M. J., & Collins, R. L. (in press). Ethnic variation in women and men's drinking. In R. W. Wilsnack & S. C. Wilsnack (Eds.), *Gender and alcohol.* New Brunswick, N. J.: Rutgers Center of Alcohol Studies.

Glantz, M. D., & Backenheimer, M. S. (1988). Substance abuse among elderly women. *Clinical Gerontologist, 8*, 3–25.

Glynn, R. J., Bouchard, G. R., LoCastro, J. S., et al. (1986). Aging and generational effects on drinking behaviors in men: Results from the Normative Aging Study. *American Journal of Public Health, 75*, 1413–1419.

Gomberg, E. S. L. (1990). Drugs, alcohol, and aging. In L. T. Kozlowski, H. M. Annis, H. D. Cappell, F. B. Glaser, M. S. Goodstadt, Y. Israel, H. Kalant, E. M. Sellers, & E. R. Vingilis (Eds.), *Research advances in alcohol and drug problems* (pp. 171–213). New York: Plenum.

Gomberg, E. S. L. (June, 1992). *Gender differences among older alcoholics in treatment.* Paper presented at the Annual Meeting, Research Society on Alcoholism, San Diego, CA.

Gomberg, E. S. L. (1993). *Adult to elderly issues.* Paper presented to the Working Group for Prevention Research on Women and Alcohol, Prevention Research Branch, National Institute on Alcohol Abuse and Alcoholism, Bethesda, Maryland.

Gomberg, E. S. L., & Lisansky, J. M. (1984). Antecedents of alcohol problems in women. In S. C. Wilsnack & L. J. Beckman (Eds.), *Alcohol problems in women: Antecedents, consequences, and intervention* (pp. 233–259). New York: Guilford.

Goodwin, D. W. (1976). *Is alcoholism hereditary?* New York: Oxford University Press.

Graham, K. (1986). Identifying and measuring alcohol abuse among the elderly: Serious problems with existing instrumentation. *Journal of Studies on Alcohol, 47*, 322–326.

Graham, K., Carver, V., & Brett, P. J. (in press). Alcohol and drug use by older women: Results of a national survey. *Canadian Journal on Aging.*

Graham, K, Saunders, S. J., Flower, M. C., Timney, C. B., White-Campbell, M., & Pietropaolo, A. Z. (in press). *Addictions treatment for older adults: Evaluation of an innovative client-centered approach.* New York: Haworth Press.

Grant, B. F., Harford, T. C., Chou, P., Pickering, R., Dawson, D. A., Stinson, F. S., & Noble, J. _____ (1991). Epidemiologic Bulletin No. 27: Prevalence of DSM-III-R alcohol abuse and dependence: United States, 1988. *Alcohol Health and Research World, 15*, 91–96.

Haavio-Mannila, E. (March, 1991). *Impact of colleagues and family members on female alcohol use.* Paper presented at the Symposium on Alcohol, Family and Significant Others, Social Research Institute of Alcohol Studies and Nordic Council for Alcohol and Drug Research, Helsinki, Finland.

Hammer, T., & Vaglum, P. (1989). The increase in alcohol consumption among women: A phenomenon related to accessibility or stress? A general population study. *British Journal of Addiction, 84*, 767–775.

Hartka, E., Johnstone, B. M., Leino, V., Motoyoshi, M., Temple, M., & Fillmore, K. M. (1991). A meta-analysis of depressive symptomatology and alcohol consumption over time. *British Journal of Addiction, 86*, 1283–1298.

Heath, A. C., Slutske, W. S., & Madden, P. A. F. (in press). Gender differences in the genetic contribution to alcoholism risk and to alcohol consumption patterns. In R. W. Wilsnack & S. C. Wilsnack (Eds.), *Gender and alcohol.* New Brunswick, N. J.: Rutgers University Center of Alcohol Studies.

Herd, D. (1991). Drinking problems in the black population. In W. B. Clark & M. E. Hilton (Eds.), *Alcohol in America: Drinking practices and problems* (pp. 308–328). Albany: State University of New York Press.

Hesselbrock, M. N., & Hesselbrock, V. (in press). Psychiatric comorbidity in alcoholic women.

In R. W. Wilsnack & S. C. Wilsnack (Eds.), *Gender and alcohol.* New Brunswick, N. J.: Rutgers Center of Alcohol Studies.

Hesselbrock, M., Meyer, R., & Keener, J. (1985). Psychopathology in hospitalized alcoholics. *Archives of General Psychiatry, 42,* 1050–1055.

Hill, S. Y. (1993). Genetic vulnerability to alcoholism in women. In E. S. L. Gomberg & T. D. Nirenberg (Eds.), *Women and substance abuse* (pp. 42–61). Norwood, NJ: Ablex Publishing.

Hilton, M. E. (1988). Trends in U.S. drinking patterns: Further evidence from the past 20 years. *British Journal of Addiction, 83,* 269–278.

Hilton, M. E. (1991). The demographic distribution of drinking patterns in 1984. In W. B. Clark & M. E. Hilton (Eds.), *Alcohol in America: Drinking practices and problems* (pp. 73–86). Albany: State University of New York Press.

Holzer, C. E. III, Robins, L. N., Myers, J. K., Weissman, M. M., Tischler, G. L., Leaf, P. J., Anthony, J., & Bednarski, P. B. (1984). Antecedents and correlates of alcohol abuse and dependence in the elderly. In G. Maddox, L. N. Robins, & N. Rosenberg (Eds.), *Nature and extent of alcohol problems among the elderly* (NIAAA Research Monograph No. 14, Department of Health and Human Services Publication No. ADM 84-1321) (pp. 217–244). Washington, DC: U.S. Government Printing Office.

Hubbard, R. W., Santos, J. F., & Santos, M. A. (1979). Alcohol and older adults: Overt and covert influences. *Social Casework: The Journal of Contemporary Social Work, 60,* 166–170.

Hurt, R. D., Finlayson, R. E., Morse, R. M., & Davis, L. J. (1988). Alcoholism in elderly persons: Medical aspects and prognoses of 216 inpatients. *Mayo Clinic Proceedings, 63,* 753–760.

Janik, S. W., & Dunham, R. G. (1983). A nationwide examination of the need for specific alcoholism treatment programs for the elderly. *Journal of Studies on Alcohol, 44,* 307–316.

Johnson, P., Armor, D. J., Polich, S., & Stambul, H. (1977). *U.S. adult drinking practices: Time trends, social correlates and sex roles.* Working Note prepared for the National Institute on Alcohol Abuse and Alcoholism. Santa Monica, CA: Rand Corporation.

Kahn, H. A., & Sempos, C. T. (1989). *Statistical methods in epidemiology* (Chapter 4: Attributable risk). New York: Oxford University Press.

Kendler, K. S., Heath, A. B., Neale, M. C., Kessler, R. C., & Eaves, L. J. (1992). A population based twin study of alcoholism in women. *Journal of the American Medical Association, 268,* 1877–1882.

Klassen, A. D., & Wilsnack, S. C. (1986). Sexual experience and drinking among women in a U.S. national survey. *Archives of Sexual Behavior, 15,* 363–392.

Kubicka, L., Csemy, L., & Kozeny, J. (March, 1991). *The sociodemographic, microsocial, and attitudinal context of Czech women's drinking.* Paper presented at the Symposium on Alcohol, Family and Significant Others, Social Research Institute of Alcohol Studies and Nordic Council for Alcohol and Drug Research, Helsinki, Finland.

LaGreca, A. J., Akers, R. L., & Dwyer, J. W. (1988). Life events and alcohol behavior among older adults. *The Gerontologist, 28,* 552–558.

LaRosa, J. H. (1990). Executive women and health: Perceptions and practices. *American Journal of Public Health, 80,* 1450–1454.

Lex, B. W. (1993). Women and illicit drugs: Marijuana, heroin, and cocaine. In E. S. L. Gomberg & T. D. Nirenberg (Eds.), *Women and substance abuse* (pp. 162–190). Norwood, N. J.: Ablex.

Liberto, J. G., Oslin, D. W., & Ruskin, P. E. (1992). Alcoholism in older persons: A review of the literature. *Hospital and Community Psychiatry, 43,* 975–984.

Lichtenberg, P. A., Gibbons, T. A., Nanna, M. J., & Blumenthal, F. (1993). The effects of age and gender on the prevalence and detection of alcohol abuse in elderly medical inpatients. *Clinical Gerontologist, 13*, 17–27.

McCrady, B. S. (1990). The marital relationship and alcoholism treatment. In R. L. Collins, K. E. Leonard, & J. S. Searles (Eds.), *Alcohol and the family: Research and clinical perspectives* (pp. 338–355). New York: Guilford.

McCrady, B. S., & Raytek, H. (1993). Women and substance abuse: Treatment modalities and outcomes. In E. S. L. Gomberg & T. D. Nirenberg (Eds.), *Women and substance abuse* (pp. 314–338). Norwood, N. J.: Ablex.

McGue, M., & Slutske, W. (September, 1993). *The inheritance of alcoholism in women.* Paper presented to the Working Group for Prevention Research on Women and Alcohol, Prevention Research Branch, National Institute on Alcohol Abuse and Alcoholism, Bethesda, Maryland.

McKim, W. A., & Quinlan, L. T. (1991). Changes in alcohol consumption with age. *Canadian Journal of Public Health, 82*, 231–234.

Midanik, L. (1983). Alcohol problems and depressive symptoms in a national survey. *Advances in Alcohol and Substance Abuse, 2*, 9–28.

Midanik, L. T., & Clark, W. B. (November, 1992). *The demographic distribution of U.S. drinking patterns in 1990: Description and trends from 1984.* Paper presented at the 120th Annual Meeting, American Public Health Association, Washington, DC.

Midanik, L. T., & Room, R. (1992). The epidemiology of alcohol consumption. *Alcohol Health & Research World, 16*, 183–190.

Miller, B. A., Downs, W. R., & Testa, M. (1993). Interrelationships between victimization experiences and women's alcohol use. *Journal of Studies on Alcohol*, Suppl. 11, 109–117.

Mooradian, A. D., & Greiff, V. (1990). Sexuality in older women. *Archives of Internal Medicine, 150*, 1033–1038.

Moore, R. D., Bone, L. R., Geller, G., Mamon, J. A., Stokes, E. J., & Levine, D. M. (1989). Prevalence, detection, and treatment of alcoholism in hospitalized patients. *Journal of the American Medical Association, 261*, 403–407.

Moos, R. H., Brennan, P. L., & Moos, B. S. (1991). Short-term processes of remission and nonremission among late-life problem drinkers. *Alcoholism: Clinical and Experimental Research, 15*, 948–955.

Mulford, H. A. (1977). Women and men problem drinkers: Sex differences in patients served by Iowa's community alcoholism centers. *Journal of Studies on Alcohol, 38*, 1624–1639.

National Institute on Alcohol Abuse and Alcoholism. (1980). *Alcoholism and alcohol abuse among women: Research issues* (NIAAA Research Monograph No. 1, U.S. Department of Health, Education and Welfare Publication No. ADM 80-835). Washington, DC: U.S. Government Printing Office.

National Institute on Alcohol Abuse and Alcoholism. (1986). *Women and alcohol: Health-related issues* (NIAAA Research Monograph No. 16, Department of Health and Human Services Publication No. ADM 86-1139). Washington, DC: U.S. Government Printing Office.

National Institute on Alcohol Abuse and Alcoholism. (1991). *Alcohol Health and Research World* (Special Focus: Alcohol and Sexuality), *15* (2).

Norris, J. (September, 1993). *Alcohol consumption and female sexuality: A review.* Paper presented to the Working Group for Prevention Research on Women and Alcohol, Prevention Research Branch, National Institute on Alcohol Abuse and Alcoholism, Bethesda, Maryland.

O'Farrell, T. (1990). Sexual functioning of male alcoholics. In R. L. Collins, K. E. Leonard, & J. S. Searles (Eds.), *Alcohol and the family: Research and clinical perspectives* (pp. 244–271). New York: Guilford.

Olenick, N. L., & Chalmers, D. K. (1991). Gender-specific drinking styles in alcoholics and nonalcoholics. *Journal of Studies on Alcohol, 52*, 325–330.

Rathbone-McCuan, E., & Roberds, L. A. (1980). Treatment of the older female alcoholic. *Focus on Women: Journal of Addictions and Health, 1*, 104–129.

Rathbone-McCuan, E., & Triegaardt, J. (1979). The older alcoholic and the family. *Alcohol Health and Research World, 3* (4), 7–12.

Robbins, C. A. (1991, January). Social roles and alcohol abuse among older men and women. *Family & Community Health*, 37–48.

Robins, L. N., Helzer, J. E., Przybeck, T. R., & Regier, D. A. (1988). Alcohol disorders in the community: A report from the Epidemiologic Catchment Area. In R. M. Rose & J. Barrett (Eds.), *Alcoholism: Origins and outcome* (pp. 15–29). New York: Raven Press.

Rosin, A. J. & Glatt, M. M. (1971). Alcohol excess in the elderly. *Quarterly Journal of Studies on Alcohol, 32*, 53–59.

Rounsaville, B., Dolinsky, Z., Babor, T., & Meyer, R. (1987). Psychopathology as a predictor of treatment outcome in alcoholics. *Archives of General Psychiatry, 44*, 505–513.

Schuckit, M. A. (1982). A clinical review of alcohol, alcoholism, and the elderly patient. *Journal of Clinical Psychiatry, 43*, 396–399.

Schuckit, M. A. (1985). The clinical implications of primary diagnostic groups among alcoholics. *Archives of General Psychiatry, 42*, 1043–1049.

Schuckit, M. A. Atkinson, J. H., Miller, P. L., & Berman, J. (1980). A three year follow-up of elderly alcoholics. *Journal of Clinical Psychiatry, 41*, 412–416.

Schuckit, M. A., Morrissey, E. R., & O'Leary, M. R. (1978). Alcohol problems in elderly men and women. *Addictive Diseases: An International Journal, 3*, 405–416.

Seppa, K., Koivula, T., & Sillanaukee, P. (1992). Drinking habits and detection of heavy drinking among middle-aged women. *British Journal of Addiction, 87*, 1703–1709.

Stall, R. (1986). Change and stability in quantity and frequency of alcohol use among aging males: A 19-year follow-up study. *British Journal of Addiction, 81*, 537–544.

Temple, M. T., & Leino, E. V. (1989). Long-term outcomes of drinking: a 20-year longitudinal study of men. *British Journal of Addiction, 84*, 889–899.

U.S. Bureau of the Census. (1992). *Statistical Abstract of the United States, 1992* (Table No. 12, p. 14). Washington, DC: U.S. Government Printing Office.

Vannicelli, M. (1984). Treatment outcome of alcoholic women: The state of the art in relation to sex bias and expectancy effects. In S. C. Wilsnack & L. J. Beckman (Eds.), *Alcohol problems in women: Antecedents, consequences, and intervention* (pp. 369–412). New York: Guilford.

Williams, C. N., & Klerman, L. V. (1984). Female alcohol abuse: Its effects on the family. In S. C. Wilsnack & L. J. Beckman (Eds.), *Alcohol problems in women: Antecedents, consequences, and intervention* (pp. 280–312). New York: Guilford.

Williams, G. D., & DeBakey, S. F. (1992). Changes in levels of alcohol consumption: United States, 1983–1988. *British Journal of Addiction, 87*, 643–648.

Williams, G. D., Shaw-Taylor, Y., DeBakey, S., Dufour, M., & Bertolucci, D. (1993). Drinking status and knowledge of risks of heavy drinking: 1985 and 1990 health promotion and disease prevention questionnaire, National Health Interview Survey. Washington, DC: Alcohol Epidemiological Data System, Cygnus Corporation.

Williams, G. D., Stinson, F. S., Clem, D., & Noble, J. (December, 1992). *Apparent per capita alcohol consumption: National, state, and regional trends, 1977–1990.* Surveillance Report No. 23. Rockville, MD: National Institute on Alcohol Abuse and Alcoholism.

Wilsnack, R. W. (1992). Unwanted statuses and women's drinking. *Journal of Employee Assistance Research, 1*, 239–270.

Wilsnack, R. W., & Cheloha, R. (1987). Women's roles and problem drinking across the lifespan. *Social Problems, 34*, 231–248.

Wilsnack, R. W., Harris, T. R., & Wilsnack, S. C. (June, 1993). *Changes in U.S. women's drinking: 1981–1991.* Paper presented at the 19th Annual Alcohol Epidemiology Symposium of the Kettil Bruun Society for Social and Epidemiological Research on Alcohol, Krakow, Poland.

Wilsnack, R. W., & Wilsnack, S. C. (June, 1990). *Husbands and wives as drinking partners.* Paper presented at the 16th Annual Alcohol Epidemiology Symposium of the Kettil Bruun Society for Social and Epidemiological Research on Alcohol, Budapest, Hungary.

Wilsnack, R. W., & Wilsnack, S. C. (1992). Women, work, and alcohol: Failure of simple theories. *Alcoholism: Clinical and Experimental Research, 16,* 172–179.

Wilsnack, R. W., Wilsnack, S. C., & Klassen, A. D. (1984). Women's drinking and drinking problems: Patterns from a 1981 national survey. *American Journal of Public Health, 74,* 1231–1238.

Wilsnack, R. W., Wilsnack, S. C., & Klassen, A. D. (1987). Antecedents and consequences of drinking and drinking problems in women: Patterns from a U.S. national survey. In P. C. Rivers (Ed.), *Alcohol and addictive behavior* (Nebraska Symposium on Motivation, Vol. 34) (pp. 85–158). Lincoln: University of Nebraska Press.

Wilsnack, R. W., & Wright, S. I. (August, 1991). *Women in predominantly male occupations: Relationships to problem drinking.* Paper presented at the Annual Meeting of the Society for the Study of Social Problems, Cincinnati, OH.

Wilsnack, S. C. (1984). Drinking, sexuality, and sexual dysfunction in women. In S. C. Wilsnack & L. J. Beckman (Eds.), *Alcohol problems in women: Antecedents, consequences, and intervention* (pp. 189–227). New York: Guilford.

Wilsnack, S. C. (1991a). Barriers to treatment for alcoholic women. *Addiction and Recovery,* July/August 1991, 10–12.

Wilsnack, S. C. (1991b). Sexuality and women's drinking: Findings from a U.S. national study. *Alcohol Health and Research World, 15,* 147–150.

Wilsnack, S. C., Klassen, A. D., Schur, B. E., & Wilsnack, R. W. (1991). Predicting onset and chronicity of women's problem drinking: A five-year longitudinal analysis. *American Journal of Public Health, 81,* 305–318.

Wilsnack, S. C., Klassen, A. D., Vogeltanz, N. D., & Harris, T. R. (May, 1994). *Childhood sexual abuse and women's substance abuse: National survey findings.* Paper presented at the Conference on Psychosocial and Behavioral Factors in Women's Health, American Psychological Association, Washington, DC.

Wilsnack, S. C., & Wilsnack, R. W. (1993). Epidemiological research on women's drinking: Recent progress and directions for the 1990s. In E. S. L. Gomberg & T. D. Nirenberg (Eds.), *Women and substance abuse.* Norwood, N. J.: Ablex.

Wilsnack, S. C., Wilsnack, R. W., & Klassen, A. D. (1986). Epidemiological research on women's drinking, 1978–1984. In National Institute on Alcohol Abuse and Alcoholism, *Women and alcohol: Health-related issues* (NIAAA Research Monograph No. 16, Department of Health and Human Services Publication No. ADM 86-1139) (pp. 1–68). Washington, DC: U.S. Government Printing Office.

Zeiss, A. M. (1982). Expectations for the effects of aging on sexuality in parents and average married couples. *Journal of Sex Research, 18* 47–57.

Zimberg, S. (1974). The elderly alcoholic. *Gerontologist, 14,* 221–224.

Zisook, S., Shuchter, S. R., & Mulvihill, M. (1990). Alcohol, cigarette, and medication use during the first year of widowhood. *Psychiatric Annals, 20,* 318–326.

18

Elderly Homeless
Alcoholic Careers

EARL RUBINGTON

People become homeless at different points in their life cycles, at different stages of their drinking patterns, and under specific social and economic conditions. When and how they become homeless bears heavily on how they adapt to their situation. And, as homeless people age and change, so do their situations. This chapter deals with how aging people deal with their problems of homelessness and alcoholism.

FOUR SOCIAL TYPES

Cumulative and recurrent crises are constant features of the homeless alcoholic lifestyle. Examples from the sobriety-intoxication cycle include obtaining alcoholic beverages, finding places to drink and people to drink with, sleeping it off, and coping with hangover and withdrawal symptoms. Examples from the outcast's predicament include coping with social punishments such as exploitation, insult, injury, denial of social and medical services, and arrest. Examples from sheer survival include finding food, shelter, work, and money.

In the course of experiencing recurrent crises, all homeless alcoholics come into contact, both voluntary and involuntary, with people in similar circumstances, and with agencies of social control such as jails, shelters, and treatment facilities of various kinds. Over time, they evolve one of four ways of adapting to the exigencies of their situation as homeless alcoholics. They adopt the social roles of the *mixer*, the *company man*, the *regular guy*, and the *loner*.

Since Knight's (1938) formulation of essential and reactive alcoholics, researchers have sorted alcoholics into early-onset problem drinkers and late-onset problem drinkers. Similarly, researchers such as Pittman and Gordon (1958) have differentiated those who entered the ranks of the homeless earlier in the life cycle from those who joined up much later in life. Combining onset of problem drinking with entry into homelessness yields four types. *Loners* become homeless and alcoholic very early in their lives. Early-onset problem drinkers who become homeless later in life are *company men*.

Regular guys enter the homeless ranks early in life only to become problem drinkers later on. *Mixers* are latecomers to both homelessness and alcoholism.

The Loner

Often products of broken or disturbed homes, instant relief for tensions came to them with their first experiences with drinking. Mostly high school dropouts, they began to fend for themselves very early in life. Examples of the undersocialized (Bacon, 1944; Straus, 1946; Pittman & Gordon, 1958), they find employment, companionship, and congenial drinking in an all-male social world. Loners, after a while, get sorted into two categories: those who prefer to drink alone and those who when drinking become combative. In the first instance they go out of their way to avoid the company of other drinkers. In the second instance, once they establish their irascible reputation, other drinkers go out of their way to avoid them.

As crises of homelessness and alcoholism recur, loners cannot or will not draw upon peer support. As a result, they spend sober periods in social control agencies, drinking periods in social isolation. Homeless alcoholics, over time, must manage career problems as their dependency on alcohol deepens. Loners turn to agencies for help rather than to their fellow homeless people in a pattern that Straus (1974) has called "institutional dependency."

Frank Moore (Straus, 1948, 1974) lived a rather long life as a loner. His father committed suicide when he was two. His mother abandoned him shortly thereafter. His grandfather raised him until he quit high school to join the Navy. After 4 years in the Navy, he enlisted in the Army for the next 4 years. For committing a serious offense he was sentenced to the federal prison at Alcatraz where he served 5 years. Discharged from Alcatraz at 27, he spent the rest of his life either in jail or a state hospital, usually after being found drunk in public. In some of these state hospitals he worked as an orderly or attendant (in the Navy he had been a pharmacist's mate). He also worked as a freight handler, furniture mover, kitchen helper, and on railroad labor gangs ("gandy dancer"). In the 50 years after Alcatraz, he served 133 sentences in 16 different county jails. Similarly, he was a patient 147 times in nine state hospitals. Twice he was a patient in an alcoholic rehabilitation center. Finally, he was a resident in seven different men's shelters a total of 13 times. He was a spree drinker who rarely sought the company of other alcoholics. A number of his arrests came about after he had been in fights. Much of his assaultiveness may well have taken place during blackouts since he often could not remember how and why he came to be incarcerated. But unlike many other loners, Moore lived a comparatively long life, dying at age 72.

The Company Man

Company men combine late entry into homeless living with early-onset problem drinking. Despite their increased heavy drinking, they marry, raise families, and hold jobs. Ultimately, increased dependency on alcohol ruptures ties to family and work. Consequently, they become overexposed to all the many crises of heavy drinking. Despite exposure to these dilemmas, they look at their new world through the eyes of the conventional community. Thus, although they are *in* the world of homeless alcoholics, they are not *of* that world. Despite considerable contact with other homeless alcoholics in tuberculosis sanitaria, jails, and other agencies, they do not identify with the inhabitants of their world. They are not in the same category with their involuntary associates, whom they regard as worthy objects of disgrace. And whenever they are patients, inmates, residents, or clients of control agencies, they define all people in that category (save themselves) from the point of view of the agency's staff.

Grady (Rubington, 1964) married, raised a large family, separated from his wife, and began drinking heavily. While a truck driver, he stopped regularly at a local tavern to buy a round of drinks for the house, thereby ensuring reciprocity. He had many acquaintances in the local homeless alcoholic community but few friends. Similarly, he was well known to the police, being listed in their "red book" of men who had 50 or more arrests for public drunkenness.

After several years of homelessness and heavy drinking, he contracted tuberculosis. He spent 29 months in a sanitarium only to resume drinking after discharge. On the advice of a physician at an outpatient alcoholism clinic, he became a resident of a halfway house for chronic drunkenness offenders. He regained his sobriety and later "graduated" from the halfway house. Yet all during his stay, he had little regard for his fellow residents or for the staff counselors. He deferred only to the director of the halfway house and the director of the mission in which the halfway house was located. He complied with halfway house rules, disclosed little about himself during group meetings, and rejected both the disease conception of alcoholism (he drank because he wanted to, not because he needed to) and his fellow residents (to him they were all "bums"). Later he assumed the post of night watchman in the mission and became in the eyes of most other people a "reformed drunk" (a person who believes he regained sobriety on his own and who cannot tolerate drunks).

Down through the years, participants in the homeless man's subculture have looked down on "mission stiffs" (Anderson, 1923). When "down and out," homeless men recognize that they may have to rely some time on rescue missions for food, clothing, and shelter. In exchange, they must attend religious services. While it's all right to get help from missions, it is not all right to make a habit of it. Anyone who does so regularly gets called a "mission stiff." Lowlier than the "mission stiff," however, is the person who ends up working for the mission.

The company man is the equivalent of the "mission stiff." While a jail inmate, a patient in an alcoholism treatment center, or a halfway house resident, a company man gives considerable lip service to the agency's definition of the situation, particularly as the staff presents it. Thus, at the very outset of the agency career whether inmate, patient, or resident, the company man expresses gratitude for being helped, exhibits exemplary compliance with agency rules, and quickly accepts agency definitions of the situation. The company man goes out of his way to differentiate himself from other inmates, patients, clients, or residents. They are only in the place to "get the wrinkles out of their bellies" or to "dry out" while he is there to "straighten out."

The Regular Guy

Regular guys are early entrants into homelessness whose problem drinking emerges much later in their homeless careers. They enter the homeless way of life much earlier than the other types. They become socialized earlier and much more intensively into the homeless subculture. Like the hobo (Anderson, 1923), they learn the language, skills, rules, and ideology of the homeless subculture. Among other things, they learn where to find work; places where one can obtain free food and a night's lodging; places to sleep; and people, places, and things to avoid. In time, as drinking comes to interfere with work, additional learning takes place. This learning centers around drinking ritual as well as how to cope with the aftermath of heavy drinking. Drinking-centered repertoire teaches how to act in taverns, people with whom it is safe to drink, how to drink when in the company of a "live one" (host of the drinking party whether in a room, tavern, or on the street), and how to protect associates who may become intoxicated. And, as a man passes through the various stages in the homeless alcoholic career from "lush" to "wino" to "Skid Row bum," another body of information on how to act comes his way from a different set of associates (Jackson & Connor, 1953; Peterson & Maxwell, 1958; Rooney, 1982, 1961; Rubington, 1962).

Central to regular guys are their ties to one another. Associates in a number of situations, including drinking groups such as bottle gangs (Rooney, 1961; Rubington, 1968), develop the conception of a regular guy. A person so identified subscribes to the norms of sharing, mutual aid, and above all, the ethic of reciprocity. As a consequence, whether on the street, in jail, in treatment, or in a halfway house, regular guys know the accepted definition of their situation and what each can expect from the others. And, other things equal, the longer one has lived the homeless life, the more set one becomes in these ways. The other side, of course, is that the longer one has been accustomed to living by one's wits as well as the ground rules of the homeless way of life, the harder it is for one to make an exit from it.

Marilyn Fish, a key informant for a recent study of the Austin, Texas, homeless subculture (Snow & Anderson, 1993), exemplifies the regular guy. The authors first met her in an alley near the Salvation Army giving out discarded burritos to people. She knew what it was like to go hungry. During her subsequent 25 contacts with the authors, she described the kinds of relationships street drinkers develop. Joining a bottle gang typifies instrumental relationships, usually short-term. Sleeping outdoors for mutual protection against predators or police exemplifies relationships that are both long-term and social-emotional.

In either case, Austin street drinkers were much older than the other street people and had a more extensive range of acquaintances. They were more apt to accept their identity as street people, less apt to take a job with the Salvation Army. Such a job would have put them in a position of authority over people with whom they had only recently been companions in misery. Thus, despite the fact that over the years they have become more dependent on alcohol, unlike the other social types, regular guys become more rather than less dependent on other regular guys. And so, whether patients, inmates, or residents, they continue to orient themselves to the world from the perspective of street people. Such ties as they do develop are primarily with their associates rather than with any of the agencies that service, control, or treat homeless alcoholics.

The Mixer

Mixers, for the most part, are people whose problem drinking and entry into homelessness both occurred much later in their life cycle. Drastic upsets, such as loss of a job, death of a spouse, physical disability, or severe illness trigger descent into home-lessness. Binge drinking, a frequent concomitant of these personal disasters, only speeds up a person's drop in status. The rapidity of the status fall precipitates culture shock. Mixers compare their situation in the immediate present with where they were and what they were just the day before, as it were. The suddenness of their change in status creates the juxtaposition of perspectives that makes them mixers.

Regular guys, for example, have had a rather lengthy and gradual introduction to the folkways of homelessness. In addition, they are much more likely to have a larger number of people in the same situation teaching by instruction or by example on how to "get by," how to "make it." Mixers, by contrast, see little similarity between themselves and the other passengers in the boat.

Mixers feel that they have "known something better." And there is something they want to get back to along with something they very much wish to avoid, namely falling any further down. The contrast between where they now are and where they would very much like to return to has caused numerous students of alcoholism to mark mixers as perhaps the best candidates for exiting homelessness by way of alcoholism rehabil-itation (Henderson, 1954).

Miles (Cohen & Sokolovsky, 1989) became one of the chief fry cooks in a New York seafood restaurant. By his late forties, he had an apartment in the Bronx and was living with a woman who worked for the electric company. In 1972, he had several heart attacks and the restaurant closed. Without a job and in poor health, he went on a series of periodic drunks. He lost his apartment and then began moving from one SRO hotel to another. Then he began taking day labor jobs, working summer resorts, and drinking more in the winter, a pattern common to older homeless men. He also began to spend more time in shelters for older men such as Camp La Guardia in upstate New York.

His last stay at Camp La Guardia precipitated a crisis. A man named Paco befriended him, saying he could help him get an apartment in the Bronx. Back in New York, Miles cashed his Social Security check, paid off some loans, and went to meet Paco. Paco promptly hit him over the head with a bottle and relieved him of the remaining $350. Miles had told social workers some time before this that "I refuse to sleep on the Bowery." Despite his long period of homelessness he had only slept twice on the Bowery. He also refused to panhandle. He avoided the Men's Shelter on the Bowery because the last time he had gone there for assistance, a drug addict had assaulted him. Before when "carrying the stick" (walking the streets all night), he had slept alone. After Paco's assault, he joined three other older men who slept together in a park just off the Bowery. One of the men introduced him to redeeming discarded and empty soda cans.

Now 63, Miles joined these three other older black men to drink together in the evening after their daily pursuits and to protect each other from the "hawks" (younger black men who prey on older men). Thus, rather rapidly, Miles had learned some of the basic survival strategies of older men while at the same time orienting himself to finding work again as a fry cook. He had now entered that phase of his career as a mixer, one who is reluctantly adapting to the realities of his present situation with the aid of associates while at the same time looking to return to his prior status as an independent and self-sustaining adult.

CONTINGENCIES IN HOMELESS ALCOHOLIC CAREERS

Mixers, company men, regular guys, and loners adapt to the exigencies of their situation by differential reliance on alcohol, associates, and agencies. How they manage their later career problems and whether they exit the career varies with their style of coping. In the later stages of their careers they manage drinking problems by resignation, cessation, or cycling. Those who continue to drink define themselves as "hopeless cases." Those who stop drinking literally "burn out" (they believe that their bodies can no longer take it), and stop on their own or with some kind of treatment. Those who cycle plan for intervals of sobriety between drinking bouts.

Elderly homeless alcoholics learn how to deal with their problems. How they define and respond to those problems depends heavily on how they have learned to cope. The point at which they became problem drinkers and homeless persons shapes their chances of becoming mixers, company men, regular guys, or loners. All four of these coping strategies can lead to being homeless alcoholics. They also indicate degrees of involvement with homeless alcoholic subculture.

Homeless alcoholic subculture provides an ideology for interpreting experiences with alcohol, rules for dealing with associates as well as agencies, skills for solving the dual problems of homelessness and alcoholism, and self-definitions that avert or mititage societal rejection. Over the past 100 years there have been changes in both the circumstances and the social definitions of homelessness. Changes in the economy, in ecology, and in agency policies toward homeless alcoholics became major contingencies influencing how homeless alcoholics managed their later career problems. These changes made significant differences in the size of homeless alcoholic populations, the character of their settlements, and how agencies of social control defined and responded to them. The size and characteristics of the pool of potential associates in homeless living along with the ratio of control agencies (criminal justice, service, and treatment) bear heavily on the extent and degree to which they adopted roles as mixers, company men, regular guys, or loners.

Four periods in U.S. history (1893–1920, 1920–1945, 1945–1970, and 1970–1993) show how changes in economy, ecology, and policies influenced both the pool of potential associates and the ratio of criminal justice, service, and treatment agencies. These changes altered the situation of homelessness, the numbers and kinds of recruits to homeless living, and the kinds of responses to that situation that homeless subculture afforded.

In the 1893–1920 period, railroads aided development of the manufacturing economy. Unattached young men ("hobos") rode trains illegally in order to work on the country's frontiers. They harvested crops, cut timber, and laid railroad track. During the off season, they "wintered over" in densely populated bachelor neighborhoods. They worked hard, they played hard, and they drank hard. And they sought to distinguish themselves from "tramps" who traveled but didn't work, and "bums" who neither traveled nor worked. Most people lumped all three types into the feared and hated "tramp" category. Criminal justice agencies came into the most frequent and repressive contact with homeless men during this period. Frequent exposure to repression alienated homeless men from conventional society at the same time that it solidified their ties to one another. These experiences at work, in jails, and in drinking situations established and sustained the basic components of the homeless alcoholic subculture.

Though hobos in time could descend in this social system to the level of tramps, later of bums, through combinations of disaster, disability, and drinking, few of them saw alcoholism as a kind of illness. The main treatment for alcoholism in homeless men's quarters came infrequently to a tiny minority through religious redemption in Skid Row rescue missions.

In the 1920–1945 period the demand for migratory workers declined. Mechanization of agriculture reduced the need for hobos at the same time that further development of manufacturing stimulated demand for an urban, unskilled casual labor supply. Resident working men ("home guards") supplanted hobos in the homeless men's neighborhoods. They moved into bachelor living arrangements (rooming houses, working men's hotels, cage hotels with cubicles and dormitories) in many large and middle-sized cities. The depression of the 1930s sent thousands of unemployed men to these same neighborhoods. Cities responded by building municipal lodging houses to accommodate the hordes of unemployed men, single and married alike, who were looking for work. Sutherland and Locke (1936) described the influx as the "new homeless" and coined the term "shelterization" to describe the process whereby despondent men adopted the drinking practices of the traditional homeless. If some unemployed men brought their alcoholism with them as they migrated to the shelters, others came by it in time through adoption of the heavy-drinking norms of homeless men. In large and middle-sized cities these service agencies outnumbered police and treatment responses. In smaller cities and rural areas unemployed homeless men looking for work were regarded as vagrants or tramps and were treated harshly by police.

The post-war period, 1945–1970, contains some paradoxes. Post-war prosperity along with welfare state entitlements reduced population density in traditional homeless men's areas. At the same time, the sight of numerous drunken men on Skid Row streets spread the stereotype of the alcoholic as derelict. The young alcoholism movement, seeking to break down this negative stereotype, showed that most male alcoholics in treatment had homes, wives, families, and jobs (Straus & Bacon, 1951). Demographic research, financed by urban renewal movements, refuted the derelict stereotype with its findings that one-third of Skid Row residents were abstainers and that only one-third were chronic alcoholics (Caplow, Lovald, & Wallace, 1958; Temple University, 1960; Bogue, 1963). Ethnographic research showed both social organization as well as variation among types of drinkers in the homeless world (Straus & McCarthy, 1951; Jackson & Connor, 1953; Peterson & Maxwell, 1958; Rooney, 1961; Wallace, 1965; Rubington, 1962, 1968). In 1950, the Salvation Army added professional alcoholism rehabilitation to its many Men's Service Centers across the country (McKinley, 1980) and a variety of counseling and treatment services for homeless alcoholics appeared. Though there was a slight increase in treatment facilities, service agencies remained fairly constant. By contrast, arrests for public drunkenness continued to mount as the criminal justice response to homeless alcoholics peaked.

The economic, ecological, and social policy changes of the 1970–1993 period altered the characteristics of homeless alcoholics, their participation in homeless alcoholic subculture, their contacts with agencies of social control, and their later careers. The shift from a predominantly manufacturing economy to a service economy further reduced the need for unskilled manual labor. Declining demand for unskilled labor coupled with gentrification changed the ecology of numerous cities. As condominiums replaced such low-cost housing as SRO hotels, homeless men's areas began to disappear entirely or shrink in size, with residents dispersing to smaller pockets elsewhere in the city (Miller, 1982). Researchers had all ready begun to note in the late 1960s not only the gradual disappearance of Skid Row but also a change in the age and ethnic status of new migrants (Bahr, 1967; Rubington, 1971). Unemployed young blacks, some of them drug addicts, took up residence in places like New York's Bowery. These migrants to homeless areas did not adopt any of the traditional and accepted ways of the older men's homeless subculture. Their appearance increased the level of risk and apprehension (as Miles pointed out) and caused many older residents to move out.

Concurrently, passage of the Hughes bill in 1970 mandated official change in the definition of alcoholism. *Hughes* specified that alcoholics were now to be seen as sick people, as the alcoholism movement had long argued (Anderson, 1942). The bill (*Alcohol and Health*, 1973) marked the beginnings of a revolution in the definition of and responses to alcoholics. Public drunkenness, long defined as a crime, was now to be seen as the symptom of an illness called alcoholism. The bill established the National Institute on Alcoholism and Alcohol Abuse and gave vast sums of money to the 50 states for research, education, and treatment of alcoholism. Some 35 states adopted the provisions of the Model Alcohol and Intoxication Control act. All of them decriminalized public drunkenness. Many of them also established detoxification centers and a network of comprehensive alcoholism treatment services. The Act's drafters saw detox not only as the replacement for the drunk tank but as the agency that would become the entry point into recovery from alcoholism for the typical chronic drunkenness offender.

Federal monies, third-party payments for treatment, and growing acceptance of the disease concept of alcoholism simply spurred further growth in the national network of alcoholism treatment services, private as well as public. Homeless alcoholics had always made their own use of the circuit of agencies in their areas that either serviced, treated, or incarcerated them. *Hughes* simply expanded both agencies and circuits.

The 1980s brought recession, cutbacks in social services, further depletion of low-cost housing stock, and the rediscovery of the homelessness problem. The "new homeless," consisting of deinstitutionalized mental patients, drug addicts, runaway youth, whole families, and single-parent mothers now joined with the "traditional" homeless (alcoholics) to constitute a population estimated to be anywhere from 250,000 to 3,000,000 (Rossi, 1988). As during the depression of the 1930s, shelters and soup kitchens once again sprang up across the country. In 1988 Congress passed the McKinney Act which disbursed millions of dollars to the cities to aid the homeless. Since experts had estimated that substance abusers constituted anywhere from 30% to 50% of the homeless, a diverse set of agencies came into being to aid homeless alcoholics. In addition to detox centers and residential treatment centers like halfway houses, some of the agencies offered a variety of specialized services to homeless alcoholics such as drop-in centers, sobering-up stations, storefront counseling, "wet" hotels, and alcohol-free residences (Rubington, 1986; Schutt & Garrett, 1992; Argeriou & McCarty, 1990).

Despite considerable regional variation, decreases in public drunkenness went along with increased expansion of agencies now servicing homeless alcoholics. In 1965 there were approximately 2 million arrests for public drunkenness; in 1989, drunkenness arrests had dropped to 822,500 (Collins, 1991). The decrease was very likely a combination of decreased prevalence (attrition in the ranks of the homeless alcoholics), shifts in police policies, and increased tolerance for drunkenness. Thus, in some areas where criminal justice agencies focused attention elsewhere, agencies that either serviced or treated homeless alcoholics multiplied. In previous periods, police agency responses outnumbered service or treatment responses. During that time, the ratio of agencies as well as the sheer frequency of contacts favored criminal justice over service or treatment responses. At the present time, in many urban areas there has been an expansion of service and treatment agencies for homeless alcoholics. Thus, a smaller number of homeless alcoholics are now making both more extended as well as more frequent use of the variety of agencies that the alcoholism and the homelessness movements have brought into being. What was a "revolving door" jail before *Hughes* (Pittman & Gordon, 1958) has become a "spinning door" detox after *Hughes* (Room, 1976; Fagan & Mauss, 1978).

MANAGING THE LATER STAGES OF THE CAREER

As homeless alcoholics age, they respond to their situation much as aging people generally do. As the circle of acquaintance diminishes over time, the frequency, intensity, and variety of their contacts with a smaller social circle increases. Outsiders have always commented that relations among homeless alcoholics are generally transitory, superficial, and short-lived. Similarly, outsiders also contend that their relations are primarily instrumental, materialistic, and heavily focused on their immediate, short-term, yet pressing needs. But, of course, these are characteristically the universal responses of people with few resources.

Nonetheless, as Cohen and Sokolvsky (1989) show, Bowery men like others divide up categories of people with whom they come into contact as friends, associates, and acquaintances. They further distinguish three networks of social exchange: one pattern when parties to the relationship are alternately givers and takers, one where they are predominantly givers, and a third where they are predominantly takers. This network is probably composed of regular guys, based as it is on a nexus of social exchange. By contrast, most exchanges taking place when one of the parties is an older "loner" are more apt to be based solely on a cash nexus.

The ethic of reciprocity, a cardinal norm among homeless alcoholics, centers more and more, as they age, around all of the contingencies of drinking such as obtaining alcohol, consuming it, and then handling the effects of overconsumption. Despite their frequent contact with agencies, whether voluntary or involuntary, regular guys distrust agencies, seek to keep their distance from them whenever possible, and look to each other for assistance of one kind or another. Building trust in caregivers takes considerable time. As one recent study shows, compared with social service referrals to a drop-in center, police referrals were less apt to use the services of the center and less apt to accept center referrals for continued treatment (Bonham, 1992).

Assistance from associates generally includes watching out for a drinking partner who has become intoxicated, helping others through withdrawal distress (getting drinks for them when they are "rum-sick"), getting them out of harm's way, taking them to detox, removing them from the streets so they won't get arrested, and sometimes placing them in the streets so police will arrest them (another way of obtaining shelter, treatment, or medical attention).

Like so many Americans, old or young, a streak of independence exists among regular guys. This lends itself to one typical outcome of homeless alcoholic careers: resignation. Untold members of older homeless men who have not come to the attention of agencies (as well as many who have) have accepted their lot. Eschewing assistance, they prefer to go on drinking until they die from any of the complications of alcoholism, or the assorted health hazards of homeless living, such as death from chronic diseases, accidents, exposure, or violence. It is a moot question whether the population of homeless alcoholics is getting smaller while the percentage of the elderly among them is increasing. But if this should turn out to be the case, then it may well be because of increased medical services available to homeless alcoholics in detox as well as elsewhere and the additional possibility that the disease concept of alcoholism has begun to make some inroads among this category of hard-line disbelievers.

Spontaneous as well as social recoveries from alcoholism do occur among segments of the homeless alcoholic population. While some unknown number change drinking patterns, still others may go on to either maintain or regain control over their drinking. Some may even "mature out" of their alcoholism. Among abstainers in his sample, Bogue (1963) found that 60% had stopped drinking on their own, that 15% stopped drinking after being sick, and that the remaining 25% sobered up after joining AA or having some kind of medical of psychological treatment. Both Grady and Marilyn Fish, aforementioned prototypes of "company man" and "regular guy" respectively, both regained their sobriety after treatment for tuberculosis. Cohen and Sokolovsky (1989:101) report a most unusual spontaneous recovery. Ronnie "simply decided that life on the street as a drunk was too dangerous." He got tired of losing all of his money either from going on month-long drinking binges or being robbed in his hotel. So he broke all of his wine bottles, went through a week of withdrawal in his cage hotel room. Once sober, he left. And for the next 10 years Ronnie never stayed in a Bowery hotel again. He slept only in secret places he had found elsewhere in the city. But he continued to work on the Bowery as a runner, getting anything older men in the hotels needed except alcoholic beverages. Where Bogue's abstainers renounced alcoholism while continuing to live in the traditional homeless men's area, Ronnie gave up drinking but stayed homeless off Skid Row.

Wiseman (1970) said there are only three ways of leaving Skid Row: death, forming a relationship with a woman, or becoming a worker in an alcoholic rehabilitation agency. Since regular guys have the closest ties along with the longest involvement with homeless living, they stand the slimmest chances of getting off Skid Row. But once again, this may well change when the specific situation in which they find themselves gets taken into account. In homeless men's habitats where demands for casual labor still exist (as in many of the western and southwestern states) and where homeless men's habitats have reputations for violence as well as overexposure to repressive police practices, only the hardiest of homeless alcoholics will survive in these circumstances.

By way of contrast, in northeastern sections of the country where a variety of rehabilitative agencies have come into being, a rather slow process of resocialization may take place among older regular guys. When some of their associates die or leave the scene for one reason or another and their own contact with help agencies begins to increase, some slow changes in their way of life may take place. Sadd (1985), for example, reports how some older homeless alcoholics who continued to return to social detox begin to regard the place as a home and to look upon some of the staff members as significant others.

There are two conceivable outcomes for those clients who develop these attachments over time. First, the staff becomes greatly concerned about the various health problems of the client. Second, they begin to encourage the client to adopt their definition of the client's situation rather than the way the client's former associates would have defined it. A consequence of some of these instances is the gradual "maturing out" of alcoholism. Slowly, over time they increase the length of time between drinking bouts while they shorten the duration of drinking bouts (reverse tolerance aids the staff cause here). And, most importantly, they come to regard the aftermath of drinking bouts as unnecessary and avoidable suffering rather than the price one pays for self-indulgence.

To the extent that the agency circuit has expanded, homeless alcoholics will continue to use agencies for their immediate rather than the agency's long-range purposes. Just as they have in the past learned how to "do time" in jails and other correctional institutions, they have already learned how to comport themselves when they are clients of detoxification centers (Rubington, 1991) as well as some of the newer agencies. Thus, a dwindling supply of regular guys will make up the bulk of those clients who return regularly to detox, ostensibly for treatment, but actually for shelter (Finn, 1985; Rodin, Pickup, Morton, & Keatinge, 1986).

Company men and mixers stand to profit most from their use of detoxification services, if only because they are very recent and reluctant entrants into homelessness and because their contact with other homeless alcoholics is either sparse, unrewarding, or both. As a consequence, they are and will be in a much better position to adopt, in time, the staff's definition of their drinking problem and the best ways of dealing with it.

Several researchers have called into question the view, held largely by Skid Row ethnographers, that alcoholism follows rather than precedes homelessness (Cohen & Sokolovsky, 1989). Similarly, other researchers have found that shelter residents became alcoholics before they became homeless (Welte & Barnes, 1992). And still others argue that the most frequent and most difficult alcoholic cases are the essential alcoholics (Zucker, 1987). Considerable evidence seems to be emerging that suggests that a larger proportion of alcoholics will be coming from these sources. If there is a shift and loners come to predominate in the population of homeless alcoholics, then the prospects for long-term sober treatment outcomes seem rather dim.

SUGGESTIONS FOR FUTURE RESEARCH

The term *career* implies that at different points in time changes of various kinds may be regularly anticipated. This chapter has argued that homeless alcoholics adopt one of four strategies to cope with the stresses of homelessness and alcoholism. As they age and as their dependence on alcohol increases, mixers, company men, regular guys, and loners fashion four different patterns of reliance on associations with other homeless alcoholics and on agencies of social control. These patterns ought to result in observable differences and results. What follows below are a few suggestions on how to discover these patterns and note what differences, if any, they may make.

A longitudinal study of clients' contacts with agencies puts this chapter's argument to the test. The development of management information system forms now in use in many agencies makes it possible to track clients of service and treatment agencies. Thus, a longitudinal study draws three cohorts of detox clients, men in their forties, fifties, and sixties. Researchers then contact clients in the three cohorts, interview them, and establish whether they are mixers, company men, regular guys, or loners. On the anniversary of clients' entries into the study, researchers check the frequency and variety of agency contacts during the previous study year. This study makes it possible to classify the kinds of agency contacts and to establish the relationship of agency contacts and outcomes to social types.

A second study follows the example of the classic Skid Row ethnographies (Wallace, 1965; Spradley, 1970; Wiseman, 1970; Regier, 1979). A field worker conducts participant observation in a detox center. The principal goal of this research is to establish patterns of staff-client interaction and to ascertain the influence of the four social types on length of stay, type of discharge, and acceptance or rejection of post-detox referrals.

Two other studies concern termination of older homeless alcoholic careers. The first study compares death rates in three different cities according to the predominant kind of agency responding to homeless alcoholics. Death rates for the previous 10 years will be compared in all three cities. This study tests the hypothesis that social policy and death rates of homeless alcoholics are related: The more repressive the social policy, the younger the age at death, and the greater the number of deaths attributed to violence.

The second study seeks by means of snowball sampling to obtain a number of former homeless alcoholics who are over 50 and who have stopped drinking on their own (Tuchfield, 1981). The presumption here is that a considerable number of homeless alcoholics rarely if ever come to the attention of the three kinds of agencies. This study seeks to establish if there is a relationship between spontaneous recovery and social type.

SUMMARY AND CONCLUSIONS

For over 100 years people have paid a good deal of attention to unattached men who have lived outside the boundaries of conventionality. During that time, various studies have painted a picture of them that differs considerably from popular negative stereotypes. The social science portrait describes the situation they face and how they try to come to terms with it. These men face a set of problems in common. They devise collective solutions to the common problems of homelessness and alcoholism. How they rely on alcohol, other alcoholics, and social control agencies bears directly on how they pursue their careers as homeless alcoholics. As the pool of potential associates begins to shrink while treatment and service agencies begin to outnumber criminal justice responses, coping styles change. This chapter suggests that with the slow demise of the homeless alcoholic subculture, the number of regular guys in the ranks of homeless alcoholics will shrink. In the future, the ways of becoming and being a homeless alcoholic will also very likely change. If more routes out of both homelessness and alcoholism continue to open up, mixers and company men are much more apt to take them than loners.

References

Alcohol and Health. (1973). Report from the Secretary of Health, Education and Welfare. New York: Charles Scribner's Sons.

Anderson, D. (1942). Alcohol and public opinion. *Quarterly Journal of Studies on Alcohol, 3*, 392.

Anderson, N. (1923). *The hobo*. Chicago: University of Chicago Press.

Argeriou, M., & D. McCarty (Eds.). (1990). *Treating alcoholism and drug abuse among homeless men and women*. New York: Haworth Press, 1990.

Bacon, S. D. (1944). Inebriety, social integration and marriage. *Quarterly Journal of Studies on Alcohol, 5*, 86–125, 303–339.

Bahr, H. M. (1967). The gradual disappearance of skid row. *Social Problems, 15*, 41–45.

Blumberg, I., Hoffman, F. H., LoCicero, V. J., Niebuhr, H. Jr., Rooney, J. F., Shipley, T. E. Jr. (1961). The men on skid row: A study of Philadelphia's homeless man population. Lithographed. Philadelphia: Department of Psychiatry, Temple University School of Medicine, for the Greater Philadelphia Movement and the Redevelopment Authority of the City of Philadelphia.

Bogue, D. J. (1963). *Skid row in American cities*. Chicago: University of Chicago Press.

Bonham, G. S. (1992). Recruitment of homeless men with alcohol and drug problems into case management. *Alcoholism Treatment Quarterly, 9*, 57–77.

Caplow, T., K. A. Lovald, & S. E. Wallace. (1958). *A general report on the problem of relocating the population of the lower loop redevelopment area*. Minneapolis: Minneapolis Housing and Redevelopment Authority.

Cohen, C. I., & J. Sokolovsky. (1989). *Old men of the bowery*. New York: Guilford Press.

Collins, J. J. (1991). Drinking and violations of the criminal law. In D. J. Pittman & H. R. White (Eds.), *Society, Culture and Drinking Patterns Reexamined* (pp. 650–660). New Brunswick: Rutgers Center of Alcohol Studies.

Fagan, R. W., Jr., & A. L. Mauss. (1978). Padding the revolving door: An initial assessment of the Uniform Alcoholism and Intoxication Act in practice. *Social Problems, 26*, 232–247.

Finn, P. (1985). Decriminalization of public drunkenness: Response of the health care system. *Journal of Studies on Alcohol, 46*, 7–23.

Henderson, R. M. (1954). The skid row alcoholic. *Proceedings of the First Annual Alberta Conference on Alcohol Studies. August 30 September 2, p. 92*

Jackson, J. K., & Connor, R. (1953). The Skid Row Alcoholic. *Quarterly Journal of Studies on Alcohol, 14*, 468–486.

Knight, R. P. (1938). Psychoanalytic treatment in a sanatorium of chronic addiction to alcohol. *Journal of the American Medical Association, 111*, 1443–1448.

McKinley, E. H. (1980). *Marching to glory: The history of the Salvation Army in the United States of America 1880–1980*. New York: Harper & Row.

Miller, R. J. (1982). *The Demolition of Skid Row*. Lexington: Lexington Books.

Peterson, W. J., & Maxwell, M. A. (1958). The Skid Row "Wino." *Social Problems, 5*, 308–316.

Pittman, D. J., & C. W. Gordon. (1958). *The Revolving Door*. New Haven: Yale Center of Alcohol Studies.

Regier, M. C. (1979). *Social Policy in Action*. Lexington: D. C. Health.

Rodin, M. B., L. Pickup, D. R. Morton, & C. Keatinge. (1986). Gimme shelter: Perspectives on chronic inebriates in detoxification centers. In D. J. Strug, S. Priyadarsini, & M. M. Hyman, (Eds.), *Alcohol Interventions* (pp. 81–96). New York: Haworth Press.

Room, R. (1976). Comment on the Uniform Alcoholism and Intoxication Treatment Act. *Journal of Studies on Alcohol, 37*, 113–144.

Rooney, J. F. (1982). *Career patterns in Skid Row*. Unpublished paper.

Rooney, J. F. (1961). Group processes among Skid Row winos: A reevaluation of the undersocialization hypothesis. *Quarterly Journal of Studies on Alcohol, 22*, 444–460, 470.

Rossi, P. (1988). *Down and out in America: The origins of homelessness.* Chicago: University of Chicago Press.

Rubington, E. (1991). The chronic drunkenness offender: Before and after decriminalization. In D. J. Pittman & H. R. White (Eds.), *Society, culture and drinking patterns reexamined* (pp. 733–752). New Brunswick: Rutgers Center of Alcohol Studies.

Rubington, E. (1986). Staff culture and public detoxes. In D. J. Strug, S. Priyadarsini, & M. M. Hyman (Eds.), *Alcohol interventions* (pp. 97–128). New York: Haworth Press.

Rubington, E. (1971). The changing Skid Row scene. *Quarterly Journal of Studies on Alcohol, 32*, 123–135.

Rubington, E. (1968). The bottle gang. *Quarterly Journal of Studies on Alcohol, 29*, 943–955.

Rubington, E. (1964). Grady "Breaks Out." *Social Problems, 11*, 372–380.

Rubington, E. (1962). "Failure" as a heavy drinker: The case of the chronic drunkenness offender on Skid Row. In D. J. Pittman & C. R. Snyder (Eds.), *Society, culture and drinking patterns,* (pp. 146–153). New York: John Wiley.

Sadd, S. (1985). The revolving door revisited: Public inebriates' use of medical and nonmedical detoxification services in New York City. In F. D. Wittman (Ed.), *The homeless with alcohol-related problems* (pp. 12–16). Rockville, MD: U.S. Department of Health and Human Services.

Schutt, R. K., & G. R. Garrett. (1992). *Responding to the homeless: Policy and practice.* New York: Plenum Press.

Snow, D. A., & L. Anderson. (1993). *Down on their luck.* Berkeley: University of California Press.

Spradley, J. P. (1970). *You owe yourself a drunk.* Boston: Little Brown.

Straus, R. (1974). *Escape from custody.* New York: Harper & Row.

Straus, R. (1948). Some sociological concomitants of excessive drinking as revealed in the life history of an itinerant inebriate. *Quarterly Journal of Studies on Alcohol, 9*, 1–52.

Straus, R. (1946). Alcohol and the homeless man. *Quarterly Journal of Studies on Alcohol, 7*, 360–404.

Straus, R., & S. D. Bacon. (1951). Alcoholism and social stability. A study of occupational integration in 2,023 male clinic patients. *Quarterly Journal of Studies on Alcohol, 12*, 231–260.

Straus, R., & R. G. McCarthy. (1951). Nonaddictive pathological drinking patterns of homeless men. *Quarterly Journal of Studies on Alcohol, 12*, 601–611.

Sutherland, E. H., & H. J. Locke. (1936). *Twenty thousand homeless men.* Philadelphia: J. B. Lippincott.

Tuchfield, B. S. (1981). Spontaneous remission in alcoholics: Empirical observations and theoretical implications. *Journal of Studies on Alcohol, 42*, 626–641.

Wallace, S. E. (1965). *Skid Row as a way of life.* Ottowa Bedminster Press.

Welte, J. W., & G. M. Barnes. (1992). Drinking among homeless and marginally housed adults in New York state. *Journal of Studies on Alcohol, 53*, 303–315.

Wiseman, J. P. (1970). *Stations of the lost.* Englewood: Prentice-Hall.

Zucker, R. A. (1987). The four alcoholisms: A developmental account of the etiologic process. In *Nebraska Symposium on Motivation,* Vol. 34 (pp. 27–83). Lincoln: University of Nebraska Press.

19

Black and White Older Men:
Alcohol Use and Abuse

EDITH S. LISANSKY GOMBERG
AND BELINDA W. NELSON

BLACK MALE DRINKING

The criteria for heavy or abusive drinking vary from one epidemiological study to another and include quantity/frequency measures, alcohol-related problems, and diagnoses of alcohol abuse or dependence. Whatever the criteria, it is clear that the age trajectory for black heavy drinking is not the same as the age trajectory for white heavy drinking. As is shown in Table 19.1, white males show a peak of heavy, problematic drinking early in life, in late adolescence and in their twenties, and the percentage of heavy drinkers declines with each decade. Black males, on the other hand, show *less* heavy drinking than whites early in life, but the rate of heavy drinking peaks in midlife. Both Caetano (1984) with a sample from San Francisco, and Robins et al. (1988) with a national sample, report the peak of heavy male drinking to begin with black men in their thirties. In both of these studies, black men not only peak in heavy drinking from age 30 on, they also surpass white rates of heavy drinking from age 30 on. Herd (1990) reports the peak of heavy black male drinking as occurring in their thirties, but black men do not surpass the rates of heavy drinking of white men until they reach their fifties.

Among the elderly men 60 years of age and older, Herd (1990) and Robins et al. (1988) both report more alcohol disorder among black than among white elderly men. Although drinking patterns and amounts are reported as reasonably similar, black men report more alcohol-related problems than do white men (Wahrheit et al., 1989; Herd, 1994). A study conducted in the southern states (Blazer et al., 1987) found rural, middle aged black men to have higher rates of alcohol abuse and dependence than black or white urban men of the same age.

The clinical studies (Table 19.2) show little agreement: Some are comparisons of younger and older black alcoholic patients, some are black/white comparisons, and some are comparisons of white, Puerto Rican, and black alcoholics. The samples vary widely and include subjects drawn from hospitals, outpatient clinics, and substance abuse counseling centers. On one point, two studies report results that flatly disagree: One investigator reports earlier onset for black alcoholics (Viamontes & Powell, 1974),

Table 19.1. Studies of White/Black Males' Alcohol Use and Abuse: Epidemiological Studies

Authors	Age Group	Sample	Criteria: Heavy Drinking/Abuse	Results
Cahalan, Cisin, & Crossley, 1969	21–60+	National: white males = 1082, black males = 82	3+ drinks daily	"White and Negro men varied little in their rates of drinking." Heavy drinking: 22% of white men, 19% of black men
Klatsky, Friedman, Sieglaub, & Gerard, 1977	15–79	California HMO: white males = 34,360; black males = 5031	6–9 drinks daily	Heavy drinking: 4.2% of white men and 4.4% of black men. Men 60+: 3.8% of white men and 2.1% of black men
Lipscomb, Trocki, 1981	18–60+	California community study: black	Recent episode: mean = 12.1 drinks. Drinking consequences scale: 2.9	8% self-identified as problem drinkers. Those 60+: 55% abstainer, 26% infrequent, 17% frequent, and 3% heavy drinkers
Dunham, 1981	60+	Miami community study: 43 blacks	"alcohol-related illnesses and problems"	Higher rates of alcohol-related illnesses and problems: black drinkers over-represented
Caetano, 1984	18–59	California community study: whites = 1047; blacks = 468	5+ drinks at a sitting; once a week or more	Percent of frequent heavier drinkers *Whites* *Blacks* 18–29 29% 17% 30–39 15% 30% 40–49 17% 21% 50–59 16% 17%
Blazer, Crowell, & George, 1987	18–65+	Rural South community study: whites = 2399; blacks = 1395; (46% male)	DSM III criteria for alcohol abuse/dependence	Rural black men more likely to meet DSM III criteria than black urban or white urban men. Six months prevalence: 7.6% of rural whites and 21.5% of blacks in age group 45–64
Robins, Helzer, Pryzbeck, & Regier, 1988	18–60+	National ECA study (NIMH): white males = 2826; black males = 1547	Diagnostic Interview Schedule: diagnosis alcohol abuse or dependence	Rates of alcohol disorder (lifetime): *White* *Black* 18–29 29% 13% 30–59 24% 32% 60+ 13% 24%
Robins, 1989	18–60+	Same as above	Same as above	Lifetime prevalence of alcohol disorder: *White* *Black* under 45 32% 21% 45–59 22% 36% 60+ 17% 26%

Reference	Age	Sample	Definition	Findings
Warheit, Auth, & Black, 1989	18–50+	Florida community study: white males = 767; blacks = 296	Problem drinking: symptoms of excess/dependence, social consequences and physical health sequelae	For 60+ males: Daily use of alcohol: whites 2.0%; blacks: 4.1%. Alcohol dependence index: whites 1.95; blacks 3.26. Health problems: whites .23; blacks .62. Social consequences: whites .82; blacks 1.28
Molgaard, Nakamura, Stanford, Peddecord, & Morton, 1990		California community study: white males = 382; blacks = 299	"Severe" drinking: 2+ six-packs of beer and/or 8+ glasses of wine or liquor	"Severe" drinking: 10.0% of white males; 14.3% of black males under age 40. Over age 40: 8.8% of white males; 12.2% of black males
Herd, 1990	18–60+	National: white males = 743; black males = 723	Frequent heavier drinker: at least 5 drinks at a sitting, once a week or more	Frequent heavier drinking *White* *Black* 18–29 31% 16% 30–39 21% 17% 40–49 19% 14% 50–59 17% 20% 60+ 4% 5%
Herd, 1991	same	same	same	Relationship between alcohol-related problems and income. Whites: problems drop at middle income and increase at higher income levels. Blacks: as income increases, rate of problems decline
Herd, 1994	same	same	same	Black men experience higher rates of alcohol-related problems than white men despite similar rates of drinking and drunkenness
Williams & Debakey, 1992	18 and older	1983 and 1988 National Health Interview surveys. 1983: N = 22,418 1988: N = 43,800	Abstention, light, moderate, and heavier drinking. Heavier = 2 + drinks per day/ 14+ per week.	Both black and white respondents, both sexes, decreased in percentage of heavier drinkers but only among whites was there a complementary increase in percentage of abstainers
Welte & Barnes, 1992	18–50+	412 homeless and marginally housed adults. Blacks: 52% of sample.	Questions on frequency/quantity 5–11 drinks, (12+ a day); frequency of drunkenness; specific alcohol-related problems or signs of dependence	Heavy drinking higher among blacks than whites or Hispanics

Table 19.2. Studies of White/Black Males' Alcohol Use and Abuse: Clinical Studies

Authors	Age Group	Sample	Research Interest	Results
Viamontes & Powell, 1974	Mean age of black men = 37.0; Mean age of white men = 46.2	St. Louis hospital. N = 100 black, 100 white male patients	Demographics and drinking history	Blacks: earlier onset, younger at admission, significantly greater report of hallucinations/convulsions; no race difference in blackouts or DTs
Goldstein, Tarter, Shelly, Alterman, & Petrarulo, 1983	Mean age of black men = 41.9; white men = 45.5	Pittsburgh hospital. N = 22 white and 20 black patients	Do black alcoholics have a different response to withdrawal seizures in terms of cognitive and other neuropsychological deficits?	Black male inpatients with withdrawal seizures show more cognitive and neuropsychological impairment than white counterparts
Blum & Rosner, 1983	50 young alcoholics (20–49); 50 elderly (50–79)	New York hospital	Comparison of young/elderly alcoholics: personal, demographic and socioeconomic aspects.	Black alcoholics: 46% of younger group and 64% of elderly. Elderly: fewer single; more widowed. Younger: more appetite loss, hallucination, blackouts, and sleep difficulties
Combs-Orme, Taylor, & Eobins, 1985	1,289 black and white alcoholics, 40+	St. Louis hospital	Comparison of black/white mortality; occupational prestige	Mean age of whites at death: 53.7; of blacks: 46.9. Blacks also younger at admission. Blacks had significantly higher mortality in high-prestige occupation group
Edwards, 1985	50 males and 50 female alcoholics, 55 and older; 8 men, 9 women black	Florida counseling center case records; interview	Use of alcohol and other drugs	76% of black alcoholics report using other drugs; white alcoholics: 19%; blacks report slightly later onset
Fernandez-Pol, Bluestone, Missouri, Morales, & Mizruchi, 1986	183 black, 132 Puerto Rican patients in alcoholism treatment; mean age = 41.8	New York City hospital	Similarities and differences in drinking patterns of black and Hispanic inner-city alcoholics; Drinking History Questionnaire	Black men: less daily consumption, morning drinking; less shakes, blackouts, convulsions; and less alcohol-related marital difficulties than Puerto Rican male alcoholics

Fernandez-Pol, Bluestone, & Mizruchi, 1988	New York City general hospital	Substance abuse patterns of psychiatric patients	90 black and 81 Hispanic patients in a psychiatric unit	In order of frequency of reported abuse: cannabis, alcohol, amphetamines, cocaine, PCP, barbiturates, opioids, inhalants, hallucinogens; blacks more likely to use hallucinogens
Castaneda & Galanter, 1988	New York City hospital	Ethnic differences among detoxifying alcoholics in drinking practices, psychosocial variables, and cognitive impairment	29 black, 43 Hispanics; mean age = 40	Puerto Ricans, blacks, whites in order: more cognitive impairment, daily drinking, heaviest average amount drunk, unemployment, and lack of residence, (PR highest)
Miller & Miller, 1988	Baltimore hospital	Linkage of alcoholism to other disorders in black men	596 black patients: alcohol-related diagnosis	78% of male patients were alcohol-dependent; other diagnoses: gastritis, hepatitis, cirrhosis, pancreatitis; high incidence of hypertension
Robyak, Byers, & Prange, 1989	Florida hospital	Patterns of alcohol abuse; Alcohol Use Inventory	Mean age of 78 black alcoholics = 42.9; 78 white alcoholics = 42.8	White alcoholics: greater daily consumption; more perception of alcohol to relieve psychological distress as a consequence; blacks: alcohol as means of improving mental functioning; more serious psychoperceptual withdrawal symptoms
Kline, 1990	Five treatment facilities, Midwest residential facilities	Evaluation of race-moderated expectancy-drinking behavior associations	Mean age of 105 black alcoholics = 35.6; 70 white alcoholics = 37.4	Few race-specific expectancy-drinking behavior relations. Expectations: enhances sexuality, improves sociability, elevates mood, induces relaxation
Lee, Mavis, & Stoffelmayr, 1991	Michigan randomly selected state-supported substance abuse programs	"Problems-of-life": Do blacks show more severe life problems? Addiction Severity Index	Age range 18–45. Mean age of 227 blacks = 32.2; of 535 whites = 31.2	Youngest (18–29): fewer blacks in treatment; equal number in oldest group (45+). Blacks: greater problem severity in (a) employment support, (b) other drug use; no black/white difference in severity of medical problems

(continued)

Table 19.2. Studies of White/Black Males' Alcohol Use and Abuse: Clinical Studies (continued)

Authors	Age Group	Sample	Research Interest	Results
Buchsbaum, Buchanan, Lawton, & Schnoll, 1991	Age range 20–80. (66% female) 82% nonwhite	Virginia: medical school outpatient clinic	Alcohol use patterns in primary care population: Diagnostic Interview Schedule	Prevalence of alcohol abuse/dependence significantly greater in 3rd through 5th decade than later. More severe disorder than people in general population (ECA). Disorders diagnosed in 12% of patients; criteria for past disorder: 19%
Day, Blot, Austin, Bernstein, Greenberg, Preston-Martin, Schoenberg, Winn, McLaughlin, & Fraumeni, 1993	18–79, 871 whites, 194 blacks; oral cancer patients; controls = 979 whites, 203 blacks	Population based case-control study of oral cancer risk: four U.S. areas	Reasons for the higher incidence of oral cancer among blacks; examined known etiologic factors	Difference with respect to alcohol consumption, especially among current smokers, emerged as the most important explanatory variable. Increased risk for blacks linked to greater intake of liquor. Combined effects of very heavy smoking/ drinking increased odds ratio for blacks to 5 times that for whites

another reports later onset (Edwards, 1985). It should be noted that the former study was of all male subjects and the latter study included women alcoholics. Two studies agree that black alcoholics are younger at admission (Viamontes & Powell, 1974; Combs-Orme, Taylor, & Robins, 1985).

The higher mortality rate and younger age at death for black alcoholic men compared with white alcoholic men, reported by Combs-Orme, Taylor, and Robins (1985) is consistent with all the mortality data that show a shorter life expectancy for blacks in general. More symptoms of alcohol disorder and related illnesses are reported for black patients: hallucinations, convulsions (Viamontes & Powell, 1974) cognitive and neuropsychological impairment (Goldstein et al., 1983), blackouts, sleep difficulties (Blum & Rosner, 1983), gastritis, hepatitis, cirrhosis, pancreatitis (Miller & Miller, 1988), and oral cancer (Day et al., 1993). More use of drugs other than alcohol is reported among black patients (Edwards, 1985; Lee, Mavis, & Stoffelmayr, 1991). The various alcohol-related illnesses and symptoms reported by investigators suggest that when compared, black alcoholic men show more alcohol-related medical problems than do white alcoholic men.

Two trends in Table 19.2 are of interest. First, the age trajectory of black heavier drinking, suggested in the epidemiological studies discussed above, are supported by clinical report. Blum and Rosner (1983) report 46% of their younger alcoholic group and 64% of their elderly alcoholic group to be black. Lee, Mavis, and Stoffelmayr (1991) report fewer black men in treatment under the age of 30, but equal numbers of blacks and whites in the 45-and-over group. Buchsbaum et al. (1991) found highest prevalence of alcohol abuse and dependence to be, "significantly greater in the third through the fifth decade," in a primary health care population. The second trend, also in agreement with the epidemiological studies, is the report of more alcohol-related problems among blacks. In a number of different alcohol-related medical consequences of heavy drinking, black patients show a greater incidence; Lee, Mavis, and Stoffelmayr (1991) found greater severity among blacks in problems related to employment and to use of drugs other than alcohol.

A RECENT STUDY: BLACK/WHITE ELDERLY ALCOHOLICS

We interviewed 169 older men diagnosed as alcohol-abusing or alcohol-dependent. The group included both men in treatment facilities and men screened and diagnosed as alcoholics who were not in treatment; the majority were located in various community facilities including hospitals, outpatient clinics, and substance abuse facilities. In addition to community facilities, subjects were recruited from senior citizen housing, from newspaper advertising, from senior community centers, and from Alcoholics Anonymous. The duration of heavy or problem drinking varied among both the men in treatment and those not in treatment, but all who participated in the study reported drinking alcoholically during the last 12 months. All subjects were 55 or older.

Of the 169 men, 27 were black. While this is admittedly a small sample of black alcoholic men, it constitutes 16% of the subjects, a slightly higher proportion than the black percentage of the population in Michigan. Of the ten treatment centers from which subjects were recruited, half served a large urban area and half served surrounding suburban communities. Of the 169 respondents, three-quarters of the black men and 60% of the white men were currently in a treatment program. Interviews were conducted for almost half of the black men by black interviewers.

Measures

Preliminary screening was done with the Folstein Mini-Mental Status Examination (Folstein, Folstein, & McHugh, 1975), a brief medical and psychiatric history, and the CAGE (Ewing, 1984) and Michigan Alcoholism Screening Test (Seltzer, 1971). The study subjects were then administered a modified version of the Diagnostic Interview Schedule, Version III (Robins, et al., 1981), designed for epidemiological study of the general population, which queries about the lifetime occurrence ("Have you ever . . . ?") of psychiatric symptoms and the time of occurrence. A second interview, The Coping Strategies of Older People (MRC 2, 1990) was designed to collect information about life events, social supports, religious participation, health status, drinking history and practices, self-perception of the respondent's drinking severity, and alcohol-related consequences. A genogram classification based on questions from the Family Informant Schedule and Criteria (Mannuzza, Fyer, & Endicott, 1985) provided information about family drinking history.

Conferences with interviewers and data analysts produced two indices: an Alcohol Health Consequences Index (AHCI) and a Social-Community Consequences Index (SCCI). Both indices included items drawn from the respondent's medical history screening, the Diagnostic Interview Schedule, and MRC2 interview schedule responses.

Results

As shown in Table 19.3, the black alcoholic respondents were significantly younger, had lower occupational status and income, and were significantly more likely to be unemployed than the white alcoholic men. Marital patterns were very similar for black and white subjects, and it is of interest that when asked about family consequences of heavy drinking, there were very small, nonsignificant differences: A summary score of family consequences was 1.44 for the white subjects and 1.41 for the black subjects.

Drinking Behaviors

As shown in Table 19.4, drinking behaviors show similarities. Both whites and blacks began drinking at the same age and showed early symptoms of heavy or problem drinking in their mid to late twenties. There are some differences: The black alcoholic men report an average alcohol intake that is significantly higher than the white alcoholic men's report; lifetime daily drink average is 6.2 for the whites and 10.8 for the blacks. The black men not only consume more drinks, they show a marked preference for "hard" alcoholic beverages (distilled beverages with high alcohol content), while the white alcoholics divide evenly between a preference for "hard" beverages and beer. The two groups differ in sites of drinking: White alcoholics report most drinking in bars or at parties significantly more often than do black alcoholics, while black alco-

Table 19.3. Demographics of White and Black Elderly Alcoholics

	White (N = 142)	Black (N = 27)	p-value
Age	64.3	61.7	.05
	(55 to 84)	(55 to 77)	
Education	12.8 grade	10.4 grade	.001
Occupation status			
Semiskilled/unskilled, office/clerical	19.0%	59.3%	
Skilled	44.5%	33.3%	.001
Professional/business managerial	36.6%	7.4%	
Income level, annual			
Under $15,000	43%	78%	.002
Current employment status			
Working/laid off	24.6%	22.2%	
Retired	55.2%	33.3%	.039
Unemployed/looking for work	20.2%	44.4%	
Marital status			
Married	43.1%	40.7%	
Never married	7.3%	3.7%	n.s.
Separated/divorced/widowed	49.6%	55.5%	

holics are more likely to drink "on the street." Only 6% of the white alcoholics report drinking "on the street," but 30% of black alcoholics do.

Black alcoholic men also reported more use of drugs other than alcohol, as shown in Table 19.5. Almost 30% of black alcoholics report such usage compared with 9% of white alcoholics. Differences are also significant for self-reported drug dependence, and it is interesting that the black men report first symptomatic behavior of alcoholism at 28.5 years, and onset of drug dependence at 27 years. Queried about specific drugs, the white alcoholic males report significantly more use of prescribed psychoactive medications, possibly related to their greater access to medical care; the black alcoholics more often report use of heroin and/or cocaine.

Table 19.4. Characteristics of Drinking Behaviors

	White	Black	p-value
Positive family history	58.9%	48.2%	n.s.
Age of first drink	13.6 ± 4.6 yrs	13.8 ± 5.1 yrs	n.s.
Age of first symptom	25.6 ± 11.0 yrs	28.5 ± 13.7 yrs	n.s.
Duration of problem drinking	37.8 yrs	33.2 yrs	n.s.
Lifetime daily drink average	6.2 ± 4.2 drinks	10.8 ± 7.8 drinks	.013
Preferred beverage			
Soft: Wine or beer	45.7%	7.4%	
Hard: Scotch, Whiskey, Bourbon, or Vodka	40.1%	70.4%	.001
Other: Cordials, Aperitifs, or Cocktails	14.8%	22.2%	
Public Drinking	5.9%	29.6%	.001

Table 19.5. Drug Use Other Than Alcohol

	White (N = 142)	Black (N = 27)	p-value
Ever used drug other than alcohol	9.1%	29.6%	.003
Self-reported drug dependence	5.1%	26.1%	.001
Age at onset of drug dependence	40.4 ± 13.3	27.0 ± 12.1	.077
Age at most recent self-reported drug dependence	48.1 ± 9.0	52.3 ± 3.3	n.s.

Consequences of Heavy Drinking

Univariate differences between white and black elderly male alcoholics were examined for two classes of consequences: (a) alcohol health consequences, and (b) alcohol-related community consequences.

Alcohol Health Consequences Index

The index was comprised of 14 equally weighted items, selected from the medical history, the Diagnostic Interview Schedule, and the Coping Strategies of Older People. The items are listed in Table 19.6. Black men reported more frequent health consequences in 12 of the 14 items. White/black differences are statistically significant for items about the frequency of alcohol-related health problems, continued drinking despite knowledge of illness, feeling sick most of the time, dizziness even when not drinking, and unexplained bruises. The average score of the white alcoholics was 5.7 and for the black alcoholics 7.4, a significant difference. Alcohol-related health effects seemed more severe for the black men. Regression analyses to estimate predictor vari-

Table 19.6. Alcohol Health Consequences Index

	White	Black	p-value
Alcohol-related health problems	47.1%	69.6%	.046
Continued drinking w/knowledge	42.0%	74.0%	.005
Felt sick most time	17.6%	44.4%	.002
Dizzy w/o drinking	25.4%	48.2%	.017
Unexplained bruises	28.2%	55.6%	.005
Falls and hurt self	47.1%	55.5%	n.s.
Hospital emergency room	35.9%	51.8%	n.s.
Auto accidents	30.2%	33.3%	n.s.
Home accidents	30.2%	37.0%	n.s.
Appetite loss	47.9%	66.7%	n.s.
Talked to MD	71.1%	87.0%	n.s.
Hospitalized last 12 months	65.9%	61.5%	n.s.
Continued drinking w/injury	85.8%	94.4%	n.s.
Ever liver problems	30.5%	25.9%	n.s.
Average score	5.7	7.4	.023

Table 19.7. Regression Model—Health Consequences

	beta	S.E.	p-value
Education	−.25	.08	.003
Lifetime daily drink average	.16	.05	.003
Public drinking	1.72	.52	.001
Drug dependence	2.98	.94	.002
R-Square	.30		
Overall F	15.60		< .0001

ables were performed, and a number of variables (e.g., positive family history, preferred beverage, years of problem drinking) proved weak. Table 19.7 shows the model that was finally derived; the four variables listed are strong predictors: educational achievement, the lifetime daily drink average, drinking in public, and occurrence of drug dependence in addition to the alcoholism.

Alcohol-Related Social/Community Consequences Index

This index consists of nine items, equally weighted and selected from the Michigan Alcoholism Screening Test, the Diagnostic Interview Schedule, and the Coping Strategies of Older People, as shown in Table 19.8. The items deal with the community's response to the person's drinking and, to a limited extent, with the person's utilization of a community resource like a hospital emergency room. On all nine items, a larger proportion of black alcoholics report the social consequence, and on five of the items, the white black differences are significant. The summary score of community consequences was 3.26 for the white men and 4.37 for the black men, with a nonsignificant p value of .08. Regression analyses produced four solid predictors: educational achievement, the lifetime daily drink average, drinking in public, and race. It is of interest that three predictors work for both health and community consequences—educational achievement, the lifetime daily drink average, and the public versus the private nature of the drinking. That involvement with drugs other than alcohol may be associated with the health consequences of alcoholism makes sense; so does the visible difference in

Table 19.8. Social/Community Consequences of Alcoholism

	White (N = 142)	Black (N = 27)	p-value
Objections at work	27.5%	47.8%	.05
Lost a job	16.9%	33.3%	.048
Objections from friends	55.8%	78.3%	.043
Friends stopped visiting	14.8%	33.3%	.021
Fights while drinking	26.8%	34.8%	n.s.
Driving offenses	47.8%	65.2%	n.s.
Trouble with police	43.5%	65.2%	n.s.
Alcohol detox program	66.9%	86.4%	n.s.
Emergency room	35.9%	51.9%	n.s.
Summary score mean	3.26	4.37	n.s.

Table 19.9. Regression Model—Social/Community Consequences

Variable	Parameter Estimate	S.E.	F	Probability > F
Education	−.12	.06	4.15	.044
Lifetime daily drink average	.11	.04	8.76	.004
Public vs. private	1.24	.36	12.14	.001
Race	.97	.52	3.52	.063

R-square = .27
Overall F = 13.70
Probability > F = .0001

color, the factor of race that is associated with social consequences and the response of the community. These relationships are summarized in Table 19.9.

OTHER FINDINGS

Phasic Development of Alcoholism

The Diagnostic Interview Schedule includes questions about 20 alcohol-related behaviors and effects. With each question, the respondent is asked the approximate age at which the behavior or effect first occurred. From these responses it is possible to list, in consecutive order, the sequence of early and late indicators of alcohol-related difficulties. For the white older male alcoholics, early indicators were, in order:

1. Drank more than expected
2. Twenty drinks in one day
3. Increased chances of getting hurt
4. Drinking kept you from working/childcare
5. Couple of months with 7+ drinks daily
6. Tolerance change: drank more to get drunk

The black older male alcoholics reported the following early indicators:

1. Couple of months with 7+ drinks daily
2. Twenty drinks in one day
3. Increased chances of getting hurt
4. Two weeks with 7+ drinks a day
5. Tolerance change: drank more to get drunk
6. Drank more than expected.

The two lists of early indicators are quite similar, dealing largely with quantitative increase in the amounts of alcohol consumed. Both white and black older men mention tolerance change among early indicators. The white alcoholics do list as early indicators having their drinking interfere with work or domestic responsibilities; this is listed eighth by the black alcoholics.

The relationship between these two sets of rank orders is given by the Kendall coefficient of concordance, which equals 0.852. The p value of the coefficient is .028.

There is much similarity between the rank order of symptoms of the white and black older alcoholic men. The progression of alcohol-related behaviors is very similar. Interestingly, health problems are noted relatively late: 20th for the whites, 19th for the blacks.

Strength of Religious Beliefs

Although both groups of men report similar patterns of church attendance, there are suggestions that prayer and spirituality play a stronger role for the black men. In a list of ways of coping with daily hassles and annoyances (MRC 2, 1990), the men were asked whether they "pray for guidance and strength." Almost two-thirds of the black men responded that they did so very often; 39% of the white men responded the same way. A third of the white men, 30%, said they never prayed for guidance, compared with 7% of the black men. The p value of the chi-square calculated is .013. Another question in the Coping Strategies of Older People (MRC 2, 1990) asked about the importance of "religious or spiritual beliefs in your day-to-day life." Responses were:

	Whites	*Blacks*
Very important	44%	74%
Fairly/not too important	46%	26%
Not at all important	10%	0

The chi-square of this distribution yields a p value of .026. Both questions point to a white/black difference within these two groups of men, not so much in church participation or attendance but in the importance of religious or spiritual beliefs.

DISCUSSION

It is a cliché to say that more research is needed, but it is true of aging and alcohol use nonetheless. One neglected area of research is the study of the changes that occur in drinking during the life span. There is some interest in adolescents and patterns of change that occur when the young adult marries and/or gets a job. We also know that the percentage of people in the population who drink or who have alcohol-related problems diminishes as people age into their fifties, sixties, and seventies (Fillmore et al., 1991). In a society in which increasing numbers of people live into their seventies and eighties, we must ask who continues drinking, who starts drinking, and who drinks immoderately? Which are the patterns of good/poor adjustment of the aging process and what role does moderate alcohol consumption play in that adjustment? For that matter, which are the coping mechanisms that work best for the elderly, which worst? As is true with all other age groups, the patterns of use of alcohol, the social settings, and the attitudes and expectancies toward alcohol, can reveal a good deal about life style, adaptation, distress, and depression among older people.

There has been some comparison of drinking behaviors between white and black samples (Caetano, 1984; Caetano & Herd, 1988; Caetano, 1989; Herd, 1990; Herd, 1994). Caetano (1984) noted the different age trajectory of drinking among blacks and the different social contexts in which men drink (Caetano & Herd, 1988). Herd (1994) reported that black men experience higher rates of alcohol-related problems—which agrees with our findings. She also reported that ''rates of drinking and drunkenness are similar''—we have found higher consumption among the black elderly alcoholics. Herd (1994) concludes: ''Racial differences in the prevalence of drinking problems might be related to differences in the socio-cultural context of drinking and in the material conditions under which black and white men live'' (Herd, 1994, page 61). With this last statement, we concur. There are some reports about black drinking norms and their derivation (Herd, 1985) but there is much to learn about black views of drinking, and of aging.

Drinking. White male rates of heavy drinking peak in the age group 18 to 30 and decline slowly through the decades, but black male rates of heavy drinking do not follow the same age pattern. There are proportionately fewer heavy drinkers among black adolescents and young adults, and the rate rises in the thirties. Although both groups show precipitous declines in the percentage of heavy drinkers who are 60 and older, there are slightly more older black males who are heavy drinkers than older white males (Caetano, 1984; Robins et al., 1988; Herd, 1990). Several explanations have been offered that may account for the black heavy drinking age trajectory: (a) a historical explanation in terms of South-to-North migration; (b) a generational explanation defined in terms of access to the opportunity structure; (c) declining health status of black people at age 40 and older; (d) midlife crises and depression; (e) black cultural norms, which are more permissive about mature adult drinking than youthful drinking; (f) changes in religiosity. These hypothetical explanations have not been tested.

The clinical literature has some contradictory findings, and the samples of alcohol abusers studied are far from comparable in the different studies. By and large, however, the age trajectory suggested by the epidemiological literature is supported. A study of younger versus older alcoholics (Blum & Rosner, 1983) showed relatively fewer black alcoholics in the younger group, but blacks constitute two-thirds of the older group. Several clinical reports agree in showing a higher proportion of black alcoholics manifesting alcohol dependence symptoms, such as hallucinations and cognitive impairments, as well as alcohol-related illnesses like cirrhosis, pancreatitis, and gastritis. The findings of black ''greater problem severity'' occur in several studies; the alcohol-related problems reported by black subjects to a greater extent than white subjects include employment problems, illness, and the use of other drugs (see Table 19.2).

Reported here are the results of a recent comparison of elderly black and white male alcoholics. Despite the fact that the alcoholic men were often drawn from the same clinical settings, the demographics showed them to be significantly different in terms of education, occupation, income, and current employment status. The black respondents were somewhat younger; there were some white but no black respondents in their eighties. From the very small sample of 27 black men, some trends and hypotheses emerge, but future racial comparisons—particularly study of the consequences of chronic heavy drinking—need to be made by subjects matched at least for education, occupation, and income. This will help resolve the question of differences based on race or on socioeconomic status.

The present study suggests a number of questions.

1. Although our sample shows the black men to have a higher rate of consumption, different observations have been reported. It should be noted, however, that Herd's (1994) observation of the similarity of black/white subjects in "heavier drinking and drunkenness" was made on a general population sample and the subjects in the study reported here are diagnosable as alcoholic.

2. There are consistent reports that black men are more likely to drink in public places (parks, streets, parking lots, cars) than are white men (Caetano & Herd, 1988). The same is true for the subjects of the present study. It is not altogether clear what the implications of such public drinking are, but public drinking turns out in analysis to be a significant variable in both alcohol-related health problems and in community response to the men's drinking.

3. Consistently reported in the clinical literature and found here as well is more reported use of drugs other than alcohol by black elderly alcoholics as compared to white. To what extent this is related to street drinking per se and to greater availability of drugs is not clear.

4. The reported literature and the present study agree in showing greater alcohol-related medical and community consequences for black alcoholics in general and, in the present study, for black elderly alcoholics than for white. A recent study (Lee, Mavis, & Stoffelmayr, 1991) showed employment problems to be more severe among black alcoholics, and the present study included work-related difficulties in the community consequences index (see Table 19.8).

5. We found very little difference between white and black elderly alcoholics in reported phasic development of alcoholism. There was a good agreement as to what constituted earlier and later indicators of alcoholism.

6. There are suggestions in present findings that the strength of spirituality and religious beliefs may be greater for black older male alcoholics. If this proves to be true, it suggests a therapeutic approach that might be effective with black older problem drinkers. Those who write about treatment for black alcoholics often bring up the role of the clergy.

At this stage of knowledge, we know all too little about black problem drinking. We know all too little about the lives of older people and the choices they make about alcohol. To improve effectiveness as casefinders, diagnosticians, therapists, and preventers, we must expand our limited store of knowledge.

References

Blazer, D., Crowell, B. A., & George, L. K. (1987). Alcohol abuse and dependence in the rural South. *Archives of General Psychiatry, 44*, 736–740.

Blum, L. & Rosner, F. (1983). Alcoholism in the elderly: An analysis of 50 patients. *Journal of the National Medical Association, 75*, 489–495.

Buchsbaum, D. G., Buchanan, R. G., Lawton, M. J., & Schnoll, S. H. (1991). Alcohol consumption in a primary care population. *Alcohol and Alcoholism, 26*, 215–220.

Caetano, R. (1984). Ethnicity and drinking in northern California: A comparison among whites, blacks and Hispanics. *Alcohol and Alcoholism, 1*, 31–44.

Caetano, R. (1989) Concepts of alcoholism among whites, blacks and Hispanics in the United States. *Journal of Studies on Alcohol, 50*, 580–582.

Caetano, R., & Herd, D. (1988). Drinking in different social contexts among white, black and Hispanic men. *The Yale Journal of Biology and Medicine, 61*, 243–258.

Cahalan, D., Cisin, I. H., & Crossley, H. M. (1969). *American drinking practices*. New Brunswick, NJ: Rutgers Center of Alcohol Studies Publications Division.

Castaneda, R., & Galanter, M. (1988). Ethnic differences in drinking practices and cognitive impairment among detoxifying alcoholics. *Journal of Studies on Alcohol, 49*, 335–339.

Combs-Orme, T., Taylor, J. R., & Robins, L. N. (1985). Occupational prestige and morality in black and white alcoholics. *Journal of Studies on Alcohol, 46*, 443–446.

Day, G. L., Blot, W. J., Austin, D. F., Bernstein, L., Greenberg, R. S., Preston-Martin, S., Schoenberg, J. B., Winn, D. M., McLaughlin, J. K., & Fraumeni, J. F. (1993). Racial differences in risk of oral and pharyngeal cancer: Alcohol, tobacco, and other determinants. *Journal of the National Cancer Institute, 85*, 465–473.

Dunham, R. G. (1981). Aging and changing patterns of alcohol use. *Journal of Psychoactive Drugs, 13*, 143–151.

Edwards, D. W. (1985). An investigation of the use and abuse of alcohol and other drugs among 50 aged male alcoholics and 50 aged female alcoholics. *Journal of Alcohol and Drug Education, 30*, 24–30.

Ewing, J. A. (1984). Detecting alcoholism, the CAGE questionnaire. *Journal of the American Medical Association, 252*, 1905–1907.

Fernandez-Pol, B., Bluestone, H., Missouri, C., Morales, G., & Mizruchi, M. S. (1986). Drinking patterns of inner-city Black Americans and Puerto Ricans. *Journal of Studies on Alcohol, 47*, 156–160.

Fernandez-Pol, B., Bluestone, H., & Mizruchi, M. S. (1988). Inner-city substance abuse patterns: A study of psychiatric inpatients. *American Journal of Drug and Alcohol Abuse, 14*, 41–50.

Fillmore, K. M., Hartka, E., Johnstone, B. M., Leino, E. V., Motoyoshi, M., & Temple, M. T. (1991). The Collaborative Alcohol-Related Longitudinal Project. A meta-analysis of life course variation in drinking. *British Journal of Addiction, 86*, 1221–1268.

Folstein, M. F., Folstein, S. E., & McHugh, P. R. (1975). Mini-mental state: A practical method for grading the cognitive state of patients for the clinician. *Journal of Psychiatric Research, 12*, 189–198.

Goldstein, G., Tarter, R. E., Shelly, C., Alterman, A. I., & Petrarulo, E. (1983). Withdrawal seizures in black and white alcoholic patients: Intellectual and neuropsychological sequelae. *Drug and Alcohol Dependence, 12*, 349–354.

Herd, D. (1985). Ambiguity in black drinking norms: An ethnohistorical interpretation. In L. A. Bennett & G. M. Ames (Eds.), *The American experience with alcohol: Contrasting cultural perspectives* (pp. 149–170). New York: Plenum.

Herd, D. (1990). Subgroup differences in drinking patterns among black and white men: Results from a national survey. *Journal of Studies on Alcohol, 51*, 221–232.

Herd, D. (1991). Drinking patterns in the black population. In W. B. Clark & M. E. Hilton (Eds.), *Alcohol in America: Drinking practices and problems* (pp. 308–328). Albany, NY: SUNY Press.

Herd, D. (1994). Predicting drinking problems among black and white men: Results from a national survey. *Journal of Studies on Alcohol, 55*, 61–71.

Klatsky, A. L., Friedman, G. D., Siegelaub, A. B., & Gerard, M. J. (1977). Alcohol consumption among white, black, or Oriental men and women: Kaiser-Permanente Multiphasic Health Examination Data. *American Journal of Epidemiology, 105*, 311–323.

Kline, R. B. (1990). The relation of alcohol expectancies to drinking patterns among alcoholics: Generalization across gender and race. *Journal of Studies on Alcohol, 51*, 175–182.

Lee, J. A., Mavis, B. E., & Stoffelmayr, B. E. (1991). A comparison of problems-of-life for blacks and whites entering substance abuse treatment programs. *Journal of Psychoactive Drugs, 23*, 233–239.

Lipscomb, W. R., & Trocki, K. (1981). *Black drinking practices study report to the Department of Alcohol and Drug Programs*. Berkeley, CA: Source, Inc. Contract No. R-0034-9, A-2. 14 pp.

Mannuzza, S., Fyer, A. J., & Endicott, J. (1985). *Family Informant Schedule and Criteria (FISC)*. New York Anxiety Disorders Clinic, New York State Psychiatric Institute.

Miller, J. M., & Miller, J. M. (1988). Alcoholism in a black urban area. *Journal of the National Medical Association, 80*, 621–623.

Molgaard, C. A., Nakamura, C. M., Stanford, E. P., Peddecord, K. M., & Morton, D. J. (1990). Prevalence of alcohol consumption among older persons. *Journal of Community Health, 15*, 239–251.

MRC 2 interview schedule. *The Coping Strategies of Older People*. (1990). University of Michigan Alcohol Research Center, Ann Arbor, MI.

Robins, L. N. (1989). Alcohol abuse in blacks and whites as indicated in the Epidemiologic Catchment Area Program. In D. Spiegler. (Ed.), *Alcohol use among ethnic minorities* (pp. 63–74). Research Monograph No. 18, National Institute on Alcohol Abuse and Alcoholism, DHHS Publ. No. (ADM) 89-1436.

Robins, L. N., Helzer, J. E., Croughan, J., Williams, J. B. W., & Spitzer, R. I. (1981). *NIMH Diagnostic Interview Schedule, Version III* (May, 1981). Rockville, MD: National Institute of Mental Health.

Robins, L. N., Helzer, J. E., Przybeck, T. R., & Regier, D. A. (1988). Alcohol disorders in the community: A report from the Epidemiologic Catchment Area. In R. M. Rose & J. Barrett (Eds.), *Alcoholism: Origins and outcomes* (pp. 15–29). New York: Raven Press.

Robyak, J. E., Byers, P. H., & Prange, M. E. (1989). Patterns of alcohol abuse among black and white alcoholics. *The International Journal of the Addictions, 24*, 715–724.

Seltzer, M. L. (1971). The Michigan Alcoholism Screening Test: The quest for a new diagnostic instrument. *American Journal of Psychiatry, 127*, 1653–1658.

Viamontes, J. A., & Powell, B. J. (1974). Demographic characteristics of black and white male alcoholics. *The International Journal of the Addictions, 9*, 489–494.

Warheit, G. J., Auth, J. B., & Black, B. S. (1989). Alcohol behaviors among Southern blacks and whites: A comparative analysis. In D. Spiegler et al. (Eds.), *Alcohol use among ethnic minorities* (pp. 95–112). Research Monograph No. 18, National Institute on Alcohol Abuse and Alcoholism, DHHS Publication No. (ADM) 89-1436.

Welte, J. W., & Barnes, G. M. (1992). Drinking among homeless and marginally housed adults in New York State. *Journal of Studies on Alcohol, 53*, 303–315.

Williams, G. D., & Debakey, S. F. (1992). Changes in levels of alcohol consumption: United States, 1983–1988. *British Journal of Addiction, 87*, 643–648.

V

SUMMARY

20

Alcohol and Aging: Looking Ahead

THOMAS P. BERESFORD

A colleague who works mainly with youthful alcohol and drug abusing patients was conversing informally at a recent conference. Someone brought up the idea of alcohol abuse among elderly people. The colleague, a kind and very patient man who works with a difficult clinical population, responded, "There is no problem with elderly people. Alcohol and drug abuse are very infrequent in that age group."

Through the pages of this book, we hope the reader will have arrived at the conclusion that alcoholism, at least among older Americans, not only exists but is likely to become an increasingly more frequent health problem over the coming decades. There is no doubt that alcohol-use problems in late life have been infrequently recognized, in part because of a spuriously low frequency of alcoholism among the current elderly age cohort, but also because of the nature of alcoholism itself. It is a subtle illness that can mimic many other conditions, such as depression or anxiety disorders, that carry less social disapproval and the possibility of specific pharmacologic treatment.

Alcoholism generally, like the neutrino in particle physics, is designed not to be caught in any but the most specifically designed screening and diagnostic stratagems and by an interviewer or clinician who is dedicated to establishing the diagnosis. Alcoholism among the elderly is doubly subtle because it is more easily hidden, existing in a quieter style of living among people who remind most clinicians of a parent or a grandparent. A recent Australian study, for example, found that only about one-third of alcohol abusing, hospitalized, elderly patients were recognized by the medical staff (McInnes & Powell, 1994), a corroboration of similar data from this country (Geller et al, 1989).

PHENOMENOLOGY

But if recognition has been difficult in the past, it is good to know that we are learning more about how and where to look for alcoholism as it presents among our older population. The stereotype of an elderly, male denizen of barrooms and park benches is coming more and more to be recognized as just that. As data from the Environmental

Table 20.1. Putative Characteristics of Late Onset Problem Drinkers

Higher socioeconomic status (Glynn et al., 1988; Atkinson, 1990)
Married (Glynn et al., 1988)
Stressful life events trigger drinking increase (Finlayson et al., 1988; Wells et al., 1983
May affect women more frequently than men (Holzer et al., 1984)
May affect minorities more frequently (Gomberg, 1994)
May be related to social pressure among some elderly (Atkinson et al., 1990)
Better prognosis compared to early onset (Moos et al., 1991)
Lower frequency of family positive alcohol histories (Atkinson, 1990)
May have a more severe withdrawal syndrome than younger drinkers of similar alcohol exposure (Alling et al., 1982)
Problem drinking begins in late life (Atkinson et al., 1990; Eaton et al., 1989; Moos et al., 1991)

Catchment Area (ECA) study indicates, the predominant elderly alcoholic remains a male with a long history of drinking, but elderly women may be represented more than was previously thought. Studies of clinical populations, such as Gomberg's work (Gomberg, 1994) and that of Wilsnack and colleagues in this volume, suggest that women may be more vulnerable to beginning alcohol use problems in middle age than are their male counterparts, and that this vulnerability may continue into old age. Improving recognition patterns and providing specific therapy is a task for the near future.

Similarly, it is clear that recent-onset drinkers in late life are a common reality, not a highly unusual or infrequent aberration (Table 20.1). Clinical studies note a relationship between recent-onset alcohol problems and economic well-being, a phenomenon seen in the ECA surveys (Holzer et al., 1984; Eaton et al., 1989) that found a positive relationship between income and drinking in middle and old age.

Gomberg's data suggests, in addition, that elderly minority group members appear more vulnerable to late-life drinking than previous considerations allowed, especially in beginning and sustaining problematic alcohol use in middle and late age. Information such as this suggests that prevention methods may be productively aimed at the elderly members of special populations as well as at the young.

Finally, it is becoming more clear that an elderly alcoholic's presentation to one or another health care system or treatment facility may relate to length and severity of alcohol use, in part because of the presence or lack of economic resources lost as uncontrolled drinking progresses. This recognition can lead to better assessments of prognostic indicators that may, in turn, guide the design of appropriate treatment programs specific to patient needs.

CLINICAL DATA

Age-specific clinical phenomenology reflects, in part, an altered pharmacology of ethanol among elderly persons. But knowledge of both the normal and the toxic effects of ethanol among the elderly is still in an early state (Table 20.2). There is a clear need to establish dose-related, objective measures of intoxication among nonalcoholic elderly subjects and then to apply these to their alcoholic counterparts as a way of investigating the interactions between age and chronic, heavy alcohol use.

Similarly, alcoholism mimics an array of comorbid conditions that pose difficult diagnostic questions in this age group. As one example, the distinction between alco-

Table 20.2. Human Studies on Alcoholism and Aging

Affected by ethanol

Performance impaired among older pilots (Morrow et al., 1990)

Lessened cognitive abilities compared to non-alcoholics (Schuckit, 1982)

Stress results in increased drinking in elderly drivers (Wells et al., 1983)

Association with decreased bone mineral density in older women (Laitinen et al., 1991) and in older alcoholic men (Karantanas et al., 1991)

Normalizing of pattern reversal visual evoked potentials slowed or lost in elderly in withdrawal (Kelley et al., 1984)

Large muscle group impairment in old alcoholics only (Pendergast et al., 1990)

Altered T-1 relaxation (MR) during withdrawal related to age (Agartz et al., 1991)

Increased cerebral atrophy and increased hypointense lesions related to alcohol use associated with increased age (Hayakawa et al., 1992)

Decreased hippocampal muscarinic receptors in older alcoholics only (Hughes & Davis, 1983)

Decreased putamen muscarinic receptors in alcoholic brains; little age effect (Freund & Ballinger, 1989a)

Decreased hippocampal muscarinic and benzodiazepine receptors in alcoholic brains; little age effect (Freund & Ballinger, 1989b)

Decreased 5-HT receptor density in cortex, hippocampus, and raphe nuclei in alcoholics related to age (Dillon et al., 1991)

Unaffected by ethanol

Age-related decrease in male hormone production (Simon et al., 1992)

Relationship between MR scan changes and alcohol in elderly women (Kroft et al., 1991)

Change in stomach/duodenum prostaglandin concentration (Cryer, Lee, & Feldman, 1992)

Putamen benzodiazepine receptor density in alcoholic brains (Freund & Ballinger, 1989a)

---

holism and major depressive disorder is presently based on the clinical history alone. Alcoholism can simulate the characteristic helplessness-hopelessness-worthlessness disorder of mood along with the "biologic symptoms" of major depressive disorder such as terminal insomnia and morning depression. Although sleep studies once held out hope as a useful marker that could differentiate the two conditions, present knowledge still lacks an adequate, objectively derived biologic indicator of alcoholism versus depression in late life.

Old age brings with it increasing physical infirmity and lessened resiliency in response to toxic insults or other injuries. This results in higher frequencies of medication use among older persons than among any other age group. Because of this, elderly persons, with or without alcohol dependence, are at a higher risk of experiencing the dangers of drug interactions with alcohol. While this risk is well known among most clinicians, the interrelationship of alcohol use or dependence and the co-occurrence of addiction to other substances, especially those prescribed by physicians, remains relatively unexplored.

Lessening of cognitive abilities has always been a part of the stereotype of aging. While mild, subclinical cognitive changes may occur in some persons as a part of normal aging, clinical cognitive impairment occurs in classic dementing syndromes, such as Wernicke-Korsakoff's syndrome, Alzheimer's disease, and others. The extent to which lesser cognitive problems are caused or worsened by the extended use of alcohol among elderly persons is not clear. Few investigators now support the "premature aging" theory: that alcohol affects neurocognitive abilities in ways that advance the aging process of the brain. Others believe that alcohol works directly to injure the

Table 20.3. Differential and Interactive Effects of Age and Alcohol Use

	Age	Alcohol	Both
Sleep			
O2 desaturation episodes (Vitiello et al., 1990)	X		
Cognitive tasks			
Lack of contextual priming (Cermak et al., 1988)	X		X
Recognition of emotional themes (Oscar et al., 1990)	X		
Dichotic listening patterns (Ellis, 1990)	X		X
Neuroreceptors			
Muscarinic receptors decrease (Hughes & Davis, 1983)	X	X	
D2 receptors decrease (Govoni et al., 1988)	X		
5-HT receptors decrease (Dillon et al., 1991)		X	

brain of susceptible persons, resulting in alcoholic dementia: cognitive loss after prolonged heavy drinking and in the absence of other dementing disorders. The extent of an interaction between chronological aging of the brain and the toxicity of alcohol use is unknown. But the good news is that researchers are now thinking in terms of an alcohol/age interaction, a more complex and probably more productive model (see Table 20.3).

The genetic aspects of aging and alcohol use have until very recently focused on youthful alcohol abusers, especially those with significant family histories of use along with dependence on alcohol as one of many substances. Recent studies presented in this volume have awakened interest in the genetics of late-life alcohol use. Their focus has been on gender-specific variations, rather than familial traits, and they have shown a much higher variation among elderly women than among elderly men. If these data are correct, clinically pertinent genetic studies of variations in drinking behavior are best aimed at studying elderly women. Conversely, the development of genetically based treatments may better serve elderly men because of their low individual variation. Much will be learned in this new area of investigation.

BASIC RESEARCH

Researchers have only recently begun animal studies aimed at elucidating the mechanisms of the age/ethanol interactions seen in or hypothesized from clinical experience. In the past, basic studies in neuropharmacology and neurophysiology of alcoholism were often avoided because of the multiplicity of ethanol's effects in tissue or cellular preparations. Recent research, generally conducted without reference to aging processes, has attacked this biologic complexity through several lines of parallel study of specific neuron receptors and intracellular second messenger signaling systems. Only a few studies, however, have considered aging as a variable. Most of those that have

Table 20.4. Animal Studies on Alcoholism and Aging

LD-50 for ethyl alcohol decreases as animals age (Wiberg et al., 1970)
Older animals experience more severe withdrawal (Maier & Pohorecky, 1989; Wood et al., 1982)
Increased intoxication but less tolerance in older mice (Wood et al., 1982)
Increased sleep time after ethanol in older mice (Wood et al., 1982)
Less change in body temperature after ethanol in older mice (Wood et al., 1982)
Older rats reawaken at lower blood and brain ethanol concentrations (Ritzmann & Springer, 1980)
Lower brain ethanol concentration causes sleep in older rats (Ott et al., 1985)
Slowing of neuronal membrane functions with age and alcohol exposure (Bunting & Scott, 1989)
Decreased membrane fluidization with age after ethanol *in vitro* (Armbrecht et al., 1983)
Increased poly-phosphoinositides in young but not old mice after ethanol (Sun et al., 1987, 1992)
Decreased inhibition of GABA release by ethanol in older mice (Strong & Wood, 1984)
Decreased glutamine release after ethanol in old rats (Peinado et al., 1987)
Ethanol depolarizes old but hyperpolarizes young rat neurons (Niesen et al., 1988)
Increased muscarinic receptor density in young but not old rats after ethanol (Pietrzak et al., 1989)

done so point to a lessened resiliency or responsiveness of the aging nervous system after a toxic insult from ethanol (see Table 20.4).

Lost nervous system resiliency was the conclusion of the study by Bickford and colleagues presented in Chapter 11 of this book. Their data on the mechanism of lessened response was most interesting, however, because of the suggestion that some neurophysiologic processes affecting the pharmacodynamic effects of ethanol may be reversed through the processes of normal central nervous system aging. This phenomenon, if borne out in this and in other neurophysiologic settings, may result in a pharmacological armamentarium for elderly alcoholics that differs materially from that for younger patients.

It is clear that a strong need to define age-related mechanisms of ethanol response exists, especially with the goal of devising new pharmacological treatment approaches. To some, aging neurophysiology is regarded largely as an extension of that seen in younger persons but with lessened functional efficacy. Surprises may be in store, however, if basic research can demonstrate further alterations in the directions of physiologic mechanisms that occur with age, and that this in turn results in applying pharmacological interventions in ways that ameliorate a response to ethanol in an elderly person but have no effect or a worsening effect in a much younger person. Age- and ethanol-specific pharmacological agents may not be inconceivably distant.

TREATMENT

In the meantime, we must care for the alcoholic elderly of the present with the methods at hand. There is good beginning evidence to suggest that treatment programs for elderly alcoholics should be tailored to address age-specific needs. Atkinson (1990a) and his group have been pioneers in this line of inquiry. Perhaps their two greatest contributions have been first in the recognition that treatment settings must be tailored to the comfort of individual patients, as when they established that some older alcoholics prefer treatment with their own age group while others prefer to be in settings with younger patients. And second they recognized that while treatment settings may be a matter of preference, treatment approaches are remarkably similar: Elderly alcoholics do not do well with an aggressive, probing therapist but respond positively to a patient, supportive interpersonal style.

We have this same group (Atkinson et al., 1990b) to thank for researching and highlighting the idea that prognostic patterns appear to differentiate recent- versus early-onset elderly drinkers. This may serve to increase optimism in treating both groups: a recognition that the recent-onset drinkers will respond because of relatively intact social resources and that those early-onset drinkers with little in the way of resources will depend more heavily on treatment facilities and public and health care social support networks. Neither group is to be overlooked.

The study presented in Chapter 16 of this book by Willenbring and associates presents dramatic clinical evidence that active intervention among aging alcoholics saves lives. A brief look at his outcome data suggests that active intervention and follow-up is also much less costly than the alternative of ignoring seriously ill alcoholics who then become a burden on crisis services. Using our local hospital cost rates to estimate hospitalization expense if an active intervention service for chronically medically ill alcoholics were in operation today, the average hospitalization costs per patient would be projected to drop from $7,000 annually to about $4,000 annually, saving about $3,000 per patient or about $84,000 on average for the 28 patients Willenbring describes. At the same time the cost per patient for a group of patients left to ordinary care would rise from about $4,000 to $10,250 annually, an increase of $6,150 per patient or $172,200 on average for Willenbring's 28 control group patients. This increase in expense would obtain even though more than one in four of the control patients could be expected to die during the year. The cost savings from providing the service plus the added expense of not providing would give an estimated total of $252,560 annually, on average, for the 56 patients in Willenbring's study. While a common tendency in some quarters is to ignore aging, seriously ill, homeless alcoholics, mortality figures, cost estimates, and the dictates of human concern that Rubington describes in Chapter 18 of this volume all converge to argue for better, cheaper, more humane care for even the most difficult group of alcoholic patients.

CONCLUSION

There is much concern at the present moment that our population is aging, that as it does so it is becoming more infirm and is beginning to flood our hospitals and clinics with a high demand for services when, at the same time, health care costs have become overburdening and must be reduced. In a crisis setting such as this, it is easy to revert to stereotypes and much harder to seek complex answers to complex questions in a sound and systematic way.

Perhaps it is fitting to close this volume with a reference to the longitudinal studies of Vaillant, a unique and continuing resource that provides reliable outcome data against which to evaluate and understand both the cross-sectional data that form most of our knowledge and the not always rational social rhetoric spawned by difficult times. In *The Natural History of Alcoholism* (1983), Vaillant reported on two cohorts who formed part of an ongoing longitudinal study of male psychological health, part of which included paths into and out of alcohol dependence.

Recently, as his two cohorts moved into old age, he reported on a 50-year follow-up study of alcohol dependence (Vaillant, 1993). With the benefit of telescoping time that longitudinal prospective study can provide, he sought to answer three as yet un-answered questions that were appropriate to his data. Is alcohol abuse progressive over the life course? When does abstinence on the one hand, or controlled drinking on the other, become a stable pattern of behavior? And finally, does long-term remission, high mortality, or poor case finding explain the decline in alcoholism rates seen with in-creasing age?

His study followed 456 blue collar men and 268 male Harvard graduates and included annual histories of abstinence, controlled drinking, and problem drinking from ages 21 to 70. By the time of the 50-year follow-up in 1992, 202 of the subjects had fulfilled the DSM-III criteria for alcohol dependence. Longitudinal data from these subjects gave answers to the study questions. First, Vaillant noted that the severity of alcohol abuse, if it was present after age 45, did not increase as most progressive theories of alcoholism would have predicted. This appears congruent with data from Nordstrom and Berglund (1987), suggesting that drinking, even among heavy drinkers, wanes with the passage of the decades.

Second, even after 2 years of stable abstinence, the relapse rate to uncontrolled drink-ing was 35%. Four years of abstinence resulted, in Vaillant's view, in stable long-term remission. "Controlled drinking" subjects fared worse: Five of the 15 subjects in this category maintained controlled drinking for 10 or more years, while 7 of the remaining 10 relapsed to chronic abuse and 3 opted for total abstinence. Data such as these, viewed by either side of the controlled-drinking-versus-abstinence controversialists, can leave clinicians with at least the clear sense that alcoholism is an illness to be viewed in decades, not just months or even a few years.

Third and finally, Vaillant found, in agreement with the survey and cross-sectional data found elsewhere in this volume, that 8% of the men in his sample first abused alcohol after age 50, but by age 65, only 18% of the total alcohol-dependent sample were actively abusing alcohol. Nearly a third of the sample, 29%, had died through a combination of alcohol and cigarette abuse, a death rate three times that of the non-dependent subjects. One-fifth of the group, 19%, were abstinent, another 15% drank socially, and the fate of the remaining 19% was listed as uncertain. From these results, Vaillant concluded that three factors—abstinence, a high death rate, and socially less problematic use—all combined to lower the frequency of alcohol abuse as the subjects entered old age.

When good studies answer questions they bring us to a new plateau from which we can see further into the distance than we could before. The distance is always indistinct and a source of new curiosity. Vaillant's work, as one example among many others to be found in this book, answers some questions and asks others. If his outcome figures serve as a longitudinal baseline for understanding alcohol dependence among men in late life, what methods will allow clinicians to improve upon the baseline remission rates from alcohol dependence? Does the same natural history of late-life alcoholism, or of its recovery, apply to women as well as to men? If we are going to study outcome in elderly alcoholic people, is 3 or 4 years of prospective study too little? Can we lessen the mortality rate, and if we can, how will this affect the longitudinal course of alco-holism in this age group? We hope our readers will have entertained other questions during the course of reading this book. And we hope this volume will serve as a place from which we can begin to find new answers in the interest of health.

References

Agartz, I., Saaf, J., Wahlund, L. O., & Wetterberg, L. (1991). T1 and T2 relaxation time estimates and brain measures during withdrawal in alcoholic men. *Drug and Alcohol Dependence, 29*(2), 157–169.

Alling, C., Balldin, J., Bokstrom, K., Gottfries, C. G., Karlsson, I., & Langstrom, G. (1982). Studies on duration of a late recovery period after chronic abuse of ethanol. A cross-sectional study of biochemical and psychiatric indicators. *Acta Psychiatrica Scandinavica, 66*, 384–397.

Armbrecht, H. J., Wood, W. G., Wise, R. W., Walsh, J. B., Thomas, B. N., & Strong, R. (1983). Ethanol influenced disordering of membranes from different age groups of C57BL/NNia mice. *Journal of Pharmacology and Experimental Therapeutics, 226*, 387–391.

Atkinson, R. (1990a). Aging and alcohol use disorders in the elderly. *International Psychogeriatrics, 2*, 55–72.

Atkinson, R., Tolson, R. L., Turner, J. A. (1990b). Late versus early onset problem drinking in older men. *Alcoholism: Clinical and Experimental Research, 14*, 574–579.

Bunting, T. A., & Scott, B. S. (1989). Aging and ethanol alter neuronal electric membrane properties. *Brain Research, 501*(1), 105–115.

Cermak, L. S., Bleich, R. P., & Blackford, S. P. (1988). Deficits in the implicit retention of new associations by alcoholic Korsakoff patients. *Brain Cognition, 7*(3), 312–323.

Cryer, B., Lee, E., & Feldman, M. (1992). Factors influencing gastroduodenal mucosal prostaglandin concentrations: Roles of smoking and aging. *Annals of Internal Medicine, 116*(8), 636–640.

Dillon, K. A., Gross, I. R., Israeli, M., & Biegon, A. (1991). Autoradiographic analysis of serotonin 5-HT1A receptor binding in the human brain postmortem: Effects of age and alcohol. *Brain Research, 554*(1–2), 56–64.

Eaton, W., Kramer, M., Anthony, J. C., Dryman, A., Shapiro, S., & Locke, B. Z. (1989). The incidence of specific DIS/DSM-III mental disorders: Data from the NIMH Epidemiological Catchment Area Program. *Acta Psychiatrica Scandinavica, 79*, 163–178.

Ellis, R. J. (1990). Dichotic asymmetries in aging and alcoholic subjects. *Alcoholism: Clinical and Experimental Research, 14*(6), 863–871.

Finlayson, R., Hurt, R. D., Davis, L. J., & Morse, R. M. (1988). Alcoholism in elderly persons: A study of the psychiatric and psychosocial features of 216 inpatients. *Mayo Clinic Proceedings, 63*, 761–768.

Freund, G., & Ballinger, W. J. (1989a). Neuroreceptor changes in the putamen of alcohol abusers. *Alcoholism: Clinical and Experimental Research, 13*(2), 213–218.

Freund, G., & Ballinger, W. J. (1989b). Loss of muscarinic and benzodiazepine neuroreceptors from hippocampus of alcohol abusers. *Alcohol, 6*(1), 23–31.

Geller, G., Stokes, E. J., Levine, D. M., & Moore, R. D. (1989). Characteristics, diagnosis, and treatment of alcoholism in elderly patients. *Journal of the American Geriatric Society, 37*, 310–316.

Glynn, R. J., de Labry, L. O., & Hou, D. M. (1988). Alcohol consumption, type A behavior, and demographic variables. Results from the Normative Aging Study. *American Journal of Epidemiology, 127*(2), 310–320.

Gomberg, E. S. L. (in press). Older women and alcohol: Use and abuse. *Recent Developments in Alcoholism.*

Govoni, S., Rius, R. A., Battaini, F., Magnoni, M. S., Lucchi, L., & Trabucchi, M. (1988). The central dopaminergic system: Susceptibility to risk factors for accelerated aging. *Gerontology, 34*(1–2), 29–34.

Hayakawa, K., Kumagai, H., Suzuki, Y., Furusawa, N., Haga, T., Hoshi, T., Fujiwara, Y., & Yamaguchi, K. (1992). MR imaging of chronic alcoholism. *Acta Radiology, 33*(3), 201–206.

Holzer, C. I., Robins, L. N., Myers, J. K., et al. (1984). Antecedents and correlates of alcohol abuse and dependence in the elderly. In G. Maddox, L. N. Robins, & N. Rosenberg, (Ed.), *Nature and extent of alcohol problems among the elderly.* Rockville, MD: NIAAA/US Govt. Printing Office.

Hughes, G. J., & Davis, L. (1983). Changes in cholinergic activity in human hippocampus following chronic alcohol abuse. *Pharmacology and Biochemistry of Behavior, 1*(397), 397–400.

Karantanas, A. H., Kalef, E. J., & Glaros, D. C. (1991). Quantitative computed tomography for bone mineral measurement: Technical aspects, dosimetry, normal data and clinical applications. *British Journal of Radiology, 64*(760), 298–304.

Kelley, J. T., Pena, Y., Reilly, E. L., Overall, J. E., & Colton, G. S. (1984). Effects of age and alcohol abuse on pattern reversal visual evoked potentials. *Clinical Electroencephalography, 15*(2), 102–109.

Kroft, C. L., Gescuk, B., Woods, B. T., Mello, N. K., Weiss, R. D., & Mendelson, J. H. (1991). Brain ventricular size in female alcoholics: An MRI study. *Alcohol, 8*(1), 31–34.

Laitinen, K., Valimaki, M., & Keto, P. (1991). Bone mineral density measured by dual-energy X-ray absorptiometry in healthy Finnish women. *Calcified Tissue International, 48*(4), 224–231.

Maier, D. M., & Pohorecky, L. A. (1989). The effect of repeated withdrawal episodes on subsequent withdrawal severity in ethanol-treated rats. *Drug and Alcohol Dependence, 23*(2), 103–110.

McInnes, E., & Powell, J. (1994). Drug and alcohol referrals: Are elderly substance abuse diagnoses and referrals being missed? *British Medical Journal, 308,* 444–446.

Moos, R., Brennan, P. L., & Moos, B. S. (1991). Short-term processes of remission and nonremission among late life problem drinkers. *Alcoholism: Clinical and Experimental Research, 15,* 948–955.

Morrow, D., Leirer, V., & Yesavage, J. (1990). The influence of alcohol and aging on radio communication during flight. *Aviation Space and Environmental Medicine, 61*(1), 12–20.

Niesen, C. E., Baskys, A., & Carlen, P. L. (1988). Reversed ethanol effects on potassium conductances in aged hippocampal dentate granule neurons. *Brain Research, 445*(1), 137–141.

Norstrom, G., & Berglund, M. (1987). Ageing and recovery from alcoholism. *British Journal of Psychiatry, 151,* 382–385.

Oscar, B. M., Hancock, M., Mildworf, B., Hutner, N., & Weber, D. A. (1990). Emotional perception and memory in alcoholism and aging. *Alcoholism: Clinical and Experimental Research, 14*(3), 383–393.

Ott, J. F., Hunter, B. E., & Walker, D. W. (1985). The effect of age on ethanol metabolism and on the hypothermic and hypnotic responses to ethanol in the Fischer 344 rat. *Alcoholism: Clinical and Experimental Research, 9,* 59–65.

Peinado, J. M., Collins, D. M., & Myers, R. D. (1987). Ethanol challenge alters amino acid neurotransmitter release from frontal cortex of aged rat. *Neurobiology of Aging, 8,* 241–247.

Pendergast, D. R., York, J. L., & Fisher, N. M. (1990). A survey of muscle function in detoxified alcoholics. *Alcohol, 7*(4), 361–366.

Pietrzak, E. R., Wilce, P. A., Ward, L. C., & Shanley, B. C. (1989). A feeding regime for the study of the interaction of ethanol and aging. *Drug and Alcohol Dependence, 23*(2), 171–175.

Ritzmann, R. F., & Springer, A. (1980). Age differences in brain sensitivity and tolerance to ethanol in mice. *Age, 3,* 15–17.

Schuckit, M. A. (1982). A clinical review of alcohol, alcoholism, and the elderly patient. *Journal of Clinical Psychiatry, 43*(10), 396–399.

Simon, D., Preziosi, P., Barrett, C. E., Roger, M., Saint, P. M., Nahoul, K., & Papoz, L. (1992). The influence of aging on plasma sex hormones in men: The Telecom Study. *American Journal of Epidemiology, 135*(7), 783–791.

Strong, R., & Wood, W. G. (1984). Membrane properties and aging: *In vivo* and *in vitro* effects on synaptosomal gamma-aminobutyric acid (GABA) release. *Journal of Pharmacology and Experimental Therapeutics, 229*, 726–730.

Sun, G. Y., Huang, H. M., Lee, D. Z., Chung-Wang, Y. J., Wood, W. G., Strong, R., & Sun, A. Y. (1987). Chronic ethanol effect on acidic phospholipids of synaptosomes isolated from cerebral cortex of CB57BL/NNia mice—a comparison with age. *Alcohol and Alcoholism, 22*, 367–373.

Sun, G. Y., Navidi, M., Yoa, F. G., Wood, W. G., & Sun, A. Y. (1993). Effect of chronic ethanol administration on poly-phosphoinositide metabolism in the mouse brain: Variance with age. *Neurochemistry International, 23*, 45–52.

Vaillant, G. E. (1983). *The natural history of alcoholism*. Cambridge, MA: Harvard University Press.

Vaillant, G. E. (1993). *A 50-year follow-up of alcohol dependence*. Scientific Proceedings Summary, Annual Scientific Meeting, American Psychiatric Association, San Francisco, CA, p. 97.

Vitiello, M. V., Prinz, P. N., Personius, J. P., Nuccio, M. A., Koerker, R. M., & Scurfield, R. (1990). Nighttime hypoxemia is increased in abstaining chronic alcoholic men. *Alcoholism: Clinical and Experimental Research, 14*(1), 38–41.

Wells, P. E., Miles, S., & Spencer, B. (1983). Stress experiences and drinking histories of elderly drunken-driving offenders. *Journal of Studies on Alcohol, 44*(3), 429–437.

Wiberg, G., Trenholm, H. L., & Coldwell, B. B. (1970). Increased ethanol toxicity in old rats: Changes in LD50 *in vivo* and *in vitro* metabolism and liver alcohol dehydrogenase activity. *Toxicology and Applied Pharmacology, 16*, 718–727.

Wood, W. G., Armbrecht, H. J., & Wise, R. W. (1982). Ethanol intoxication and withdrawal among three groups of C57BL/6NNia mice. *Pharmacology and Biochemistry of Behavior, 17*, 1037–1041.

Index